Mechanical Ventilation: Physiological and Clinical Applications

Mechanical Ventilation: Physiological and Clinical Applications

Edited by Stephanie McMillan

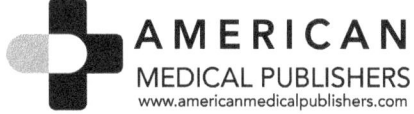

AMERICAN
MEDICAL PUBLISHERS
www.americanmedicalpublishers.com

American Medical Publishers,
41 Flatbush Avenue,
1st Floor, New York,
NY 11217, USA

Visit us on the World Wide Web at:
www.americanmedicalpublishers.com

ISBN: 978-1-63927-105-4

Cataloging-in-Publication Data

Mechanical ventilation : physiological and clinical applications / edited by Stephanie McMillan.
    p. cm.
Includes bibliographical references and index.
ISBN 978-1-63927-105-4
1. Artificial respiration. 2. Respiratory therapy. 3. Respirators (Medical equipment).
4. First aid in illness and injury. 5. Human physiology.
6. Critical care medicine. I. McMillan, Stephanie.
RC87.9 .M43 2022
616.102 5--dc23

Table of Contents

Preface

This book was inspired by the evolution of our times; to answer the curiosity of inquisitive minds. Many developments have occurred across the globe in the recent past which has transformed the progress in the field.

Mechanical ventilation is a medical method in which mechanical means are used to replace or assist spontaneous breathing. It may either involve a machine known as a ventilator or a qualified professional who may use a bag valve mask device. Mechanical ventilation may either be invasive or non-invasive in nature. It is termed invasive if an instrument is inserted inside the trachea through the mouth. Non-invasive ventilation makes use of a face or nasal mask and is used only for conscious patients. The two primary forms of mechanical ventilation are positive pressure ventilation and negative pressure ventilation. The positive pressure ventilation involves pushing air into the lungs via the airways. During the process of negative pressure ventilation, the air is sucked into the lungs by stimulating movements of the chest. Mechanical ventilation is used in severe conditions or injuries such as acute lung injury and trauma, acute severe asthma, hypotension, hypoxemia and neurological diseases. This book elucidates the concepts and innovative models around prospective developments with respect to mechanical ventilation. It outlines the processes and applications of mechanical ventilation in detail. The book will serve as a valuable source of reference for graduate and postgraduate students.

This book was developed from a mere concept to drafts to chapters and finally compiled together as a complete text to benefit the readers across all nations. To ensure the quality of the content we instilled two significant steps in our procedure. The first was to appoint an editorial team that would verify the data and statistics provided in the book and also select the most appropriate and valuable contributions from the plentiful contributions we received from authors worldwide. The next step was to appoint an expert of the topic as the Editor-in-Chief, who would head the project and finally make the necessary amendments and modifications to make the text reader-friendly. I was then commissioned to examine all the material to present the topics in the most comprehensible and productive format.

I would like to take this opportunity to thank all the contributing authors who were supportive enough to contribute their time and knowledge to this project. I also wish to convey my regards to my family who have been extremely supportive during the entire project.

Editor

Accuracy of height estimation and tidal volume setting using anthropometric formulas in an ICU Caucasian population

Erwan L'her[1,2]*, Jérôme Martin-Babau[1] and François Lellouche[3]

Abstract

Background: Knowledge of patients' height is essential for daily practice in the intensive care unit. However, actual height measurements are unavailable on a daily routine in the ICU and measured height in the supine position and/or visual estimates may lack consistency. Clinicians do need simple and rapid methods to estimate the patients' height, especially in short height and/or obese patients. The objectives of the study were to evaluate several anthropometric formulas for height estimation on healthy volunteers and to test whether several of these estimates will help tidal volume setting in ICU patients.

Methods: This was a prospective, observational study in a medical intensive care unit of a university hospital. During the first phase of the study, eight limb measurements were performed on 60 healthy volunteers and 18 height estimation formulas were tested. During the second phase, four height estimates were performed on 60 consecutive ICU patients under mechanical ventilation.

Results: In the 60 healthy volunteers, actual height was well correlated with the gold standard, measured height in the erect position. Correlation was low between actual and calculated height, using the hand's length and width, the index, or the foot equations. The Chumlea method and its simplified version, performed in the supine position, provided adequate estimates. In the 60 ICU patients, calculated height using the simplified Chumlea method was well correlated with measured height ($r = 0.78$; $\partial < 1$ %). Ulna and tibia estimates also provided valuable estimates. All these height estimates allowed calculating IBW or PBW that were significantly different from the patients' actual weight on admission. In most cases, tidal volume set according to these estimates was lower than what would have been set using the actual weight.

Conclusion: When actual height is unavailable in ICU patients undergoing mechanical ventilation, alternative anthropometric methods to obtain patient's height based on lower leg and on forearm measurements could be useful to facilitate the application of protective mechanical ventilation in a Caucasian ICU population. The simplified Chumlea method is easy to achieve in a bed-ridden patient and provides accurate height estimates, with a low bias.

Keywords: ICU, Mechanical ventilation, Height estimation

Background

Knowledge of patients' height is essential for daily practice in the intensive care unit (ICU), for either assessment of renal function [1], determination of drug doses, calculating cardiac function indices, or tidal volume setting [2]. Because it is well established that patients' lungs are well correlated with their height [3], accurate tidal volume setting should be based on ideal or predicted body weight that is functions of height and gender, rather than on actual weight to avoid acquired acute lung injury and ARDS [4–6] and to improve outcome [7].

However, height measurement is not a daily routine in all ICUs [8–11]. Although recumbent patients' height can be measured by means of a metric ribbon tape, this

*Correspondence: erwan.lher@chu-brest.fr
[1] Réanimation Médicale, CHRU de Brest – La Cavale Blanche, Bvd Tanguy-Prigent, 29609 Brest Cedex, France
Full list of author information is available at the end of the article

measurement is not always performed [12] or may lack consistency.

In fact, actual body weight is often used in routine [13], which can lead to large errors in tidal volume settings [14], especially in women and obese patients that are consistently at risk of unintentional delivery of excessive tidal volumes [7, 15–17]. Several other ICU team use height and weight estimates [9, 18, 19], but these visual estimations have yet been demonstrated as significantly inaccurate for individual observers [17, 20, 21].

In this study, we first analyzed on 60 healthy volunteers whether estimated height using various simple anthropometric formulas will agree with the exact measured height, and in second whether several formulas will help setting tidal volume in 60 mechanically ventilated ICU patients.

Methods

This prospective observational protocol was in accordance with the standards of our local ethics committee; informed consent was not deemed necessary because of the observational nature of the study.

Measurements and calculations
Height measurement
Exact height in the erect position (*actual height*) was considered the gold standard and was performed for all 60 healthy volunteers, using a standard clinical height gauge. However, such a measurement was unavailable for ICU patients and height measured with a soft tape metric ribbon in the supine position (*measured height*) was considered the standard for the 60 ICU patients; it was also measured for all healthy volunteers, as a comparison. Evaluation took also into account height provided on the healthy volunteers' ID cards (*provided height;* unavailable for most ICU patients) and the visual estimation provided by the nurse in charge of the ICU patients (*evaluated height*).

Limb measurements and height estimations
They were performed using 300- and 800-mm precision metal callipers. During the preliminary phase, on healthy volunteers, eight different limb measurements (Fig. 1) were performed, always on the right limbs, to determinate height estimation (*calculated height*) using different anthropometric formulas (Additional File 1) [22–29].

Weight measurement and calculation for ICU patients
All patients were weighted on admission using their ICU bed integrated weight scale (Total Care® P500, Hill-Rom, Batesville, IN, USA). Ideal or predicted body weight was calculated using the different height values [30, 31].

A specific computer software application was designed to facilitate height evaluation during the second phase

of the project. The choice of four equations (up from 18 used in the preliminary phase) used to evaluate height in the application took into account either accuracy and/or practical issues about the limb sections measurements.

Preliminary phase on healthy volunteers
Height and limb segment measurements were performed over a 60 healthy volunteers' cohort: four at the upper limb and four at the lower limb (Fig. 1). Height estimates are provided in Table 1.

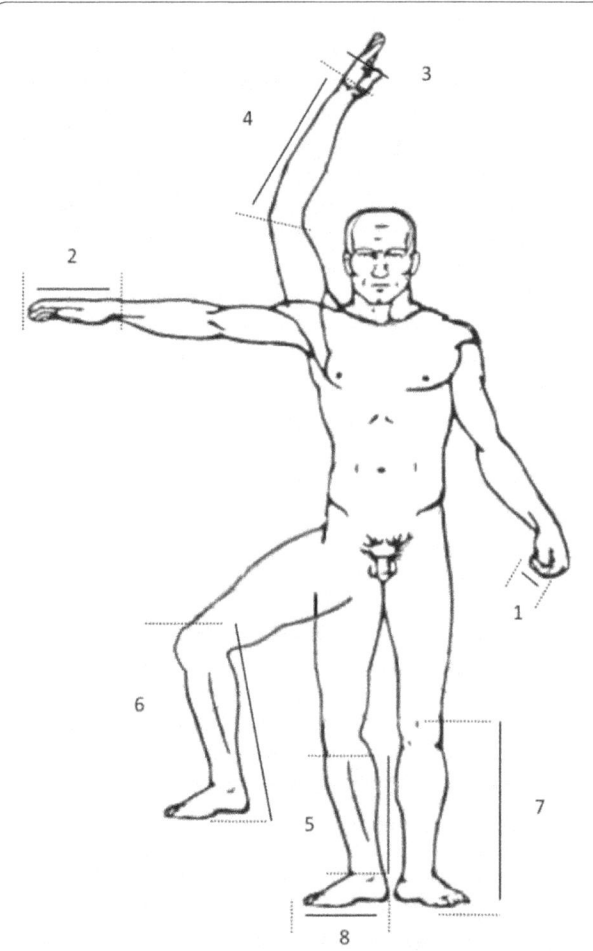

Fig. 1 Limb segment measurements. All measurements were performed using precision callipers on the right limbs. *1* index distal phalange; *2* hand length, from the IIIrd finger extremity to the wrist; *3* hand maximal width; *4* ulna, from the olecranon to the styloïd process; *5* tibia length, from the upper articular line to the extremity of the medial malleolus; *6* standard Chumlea measurement, the patient is positioned recumbent, knee raised vertically with a 90° angle between femur and tibia, and the caliper is positioned under heel and over femoral condyle of the leg; *7* simplified Chumlea measurement, the patient stays supine and the caliper is positioned under heel and over patella's upper line; *8*: foot length, from the extremity of the Ist toe to the posterior part of the heel

Accuracy of height estimation and tidal volume setting using anthropometric formulas in an ICU Caucasian...

3

Table 1 Height measurements and estimations in the healthy volunteers

Healthy volunteers (n = 59)	Measure (cm)	Correlation (r)	Bias (%) (±1.96 SD)
Actual height	*170.4 ± 8.5*	/	/
Provided height	170.2 ± 8.1	0.9633	−0.1 (2.4/−2.6)
Measured height	176.2 ± 8.5	0.9795	3.4 (5.3/1.4)
Height estimations			
Index			
I 1	164.3 ± 7.2	0.7141	−3.6 (3.4/−10.7)
I 2	167.3 ± 5.4	0.7300	−1.7 (5.0/−8.5)
Hand length			
HL 1	163.2 ± 7.7	0.7915	−4.3 (1.9/−10.4)
HL 2	160.9 ± 7.2	0.7938	−5.7 (0.3/−11.7)
HL 3	161.4 ± 5.6	0.7646	−5.3 (1.0/−11.7)
Hand width			
HW 1	155.8 ± 6.8	0.7903	−8.9 (−2.8/−14.9)
HW 2	157.7 ± 6.6	0.6962	−7.9 (−0.9/−15.0)
Ulna			
U 1	169.7 ± 8.0	0.8296	−0.4 (5.2/−5.9)
U 2	172.2 ± 8.0	0.8296	1.1 (6.6/−4.4)
U 3	171.5 ± 9.4	0.7961	0.6 (7.2/−6.0)
Tibia			
T 1	162.1 ± 6.2	0.7989	−4.9 (0.9/−10.8)
T 2	158.8 ± 8.8	0.8443	−7.1 (−1.3/−12.8)
T 3	165.6 ± 9.2	0.8501	−2.9 (2.8/−8.5)
T 4	168.1 ± 9.2	0.8501	−1.4 (4.2/−6.9)
T 5	164.7 ± 10.7	0.8287	−3.5 (3.5/−10.4)
Foot	166.2 ± 8.6	0.0269	−2.6 (11.6/−16.8)
Chumlea			
Reference Chumlea	168.9 ± 6.0	0.7894	−0.8 (5.3/−6.9)
Simplified Chumlea	168.1 ± 5.9	0.8667	−1.3 (3.9/−6.4)

Correlation coefficient r and bias: results are provided as compared with actual height; measures are provided as mean ± SD

Actual height: height measured in the erect position using a vertical calliper; provided height: height provided by the healthy volunteers; measured height: height measured in the supine position, using a soft tape metric ribbon

Index: two different formulas were used (I 1, 2); hand: five formulas were used, three based on length (HL 1–3) and two combining width and length (HW 1, 2); ulna: three formulas were tested (U 1–3); tibia: five formulas were tested (T 1–5); reference Chumlea was measured with the patient positioned recumbent, knee raised vertically with a 90° angle between femur and tibia, and the calliper positioned under heel and over femoral condyle of the leg; simplified Chumlea was measured with the patient laying supine and the calliper positioned under heel and over patella's upper line (see Fig. 1). All formulas are provided within the Additional file 1: Online Repository

Italic value indicates the reference value for height, that was measured in the erect position

Using these measurements, *calculated height* was performed using 18 different anthropometric formulas (Table 1). Complete anthropometric formulas are provided within the Additional file 1: online repository. They were chosen either because of their standard use within different domains such as geriatrics, anthropometry, and/or forensic science or because of pragmatic issues. Only a few of them are specifically dedicated to a European Caucasian population. The simplified Chumlea method was proposed by our team after several preliminary tests (*data not shown*), using the same equation but performing different measurements to better fit to ICU requirements (Fig. 1).

The four most accurate estimation indices were subsequently chosen (two for each limb segment), taking into account their accuracy (a correlation >0.75 and bias level <5 % as compared with *actual height* were considered), but also practical issues such as the measurements ease in the recumbent position; all chosen measurements had to be performed in a "one shot," using a single 1-m ruler, as a comparison with the actual height measurement that requires several steps to be performed. These four indices were integrated into the specifically dedicated software application.

Second phase on ICU patients
After the preliminary phase, weight, limb segment, and height measurements were performed in 60 consecutive mechanically ventilated ICU patients, for whom preadmission values were unknown to staff. Each patient's height was estimated by eye while the patient was lying supine. Tidal volume (Vt) and plateau pressure were recorded concomitantly.

Height and predicted body weight (PBW) estimations [30] were performed retrospectively, and no direct intervention was immediately driven taking into account these evaluations. Ideal body weight (IBW) [31] was also computed for the sake of comparison to PBW.

Statistical analysis
Anthropometric formulas have already been validated on various cohorts; however, few of them have been validated for a clinical use in our population of interest, except for the original Chumlea index [29]. For such a preliminary evaluation, a number of 60 healthy volunteers and 60 mechanically ventilated patients for more than 48 h were determined a priori.

All results are provided as mean ± SD, unless specified otherwise. Categorical variables are presented as counts. Relationship between variables was assessed using a Pearson's correlation coefficient (r) test with p value, and data were represented graphically by a scatter diagram depicting the identity line and the 95 % confidence interval (CI) for r. Method comparison and evaluation was performed using a Bland–Altman plot, taking into account the difference between the two methods on the X-axis, because all comparisons were performed considering the reference method [32]; bias (∂) plot either was reported using quantitative differences or expressed as % of difference, depending on the value type. Quantitative parameter comparisons were made using paired t test. A p value equal or below 0.05 was considered statistically significant.

All statistical analyses were performed using MedCalc® 12.4.0 software for Windows (MedCalc Inc., Ostend, Belgium).

Results
Healthy volunteers
In the 60 healthy volunteers, *actual height* was well correlated with *provided* and with *measured* heights, with a low estimation bias ($\partial = -0.1$ and 3.4 %, respectively).

Upper limb equations
Correlation was low between actual and calculated height, using either the hand's length and width, or the index equations. Correlation between *actual height* and *calculated height* using the *ulna* was considered of interest, with a low bias ($\partial = -0.4-1.1$ %).

Lower limb equations
Correlation was considered of interest whatever the tibia formulas, but with differences in terms of the estimation bias. Foot estimation was not correlated with *actual height* in our population. Height estimation using either the reference Chumlea method or the simplified one seemed to provide adequate values.

Choice of the anthropometric formulas for the second phase, within the ICU environment
Considering either the performance of the different equations or the ease of measurements at the bedside, we chose to consider U1 (ulna) and HL1 (hand length) formulas for the upper limb, T4 (tibia) and SC (simplified Chumlea) for the lower limb.

ICU patients
Patients' physiological characteristics are provided in Table 2.

Evaluated height (visual estimation) was correlated with the measured value (metric ribbon tape), with a low bias ($\partial < 1$ %). Calculated height using the simplified Chumlea method was well correlated with measured height ($r = 0.78$; $\partial < 1$ %) (Table 3).

A significant difference was observed between actual body weight (ABW), measured on ICU admittance, and either IBW or PBW. In all cases, IBW and PBW were lower than ABW.

Table 2 ICU patients' physiological characteristics

	ICU patients ($n = 59$)	P value
Diagnosis		
Cardiac arrest	18	
Coma	14	
ARDS	11	
Severe sepsis and shock	10	
ARF	4	
Other	2	
Patients' characteristics		
Sex ratio	41 male/18 female	
Actual body weight (ABW; kg)	74.4 ± 16.2	
Ideal body weight (IBW; kg)	64.1 ± 6.5	$P < 0.0001$
Predicted body weight (PBW; kg)	64.1 ± 8.8	$P < 0.0001$
Ventilatory settings		
Respiratory rate (b/min)	18 ± 3	
Plateau pressure (cmH$_2$O)	19 ± 4.5	
Vt (mL)	500 ± 56	
Vt ABW (mL/kg)	7.0 ± 1.4	
Vt IBW (mL/kg)	7.8 ± 0.8	$P < 0.0001$
Vt PBW (mL/kg)	7.9 ± 1.0	$P < 0.0001$

Results are provided as mean ± STD. A p value equal or below 0.05 was considered statistically significant

ARDS acute respiratory distress syndrome, *ARF* acute respiratory failure, *Vt* tidal volume, *ABW* actual body weight, *IBW* ideal body weight, calculated according to the Lorentz formula (ref), *PBW* predicted body weight; both reference IBW and PBW were calculated using measured height. IBW and PBW were significantly different from ABW, but without difference between each other; Vt ABW is the tidal volume that was set on the ventilator, according to the patient actual weight, measured on admission; it was significantly different from either Vt IBW or Vt PBW, without any difference between each other

IBW and/or PBW calculations using the height calculated values were well correlated with values provided using the measured height.

Tidal volume on admission was significantly higher than that suggested while using IBW and/or PBW. In all cases, tidal volume settings using calculated height (whatever the chosen formula) were below those using ABW.

Discussion
Because actual height may be difficult to obtain in all bedridden ICU patients, we compared different alternative methods to estimate height in 60 healthy volunteers and validated its usability in 60 ICU patients. Several alternative calculating methods, based on lower and upper limbs measurements, were close to the reference. When used for ventilation setting, such alternative, simple, and accurate height estimations mostly tended to decrease calculated predicted body weight, thus decreasing the risk of high tidal volume administration.

Table 3 ICU patients' height and weight estimations and calculated tidal volumes

	Measure (cm)	Correlation (r)	95 % CI for r	Bias (%) (±1.96 SD)
Measured height	169.5 ± 8.1	/	/	/
Estimated height	170.2 ± 8.1	0.77	0.64–0.86	0.4 (6.8/−6)
Height estimations				
Hand	163.3 ± 7.4	0.53	0.32–0.70	−3.8 (5.0/−12.7)
Ulna	165.2 ± 7.2	0.51	0.29–0.68	−2.6 (6.4/−11.5)
Tibia	174.2 ± 7.6	0.61	0.41–0.75	2.7 (10.9/−5.5)
Simplified Chumlea	162.2 ± 9.0	0.78	0.66–0.87	−4.5 (2.5/−11.5)
	Weight (kg)			
PBW estimations	(64.1 ± 8.8)			
Hand	58.5 ± 8.6	0.65	0.46–0.77	−10 (12.7/−32.8)
Ulna	60.2 ± 7.8	0.64	0.45–0.77	−6.6 (14.3/−27.5)
Tibia	68.4 ± 7.9	0.71	0.55–0.82	6.2 (24/−11.6)
Simplified Chumlea	57.5 ± 9.9	0.81	0.70–0.88	−12.2 (12/−36.4)
IBW estimations	(64.1 ± 6.5)			
Hand	59.7 ± 5.7	0.62	0.43–0.76	−7.2 (9.7/−24)
Ulna	60.9 ± 5.5	0.61	0.42-0.75	−5.0 (11.8/−21.8)
Tibia	67.2 ± 6.0	0.71	0.55-0.82	4.7 (19.8/−10.4)
Simplified Chumlea	59.0 ± 6.6	0.81	0.70–0.89	−8.5 (4.7/−21.6)
	Tidal volume (mL/kg)			
Vt over ABW	(7.0 ± 1.4)	/	/	/
VT over PBW	(7.9 ± 1.0)	/	/	/
Hand	8.7 ± 1.3	0.67	0.50–0.79	7.2 (24.1/−9.6)
Ulna	8.4 ± 1.3	0.69	0.53–0.81	5.0 (21.8/−11.8)
Tibia	7.4 ± 1.0	0.66	0.48–0.78	−4.7 (10.4/−19.8)
Simplified Chumlea	8.9 ± 1.7	0.84	0.74–0.90	8.5 (21.6/−4.7)
VT over IBW	(7.8 ± 0.8)	/	/	/
Hand	8.4 ± 1.0	0.71	0.55–0.82	9.6 (32.2/−13)
Ulna	8.2 ± 1.0	0.75	0.61–0.84	6.2 (28.8/−16.4)
Tibia	7.5 ± 0.8	0.74	0.60–0.84	−6.6 (13.9/−27.1)
Simplified Chumlea	8.5 ± 1.1	0.85	0.76–0.91	11.8 (31.4/−7.8)

Results are provided as mean + STD; correlation coefficient r and bias: results are provided as compared with measured height; ideal body weight is calculated according to the Lorentz formula, using the measured height; predicted body weight is calculated according to the ARDSnet tables, using the measured height

Lack of accurate height measurements in ICU patients

Despite the paucity of data, several studies suggest that height is not routinely used to set tidal volume [14, 18, 33–35] and/or that the exact patient's height is unknown as up to 40 % in ARDS patients [36]. In a UK telephone survey performed in 20 ICUs, the authors demonstrated that only 2 ICUs were using actual height for tidal volume setting [9].

When height measurements are performed, metric ribbon tape measurements are used in supine patients, even if it has proved to lack consistency in various studies [17, 20]. Such measurements have also been demonstrated to result in different height values than that would be obtained with the patient in the upright position [9]. A reason for such low performance could be that measurement is difficult to achieve by a single operator on a bed-ridden patient, especially in case of body distortion, obesity, and other physiological conditions.

In other studies, visual height estimation was the only method to be used, even if it seemed to be usually inconsistent [17, 21]. The magnitude of errors for visual estimation of height in the ICU varies from one study to the other, but several authors have depicted <41 % accuracy [20]. Most of all, experience and the level of training did not correlate well with accuracy of the estimations [17]. Such bad performance of clinicians to visually estimate physiological parameters for patients lying supine was also clearly demonstrated in the operating room, for either adults [37] or pediatrics [38], and in the emergency department [39]. In the operating room studies, marked variations were demonstrated between different observers for a single patient [37, 38].

Similar height misestimating was not observed in our study, as within a nursing study from the Netherlands [12], and measurement in supine or upright positions was well correlated in healthy volunteers. The accuracy of height measurement in such setting may be related to the fact that (1) in an experimental setting, we always try to provide the most accurate measurement, which may not always be the case in daily ICU routine measurements; (2) physical condition of healthy volunteers may have simplified measurements (no distortion, no obesity, etc.).

Alternative methods for height estimation

Numerous methods have been described to calculate patients' height indirectly, most of them being developed for anthropologic or forensic purposes. These methods used either a multiple regression approach with different bones measurements or a simple regression logistic [28]. Only a few of these simple methods have been developed for a clinical purpose and rarely in a European and Caucasian population [26].

Besides these methods, the long bone length is often considered the best indicator of stature, and knee height has been validated for stature evaluation using the Chumlea method [29] in large cohorts of mobility-impaired and bed-ridden elderly patients, close to a standard ICU population [40]. Despite promising results, knee cannot easily be raised vertically with a 90° angle between femur and tibia as in the standard method on a clinical routine [41]—especially in case of femoral venous access and/or overweight. Within all the other height estimation methods, few can yet be considered as reliable for a clinical purpose [42].

The simplified Chumlea method that is described in this article does not require such leg mobilization and can be easily achieved in supine patients by a single clinician, only using a short disposable ribbon tape, whatever the patient's morphology. It seems to provide valuable height estimation, similar to what has been demonstrated with the original version. A relationship seems to exist between actual height and the two different Chumlea estimates (Fig. 2); i.e., the difference is depending on the height (overestimation of height for higher individuals).

Potential impact of height calculation on protective ventilation implementation

Tidal volume is directly related to the exact patient height [3], and the absence of height value reference may lead to large errors in tidal volume setting [14]. The association between initial high tidal volume settings and acute lung injury or ARDS development has been clearly demonstrated [5, 6].

In numerous studies, obese patients were considered to be ventilated with higher tidal volumes than non-obese

patients [7, 15–17]. Women of shorter height are thus less likely to receive protective ventilation [43, 44]. These detrimental effects could be directly related to the fact that these categories of patients may be ventilated using actual body weight or bad estimates [13].

In some of our patients, although very few obese patients were included, 6 mL/kg of actual body weight value would be the equivalent of 10–11 mL/kg of the ARDSnet approach. In the report by Bloomfield et al. [17], using 6 mL/kg of actual body weight in some patients may have resulted in tidal volumes of 15–19 mL/kg of the ARDSnet approach (Fig. 3).

Whatever the calculation formulas that are used, tidal volume settings errors are limited, whereas height estimates are usually higher than exact height. This error also tends to limit tidal volume/kg application. While the error in terms of calculation seems to be depending on the height, for patients over 170 cm, this will always lower the estimation of required tidal volume. The clinical impact of such an approach should require a dedicated study, but the availability of height estimates that are simple, easy to use, and rapid to perform will at least enable the clinician to titrate tidal volume as safely as possible with sufficient accuracy.

A note of caution could be that if the rationale of the study is supported by RCTs showing the benefits of tidal volume reduction based on PBW, height estimates were not similarly performed within these trials, thus probably resulting in some inconsistency. The question that we addressed could make sense from a clinical point of view, whereas our technique could help standardizing height estimation using a simple, cheap, and reproducible technique.

Limitations of the study

Our study has several major limitations. The first limitation to consider should be the lack of exact height measurement for ICU bed-ridden patients. Even if metric ribbon measurements in the supine position cannot be considered as accurate as to height measurement in the erect position, it is often the only available reference for bed-ridden patients. As a matter of fact, this was the only comparable measurement that was available in our ICU survey. Second limitation could be that although height was not measured before study entry, it is unknown whether the nursing staff that was asked for visual estimation and/or metric ribbon measurements had prior knowledge of the patient's height from other sources such as the patient's family, the patient itself (rarely available at ICU admittance), or the patient's medical record and/or ID. This may have artificially enhanced the exactitude of visual estimation. Patients' position in a bed of already known length may also have bias estimation by

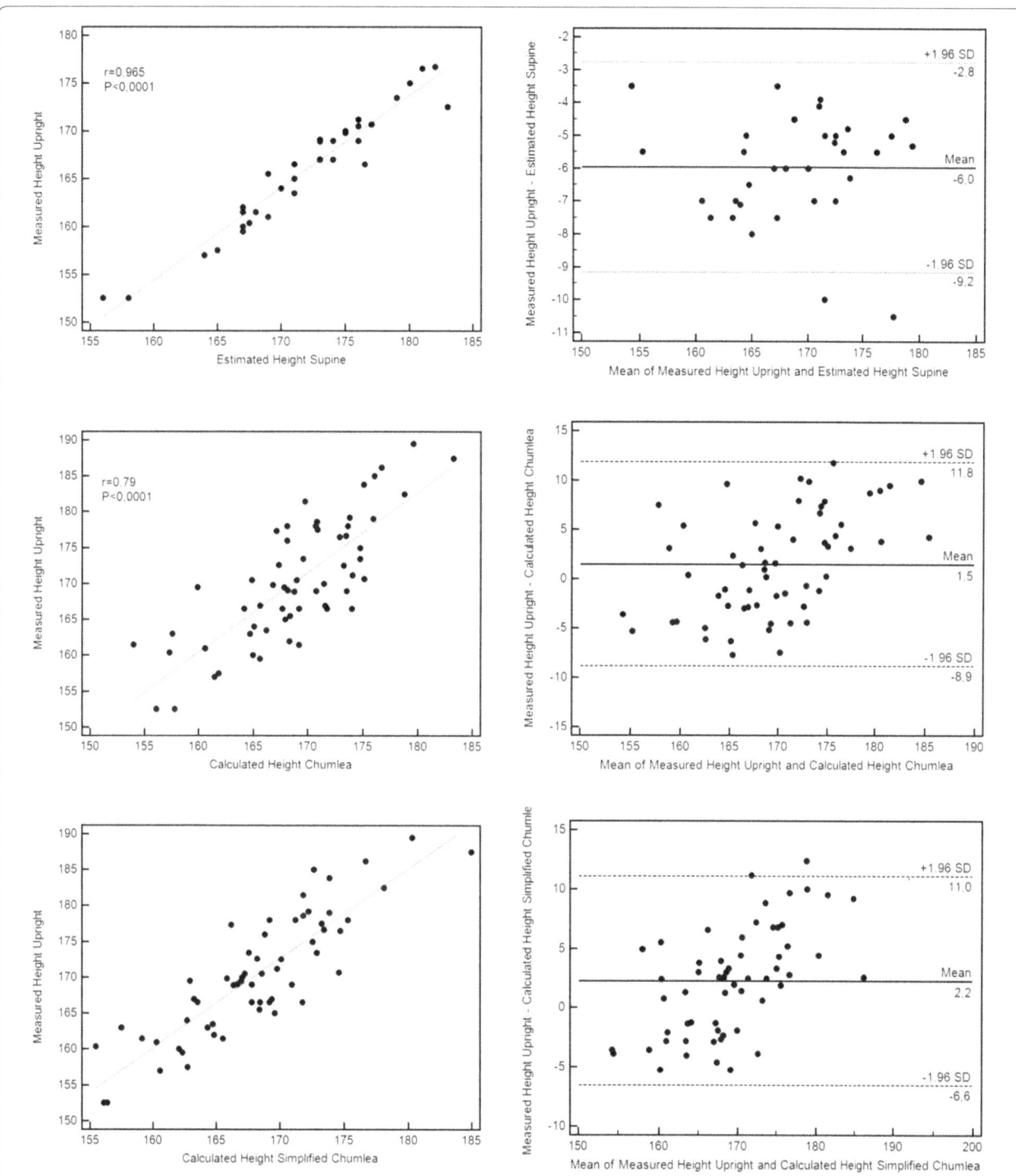

Fig. 2 Comparison of different methods for height evaluation in healthy volunteers. The *left column* represents the regression diagram of the two tested methods. The independent variable (reference value = measured height in the erect position) defines the *vertical axis*, and the dependent variable (tested method) defines the *horizontal axis*. *Dark line* represents the regression line; *r* = correlation coefficient; *P* value ≤0.05 was considered significant. The *right column* displays the scatter diagram of the differences of the two methods (Bland and Altman plot). *Dark line* represents the mean difference (estimation bias = ∂) between the two methods; *dotted line* represents the limit of agreement (plus and minus 1.96 SD) of the differences. For healthy volunteers, measured height in the upright position (reference) was well correlated with measured height in the supine position. This measured height may induce errors of 9.2 cm (2/60 volunteers with an error >10 cm). Chumlea height estimation, using either the standard or the simplified method in the supine position, was well correlated with actual height, with a low estimation bias. It may, however, induce errors from 8.9 to 11.8 cm

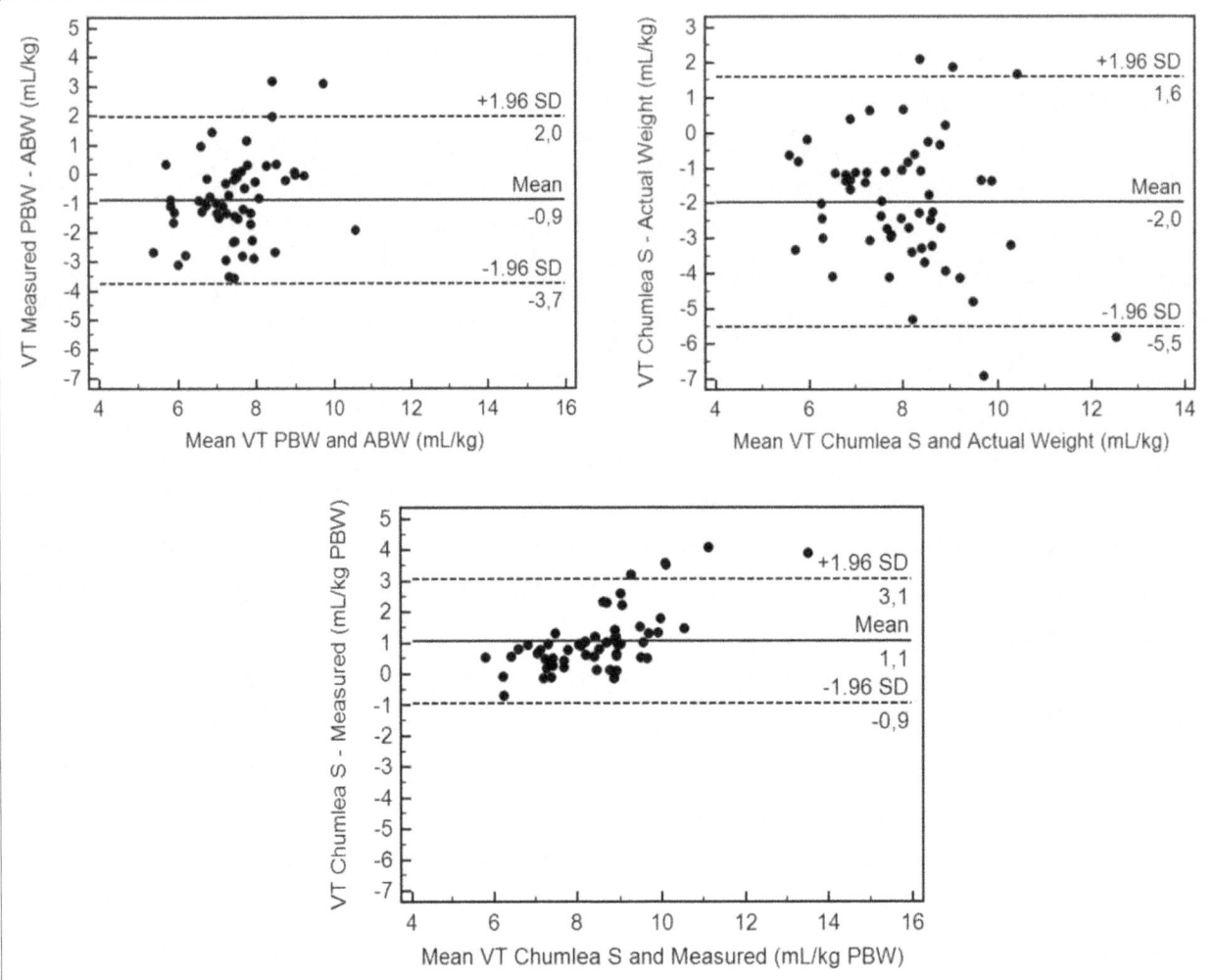

Fig. 3 Bland and Altman plot for tidal volume in ICU patients, using various measures and estimates. *VT* tidal volume, *PBW* predicted body weight, *ABW* actual body weight, *VT Measured* tidal volume set using the measured height, *VT Chumlea S* tidal volume set using the Simplified Chumlea height estimate. Tidal volume setting grandly vary while using either PBW or ABW, with as much as a 3.7 mL/kg range, whereas the mean bias remains low (−0.9 mL/kg). VT settings using either the measured PBW or its estimate (visual height estimation) are consistent. The simplified Chumlea method is consistent with the one using the measured value, generally providing a 1.1 mL/kg lower value

expert nurses. Third limitation could be that Chumlea stature prediction equations have been made specifically for defined populations [26, 29] and that other alternative methods have been developed and should be used for differing populations [45, 46]. However, such a limitation has been emphasized within the first phase of the study that was dedicated to the choice of the most accurate estimation formulas within our population of interest. Fourth limitation should be the fact that regression formula validation requires a huge cohort of patients, which is not the case within the current study. However, one should also consider that all the formulas for height estimates that were used within the study have already been validated and that the study only applies such formulas in

a different setting. Fifth and last limitation could be that our reference weight was measured on admission, while some of the patients may already have received huge amounts of intravenous fluids.

Conclusion

When actual height is unavailable in ICU patients, alternative anthropometric methods based on lower leg and forearm measurements could be useful to calculate patient's height and to facilitate the application of protective mechanical ventilation. The simplified Chumlea method is easy to achieve in a bed-ridden patient and provides accurate height estimates, with a low bias. Ulna and tibia estimates also provided valuable height estimates. All these methods are easy to perform, probably less time-consuming than standard methods, and they can also be performed with a short-length disposable tape instead of using long-lenght reusable tape, in an attempt to limit cross-contamination.

Abbreviations
ICU: intensive care unit; ARDS: acute respiratory distress syndrome; ID: identification card; ABW: actual body weight; IBW: ideal body weight; PBW: predicted body weight; CI: confidence interval; r: Pearson's correlation coefficient; ∂: bias; I 1, 2: different index measurements; HL 1–3: different hand length measurements; HW 1, 2: different hand width measurements; U 1–3: different ulna measurements; T 1–5: different tibia measurements; ARF: acute respiratory failure; Vt: tidal volume.

Authors' contributions
ELH conceived and supervised the study, analyzed the data and wrote the manuscript; JMB acquired all data and corrected the manuscript; FL conceived the study and corrected the manuscript. All authors read and approved the final manuscript.

Author details
[1] Réanimation Médicale, CHRU de Brest – La Cavale Blanche, Bvd Tanguy-Prigent, 29609 Brest Cedex, France. [2] LATIM INSERM UMR 1101, Université de Bretagne Occidentale, Brest Cedex, France. [3] Institut Universitaire de Cardiologie et de Pneumologie de Québec, Quebec, Canada.

Acknowledgements
The authors are grateful to our volunteers and patients for their participation in the study and to the entire ICU nursing staff for the technical support during the recruitment period.

Competing interests
The authors declare that they have no competing interests.

References
1. Martin JH, Fay MF, Udy A, Roberts J, Kirkpatrick C, Ungerer J, Lipman J. Pitfalls of using estimations of glomerular filtration rate in an intensive care population. Intern Med J. 2011;41:537–43.
2. Diacon AH, Koegelenberg CFN, Klüsmann KJC, Bolliger CT. Challenges in the estimation of tidal volume settings in critical care units. Intensive Care Med. 2006;32:1670–1.
3. Hepper NG, Fowler WS, Helmholz HF Jr. Relationship of height to lung volume in healthy men. Dis Chest. 1960;37:314–20.
4. Neto AS, Cardoso SO, Manetta JA, Pereira VGM, Espósito DC, Pasqualucci MDO, Damasceno MC, Schultz MJ. Association between use of lung-protective ventilation with lower tidal volumes and clinical outcomes among patients without acute respiratory distress syndrome: a meta-analysis. JAMA. 2012;308:1651–9.
5. Gajic O, Dara SI, Mendez JL, Adesanya AO, Festic E, Caples SM, Rana R, St Sauver JL, Lymp JF, Afessa B, Hubmayr RD. Ventilator-associated lung injury in patients without acute lung injury at the onset of mechanical ventilation. Crit Care Med. 2004;32:1817–24.
6. Gajic O, Frutos-Vivar F, Esteban A, Hubmayr RD, Anzueto A. Ventilator settings as a risk factor for acute respiratory distress syndrome in mechanically ventilated patients. Intensive Care Med. 2005;31:922–6.
7. Lellouche F, Dionne S, Simard S, Bussières J, Dagenais F. High tidal volumes in mechanically ventilated patients increase organ dysfunction after cardiac surgery. Anesthesiology. 2012;16:1072–82.
8. Deane AM, Reid DA, Tobin AE. Predicted body weight during mechanical ventilation: using arm demispan to aid clinical assessment. Crit Care Resusc. 2008;10:14.
9. Leary TS, Milner QJ, Niblett DJ. The accuracy of the estimation of body weight and height in the intensive care unit. Eur J Anaesthesiol. 2000;17:698–703.
10. Tremblay A, Bandi V. Impact of body mass index on outcomes following critical care. Chest. 2003;123:1202–7.
11. Schultz MJ, Wolthuis EK. Excess body weight in critically ill patients. Ann Intern Med. 2004;141:485.
12. Determann RM, Wolthuis EK, Spronk PE, Kuiper MA, Korevaar JC, Vroom MB, Schultz MJ. Reliability of height and weight estimates in patients acutely admitted to intensive care units. Crit Care Nurse. 2007;27:48–55.
13. Anzueto A, Frutos-Vivar F, Esteban A, Bensalami N, Marks D, Raymondos K, Apezteguía C, Arabi Y, Hurtado J, González M, Tomicic V, Abroug F, Elizalde J, Cakar N, Pelosi P, Ferguson ND. Ventila group: influence of body mass index on outcome of the mechanically ventilated patients. Thorax. 2011;66:66–73.
14. Kam EPY, Eslick GD, James A, Benson JP. Acute respiratory distress syndrome (ARDS) and low tidal volume ventilation: the debate about weight. Intensive Care Med. 2004;30:1502.
15. Jaber S, Coisel Y, Chanques G, Futier E, Constantin J-M, Michelet P, Beaussier M, Lefrant JY, Allaouchiche B, Capdevila X, Marret E. A multi-centre observational study of intra-operative ventilatory management during general anaesthesia: tidal volumes and relation to body weight. Anaesthesia. 2012;67:999–1008.
16. O'Brien JM, Phillips GS, Ali NA, Lucarelli M, Marsh CB, Lemeshow S. Body mass index is independently associated with hospital mortality in mechanically ventilated adults with acute lung injury. Crit Care Med. 2006;34:738–44.
17. Bloomfield R, Steel E, MacLennan G, Noble DW. Accuracy of weight and height estimation in an intensive care unit: Implications for clinical practice and research. Crit Care Med. 2006;34:2153–7.
18. Tallach R, Jefferson P, Ball DR. Mechanical ventilation for patients with ARDS: a UK survey on calculation of tidal volume. Intensive Care Med. 2006;32:176.
19. García del Moral Martín R, Morales Laborías ME, Fernández López I, Rodríguez Delgado E, Díaz Castellanos MA. Estimación subjetiva del peso y talla de los pacientes de UCI. Medidas poco aconsejables. Med Intensiva. 2013;37:50–2.
20. Hendershot KM, Robinson L, Roland J, Vaziri K, Rizzo AG, Fakhry SM. Estimated height, weight, and body mass index: implications for research and patient safety. J Am Coll Surg. 2006;203:887–93.
21. Maskin LP, Attie S, Setten M, Rodriguez PO, Bonelli I, Stryjewski ME, Valentini R. Accuracy of weight and height estimation in an intensive care unit. Anaesth Intensive Care. 2010;38:930–4.
22. Habib SR, Kamal NN. Stature estimation from hand and phalanges lengths of Egyptians. J Forensic Leg Med. 2010;17:156–60.
23. Agnihotri AK, Agnihotri S, Jeebun N, Googoolye K. Prediction of stature using hand dimensions. J Forensic Leg Med. 2008;15:479–82.
24. Krishan K, Sharma A. Estimation of stature from dimensions of hands and feet in a North Indian population. J Forensic Leg Med. 2007;14:327–32.
25. El Najjar M, McWilliams K. Forensic anthropology: the structure, morphology, and variation of human bone and dentition. Springfield: Charles C Thomas; 1978.
26. Cleuvenot E, Houët F. Proposition de nouvelles équations d'estimation de la stature applicables pour un sexe indéterminé et basées sur les échantillons de Trotter et Gleser. Bull Mém Soc Anthrop Paris. 1993;5:245–55.
27. Allbrook D. The estimation of stature in British and East African males. Based on tibial and ulnar bone lengths. J Forensic Med. 1961;8:15–28.
28. Raxter MH, Auerbach BM, Ruff CB. Revision of the fully technique for estimating statures. Am J Phys Anthropol. 2006;130:374–84.
29. Chumlea WC, Roche AF, Steinbaugh ML. Estimating stature from knee height for persons 60 to 90 years of age. J Am Geriatr Soc. 1985;33:116–20.
30. Lorentz F. Ein neuer constitutions index. Klinische Wochenschrift. 1929;8:348–51.
31. Knoben JE, Anderson PO. Handbook of clinical drug data. Hamilton: Drug Intelligence Publications; 1993.
32. Bland JM, Altman DG. Measuring agreement in method comparison studies. Stat Methods Med Res. 1999;8:135–60.
33. Umoh NJ, Fan E, Mendez-Tellez PA, Sevransky JE, Dennison CR, Shanholtz C, Pronovost PJ, Needham DM. Patient and intensive care unit organizational factors associated with low tidal volume ventilation in acute lung injury. Crit Care Med. 2008;36:1463–8.

34. Young MP, Manning HL, Wilson DL, Mette SA, Riker RR, Leiter JC, Liu SK, Bates JT, Parsons PE. Ventilation of patients with acute lung injury and acute respiratory distress syndrome: has new evidence changed clinical practice? Crit Care Med. 2004;32:1260–5.
35. Villar J, Kacmarek RM, Hedenstierna G. From ventilator-induced lung injury to physician-induced lung injury: why the reluctance to use small tidal volumes? Acta Anaesthesiol Scand. 2004;48:267–71.
36. Jia X, Malhotra A, Saeed M, Mark RG, Talmor D. Risk factors for ARDS in patients receiving mechanical ventilation for >48 h. Chest. 2008;133:853–61.
37. Coe TR, Halkes M, Houghton K, Jefferson D. The accuracy of visual estimation of weight and height in pre-operative supine patients. Anaesthesia. 1999;54:582–6.
38. Uesugi T, Okada N, Sakai K, Nishina K, Mikawa K, Shiga M. Accuracy of visual estimation of body height and weight in supine paediatric patients. Paediatr Anaesth. 2002;12:489–94.
39. Hall WL 2nd, Larkin GL, Trujillo MJ, Hinds JL, Delaney KA. Errors in weight estimation in the emergency department: comparing performance by providers and patients. J Emerg Med. 2004;27:219–24.
40. Berger MM, Cayeux M-C, Schaller M-D, Soguel L, Piazza G, Chioléro RL. Stature estimation using the knee height determination in critically ill patients. E Spen Eur E J Clin Nutr Metab. 2008;3:e84–8.
41. Hickson M, Frost G. A comparison of three methods for estimating height in the acutely ill elderly population. J Hum Nutr Diet. 2003;16:13–20.
42. Beghetto MG, Fink J, Luft VC, de Mello ED. Estimates of body height in adult inpatients. Clin Nutr. 2006;25:438–43.
43. Han S, Martin GS, Maloney JP, Shanholtz C, Barnes KC, Murray S, Sevransky JE. Short women with severe sepsis-related acute lung injury receive lung protective ventilation less frequently: an observational cohort study. Crit Care. 2011;15:R262.
44. Walkey AJ, Wiener RS. Risk factors for underuse of lung-protective ventilation in acute lung injury. J Crit Care. 2012;27(323):e1–9.
45. Hwang IC, Kim KK, Kang HC, Kang DR. Validity of stature-predicted equations using knee height for elderly and mobility impaired persons in Koreans. Epidemiol Health. 2009;31:e2009004.
46. Shahar S, Pooy NS. Predictive equations for estimation of stature in Malaysian elderly people. Asia Pac J Clin Nutr. 2003;12:80–4.

2

Aspergillus-positive lower respiratory tract samples in patients with the acute respiratory distress syndrome

Damien Contou[1,2], Matthieu Dorison[1], Jérémy Rosman[1], Frédéric Schlemmer[3], Aude Gibelin[1], Françoise Foulet[4], Françoise Botterel[4], Guillaume Carteaux[1,2], Keyvan Razazi[1,2], Christian Brun-Buisson[1,2], Armand Mekontso Dessap[1,2] and Nicolas de Prost[1,2]* (iD)

Abstract

Background: The detection of *Aspergillus* spp. in endotracheal aspirate cultures of mechanically ventilated patients may reflect either colonization or infection. However, little is known about the prevalence and the impact on outcome of respiratory tract sample positive for *Aspergillus* during the acute respiratory distress syndrome (ARDS).

Methods: We conducted a monocentric, retrospective study over a 10-year period (January 2006–December 2015) in the ICU of a university hospital. All consecutive adult patients with ARDS were included, and the diagnosis of invasive pulmonary aspergillosis was assessed using a previously validated algorithm.

Results: In total, 423 ARDS patients were included with 35 patients [8.3 %, 95 % CI (5.4–10.6)] having at least one respiratory tract sample positive for *Aspergillus* (Aspergillus+ patients) after a median delay of 3 days (1–11) following ICU admission. Comorbidities did not differ between Aspergillus+ and Aspergillus− patients except for more frequent immunosuppression in Aspergillus+ patients (40 vs. 22 %; $p = 0.02$). There was no difference between Aspergillus− and Aspergillus+ patients regarding in-ICU mortality, ventilator-free days at day 28, and incidence of ventilator-associated pneumonia, but need for renal replacement therapy was higher in Aspergillus+ patients than in others (49 vs. 27 %; $p = 0.01$). Seventeen [4.0 %, 95 % CI (2.1–5.9)] patients had putative/proven aspergillosis. After adjusting on covariates associated with ICU mortality, putative/proven aspergillosis was associated with in-ICU mortality [aOR = 9.58 (1.97–46.52); $p = 0.005$], while *Aspergillus* colonization was not [aOR = 0.64 (0.21–1.99); $p = 0.44$].

Conclusions: Eight percent of ARDS patients had *Aspergillus* spp.-positive respiratory tract cultures. These had a higher risk of mortality only when categorized as having putative or proven invasive pulmonary aspergillosis.

Keywords: *Aspergillus*, Invasive pulmonary aspergillosis, Acute respiratory distress syndrome, Immunosuppression

Background

Invasive pulmonary aspergillosis (IPA) has been reported chiefly in immunocompromised patients with prolonged neutropenia, organ and allogeneic stem cell transplantation, prolonged corticosteroids use or severe inherited immunodeficiency [1]. However, in the past decade, definite cases of IPA have also been reported in intensive care unit (ICU) patients having none of the previously defined host risk factors for IPA [2], but other associated illnesses including advanced cirrhosis [3, 4], H1N1 *Influenza* infection [5] or chronic obstructive pulmonary disease (COPD) [4–7]. In one study, the prevalence of IPA

*Correspondence: nicolas.de-prost@aphp.fr
[1] Groupe Henri Mondor-Albert Chenevier, Centre Hospitalier Universitaire Henri Mondor, DHU A-TVB, Service de Réanimation Médicale, Assistance Publique-Hôpitaux de Paris, 51, Avenue du Maréchal de Lattre de Tassigny, 94010 Créteil Cedex, France
Full list of author information is available at the end of the article

reached 6 % in a cohort of patients without malignancy hospitalized in a medical ICU [4]. Endotracheal aspirate cultures growing *Aspergillus* spp. have been recorded in 1–2 % of mechanically ventilated ICU patients having no predisposing factors and may reflect either colonization or infection [8–11]. A recent clinical algorithm developed by Blot et al. demonstrated favorable operating characteristics to discriminate *Aspergillus* respiratory tract colonization from IPA in ICU patients, whereas the European Organization for Research and Treatment of Cancer/Mycosis Study Group (EORTC/MSG) criteria failed to adequately categorize patients in the absence of conventional risk factors [1].

The acute respiratory distress syndrome (ARDS) [12] occurs in about 10 % of ICU patients and is associated with a high mortality of 35 % [13]. Respiratory tract *Aspergillus* colonization was shown to be more frequent in ARDS than in other critically ill patients [14]. An autopsy study of 64 patients with ARDS revealed that 8 of them (13 %) had died with pulmonary lesions of IPA [15]. However, the burden of IPA during ARDS has been poorly studied and little is known on the prevalence of *Aspergillus* respiratory tract colonization and IPA during ARDS, as well as on the prognosis of IPA in this setting. In this monocenter retrospective study we aimed at: (1) assessing the prevalence, (2) reporting the clinical characteristics, and (3) evaluating the impact on outcome of *Aspergillus*-positive lower respiratory tract specimen in ARDS patients.

Methods

We conducted a monocenter retrospective study in the 24-bed medical ICU of a tertiary referral center (Henri Mondor Hospital, Créteil, France). All consecutive adult (>18 years) patients admitted in the ICU for ARDS according to the Berlin definition criteria (within 48 h of admission) and receiving invasive mechanical ventilation over a 10-year period (January 2006 to December 2015) were included [12]. Exclusion criteria were as follows: previously known lung interstitial disease or tumoral infiltration, chronic respiratory failure requiring long-term oxygen therapy, pure cardiogenic pulmonary edema, mild ARDS treated with noninvasive ventilation only, proven or suspected invasive pulmonary aspergillosis under antifungal therapy upon ARDS diagnosis and patients for whom no endobronchial sampling had been obtained.

All respiratory tract samples (plugged telescoping catheter, tracheal aspirate or bronchoalveolar fluid) performed for microbiological examination were analyzed. Galactomannan antigen (GM) detection in plasma and in bronchoalveolar lavage (BAL) fluid was performed at the discretion of the managing physician. An optical

density ratio of 0.5 or greater for GM in serum and of 1.0 or greater for BAL fluid was considered positive. Chest CT scan and cerebral or facial scan were not routinely performed.

Definition of infection and categorization of patients

Patients were categorized into two groups: those with one or more respiratory tract sample positive in culture for *Aspergillus* spp. (Aspergillus+ patients) during the ICU stay and those without such positive sample (Aspergillus− patients). The former group was further split into three categories depending on the probability of IPA according to the clinical algorithm proposed by Blot et al. [16]: (A) proven IPA (microscopic analysis on sterile material: histopathologic, cytopathologic or direct microscopic examination of a specimen obtained by needle aspiration or sterile biopsy in which hyphae are seen accompanied by evidence of associated tissue damage; isolation of *Aspergillus* from culture of a specimen obtained by lung biopsy); (B) putative IPA in case of (1) *Aspergillus*-positive lower respiratory tract specimen culture (entry criterion) with (2) compatible signs and symptoms (one of the following: fever refractory to at least 3 days of appropriate antibiotic therapy, recrudescent fever after a period of defervescence of at least 48 h while still on antibiotics and without other apparent cause, pleuritic chest pain, pleuritic rub, dyspnea, hemoptysis, worsening respiratory insufficiency in spite of appropriate antibiotic therapy and ventilatory support) and (3) abnormal medical imaging by portable chest X-ray or CT scan of the lungs, and either (4a) a host risk factor (one of the following conditions: neutropenia (absolute neutrophil count <500 G/L) preceding or at the time of ICU admission, underlying hematological or oncological malignancy treated with cytotoxic agents, glucocorticoid treatment (prednisone equivalent >20 mg/day), congenital or acquired immunodeficiency) or (4b) a semiquantitative *Aspergillus*-positive culture of BAL fluid (+ or +++), without bacterial growth together with a positive cytological smear showing branching hyphae or (C) *Aspergillus* respiratory tract colonization when ≥1 criterion necessary for a diagnosis of putative IPA was not met (Tables 1, 2).

Collection of data and definitions

Demographics and clinical characteristics upon ICU admission and during ICU stay were abstracted from the medical charts of all patients. Immunosuppression was defined by one of the following conditions: neutropenia (absolute neutrophil count <500 G/L) preceding or at the time of ICU admission, underlying hematological or oncological malignancy treated with cytotoxic agents, glucocorticoid treatment (prednisone equivalent >20 mg/

Table 1 Demographics and clinical characteristics upon ICU admission of ARDS patients with (*Aspergillus*$^+$) or without (*Aspergillus*$^-$) one or more respiratory tract sample positive for *Aspergillus* spp.

	All (n = 423)	*Aspergillus*$^-$ (n = 388)	*Aspergillus*$^+$ (n = 35)	p value
Age (years)	62 (50–72)	62 (50–72)	62 (49–72)	0.82
Gender (male)	282 (67)	258 (66)	24 (69)	0.85
Previously known aspergillosis	8 (2)	7 (2)	1 (3)	0.50
Immunosuppression	100 (24)	86 (22)	14 (40)	0.023
COPD	48 (11)	44 (11)	4 (11)	>0.99
Inhaled steroids	16 (4)	15 (4)	1 (3)	>0.99
Liver cirrhosis	44 (10)	42 (11)	2 (6)	0.56
Chronic renal failure	16 (4)	15 (4)	1 (3)	>0.99
Diabetes mellitus	85 (20)	79 (20)	6 (17)	0.83
SAPS II	53 (37–69)	53 (38–70)	51 (34–68)	0.65
LODS	8 (6–12)	8 (6–12)	7 (5–11)	0.26
Main ARDS risk factors				
Pulmonary infection	202 (48)	173 (45)	29 (83)	<0.0001
Aspiration	154 (36)	147 (38)	7 (20)	0.043
Non-pulmonary sepsis	87 (21)	84 (22)	3 (9)	0.080
Drug overdose	12 (3)	11 (3)	1 (3)	>0.99
Delay first respiratory symptom—admission, days	2 (0–5)	2 (0–5)	2 (0–8)	0.41
Temperature > 38.3 °C	220 (52)	199 (51)	21 (60)	0.38
Noninvasive ventilation	69 (16)	65 (17)	4 (11)	0.63
Berlin classification				0.38
Mild	113 (27)	104 (27)	9 (26)	
Moderate	162 (38)	144 (37)	18 (51)	
Severe	148 (35)	140 (36)	8 (23)	
PaO$_2$/FiO$_2$ ratio (mm Hg)	106 (77–163)	106 (78–162)	114 (76–173)	0.84
Shock	325 (77)	297 (76)	28 (80)	0.83
Serum creatinine (μmol/L)	120 (82–180)	120 (82–177)	128 (82–207)	0.76

ARDS acute respiratory distress syndrome, *COPD* chronic obstructive pulmonary disease; continuous variables are shown as median (interquartile range 25–75); categorical variables are shown as n (%)

day for more than 4 weeks), congenital (e.g., chronic granulomatous disease, hyper-IgE syndrome [17]) or acquired (e.g., AIDS [18]) immunodeficiency. Patient initial severity was assessed using the Simplified Acute Physiology Score II (SAPS II) [19] and Logistic Organ Dysfunction (LOD) [20] scores. ARDS was categorized as mild, moderate or severe according to the lowest PaO$_2$/FiO$_2$ ratio obtained within 48 h of ICU admission [12]. Shock was defined as need for vasopressor (epinephrine or norepinephrine) at a dose higher than 1 mg/h for more than 2 h. Outcome variables included the use of adjuvant therapies for ARDS (i.e., neuromuscular blocking agents, nitric oxide inhalation, prone positioning or venovenous extracorporeal membrane oxygenation), the need for renal replacement therapy or vasopressors, the administration of corticosteroids, the number of ventilator-free days at day 28, the duration of ICU stay, the incidence of ventilator-associated pneumonia and in-ICU mortality.

All chest CT scans performed in Aspergillus$^+$ patients were reviewed by two pulmonologists (FS and NDP) blinded to the final *Aspergillus* classification and outcome. Elementary lesions including alveolar consolidation, lung nodules, ground-glass opacities, halo sign, cavitation and pleural effusion were recorded.

Patient's management

ARDS patients received mechanical ventilation using a standardized protective ventilation strategy [21, 22]. Tracheal suction was performed using a closed system. Other treatments including neuromuscular blocking agents [23], nitric oxide inhalation, prone positioning [24] and venovenous extracorporeal membrane oxygenation were administered depending on the severity of ARDS [25].

Antifungal therapy (voriconazole, caspofungin or liposomal amphotericin B) was administered at the

Table 2 Classification of ARDS patients with one or more respiratory tract sample positive for *Aspergillus* spp., according to the Blot algorithm, adapted from Blot et al. [16]

	Immunosuppression ($n = 17$)[a]	No Immunosuppression ($n = 18$)
Proven invasive pulmonary aspergillosis ($n = 1$)	1 (6)	0 (0)
Putative invasive pulmonary aspergillosis ($n = 16$)	11 (65)	5 (28)[b]
1. Aspergillus-positive lower respiratory tract specimen culture	17	18
2. Compatible signs and symptoms		
Fever refractory to at least 3 d of appropriate antibiotic therapy	3	1
Recrudescent fever after a period of defervescence of at least 48 h while still on antibiotics and without other apparent cause	1	0
Pleuritic chest pain	1	0
Pleuritic rub	0	0
Dyspnea	0	0
Hemoptysis	1	0
Worsening respiratory insufficiency in spite of appropriate antibiotic therapy and ventilatory support	6	11
3. Abnormal medical imaging by portable chest X-ray or CT scan of the lungs	17	18
4a. Host risk factors	17	0
Neutropenia (absolute neutrophil count < 0.5 G/L) preceding or at the time of ICU admission	4	0
Underlying hematological or oncological malignancy treated with cytotoxic agents	5	0
Glucocorticoid treatment (prednisone equivalent >20 mg/d and >4 weeks)	1	0
Congenital or acquired immunodeficiency	7	0
4b. Semiquantitative Aspergillus-positive culture of BAL fluid (+ or ++), without bacterial growth together with a positive cytological smear showing branching hyphae	4	6
Aspergillus respiratory tract colonization ($n = 18$)	5 (29)	13 (72)[c]

[a] Hematological malignancies ($n = 7$, including lymphoma ($n = 5$), acute leukemia ($n = 2$), one of whom required allogeneic bone marrow transplant), solid organ transplant ($n = 6$), gastric cancer ($n = 1$), HIV infection ($n = 1$), neutropenia of unknown cause ($n = 1$) and connective tissue disease under corticosteroid treatment ($n = 1$)

[b] $p = 0.018$ and [c] $p = 0.015$ (Fisher's exact test) for comparison between immunosuppressed and non-immunosuppressed patients; continuous variables are shown as median (interquartile range 25–75); categorical variables are shown as n (%)

discretion of the managing physician and not initiated on the sole basis of a positive GM in serum or in BAL fluid.

Statistical analysis

Continuous variables are reported as median [25th–75th percentiles] or mean ± standard deviation (SD) and compared as appropriate. Categorical variables are reported as numbers and percentages [95 % confidence interval (95 % CI)] and compared as appropriate. There was no imputation for missing data, except for data missing from comorbidities, which were then considered as absent. Factors associated with ICU mortality were determined by univariable and multivariable backward logistic regression analyses. Independent variables with a p value <0.10 in univariable analysis were entered into the multivariable model, with backward elimination of variables displaying a p value greater than 0.05. Interactions between variables were assessed using the Mantel–Haenszel test. Analyses were conducted using the SPSS Base 21.0 statistical software package (SPSS Inc., Chicago, IL).

Results

Prevalence of *Aspergillus*+ respiratory tract samples during ARDS

Over the 10-year study period, 423 patients were admitted for ARDS, of whom 35 [8.3 %, 95 % CI (5.4–10.6)] had at least one respiratory tract sample positive for *Aspergillus* spp. (Aspergillus+ patients) (Fig. 1; Table 1).

Among 17 (49 %) immunocompromised Aspergillus+ patients, one had proven IPA, 11 had putative IPA, and 5 were categorized as having respiratory tract colonization. Conversely, among 18 (51 %) non-immunocompromised Aspergillus+ patients, 5 had putative IPA and 13 had colonization (Fig. 1; Table 2). The overall prevalence of proven/putative aspergillosis was 4.0 % [95 % CI (2.1–5.9)].

Presentation of ARDS patients with *Aspergillus*-positive respiratory tract samples

Comorbidities did not differ between Aspergillus+ and Aspergillus− patients except for more frequent

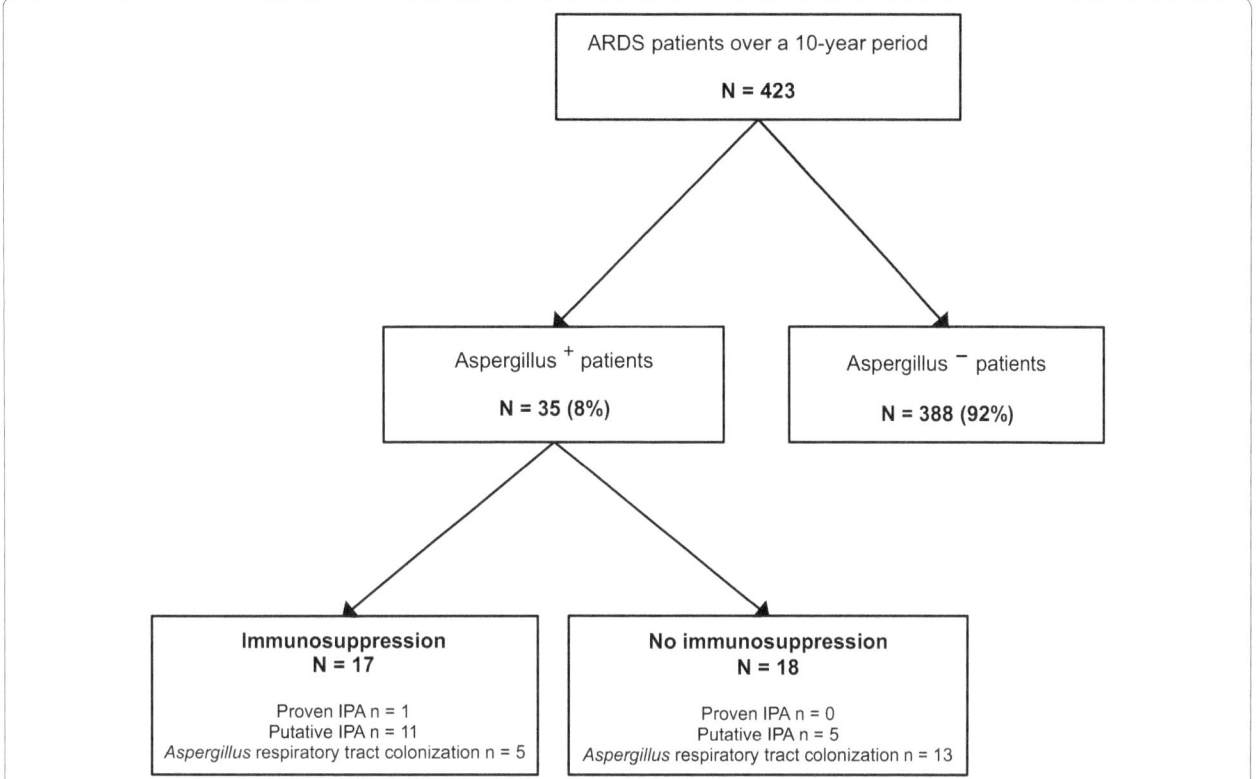

Fig. 1 Flowchart of patients with the acute respiratory distress syndrome (ARDS) included in the study. Eight percent of patients (*n* = 35) had a respiratory tract culture positive for *Aspergillus* spp., including both immunosuppressed (*n* = 17) and non-immunosuppressed (*n* = 18) patients. The diagnostic probability of invasive pulmonary aspergillosis was assessed using the algorithm of Blot et al. [16]

immunosuppression in the former group (Table 1). The two groups did not differ regarding clinical presentation and severity of illness upon ICU admission, as assessed by SAPS II, LODS and ARDS severity. Regarding the main ARDS risk factors retrieved, infective pneumonia was significantly more frequent (while aspiration pneumonitis was less frequent) in Aspergillus$^+$ patients than in others (Table 1).

Among the 35 patients of the Aspergillus$^+$ group, 27 (77 %) had a GM measurement performed in both plasma and BAL fluid. Plasma GM measurements were not significantly different between patients with proven/putative IPA and those with *Aspergillus* spp. colonization (7/15, 47 % vs. 2/12, 17 %, $p = 0.22$). In contrast, when measured in BAL fluid, GM was more frequently positive in patients with proven/putative IPA than in those with *Aspergillus* colonization (8/15, 53 % vs. 0/12, 0 %, $p = 0.003$) (Table 3).

Chest CT scans were obtained in 60 % ($n = 21/35$) of patients of the Aspergillus$^+$ group during ICU stay (Table 4; Fig. 2) and displayed no significant difference between patients categorized as having proven/putative aspergillosis ($n = 13/21$) and those with *Aspergillus*

colonization ($n = 8/21$). Of note, while lung nodules were observed in 67 % of cases, other chest CT scan patterns suggestive of IPA, including lung cavitation and halo sign, were detected in only 14 % of cases. Alveolar consolidations, consistent with the underlying ARDS, were present in 90 % of cases.

Management and outcome of ARDS patients with *Aspergillus*-positive respiratory tract samples
The median number of collected samples was 3 (2–7) per patient, and the median delay between ICU admission and the first respiratory tract sample positive for *Aspergillus* spp. was 3 days (1–11) (Table 5). There were no differences between Aspergillus$^-$ and Aspergillus$^+$ patients regarding duration of ICU stay, in-ICU mortality, number of ventilator-free days at day 28 and incidence of ventilator-acquired pneumonia and of shock. In contrast, the need for renal replacement therapy was almost twice as high in Aspergillus$^+$ patients than in others (Table 5). Within the Aspergillus$^+$ group, fifteen patients received an antifungal treatment during ICU stay (voriconazole, $n = 12$; liposomal amphotericin B, $n = 3$; caspofungin, $n = 2$; combination therapy, $n = 3$), including the sole

Table 3 Serum and bronchoalveolar lavage fluid galactomannan antigen according to the probability of invasive pulmonary aspergillosis (Blot et al. algorithm [16])

	All (n = 27)	Proven/putative aspergillosis (n = 15)	*Aspergillus* colonization (n = 12)	p value[a]
Positive serum galactomannan	9 (33)	7 (47)	2 (17)	0.22
Positive BAL fluid galactomannan	8 (30)	8 (53)	0 (0)	0.003

BAL bronchoalveolar lavage

[a] p value comes from the Fisher exact test; an optical density (OD) ratio of 0.5 or greater for galactomannan antigen in serum and 1.0 for BAL fluid was considered positive

Table 4 Chest CT scan patterns in patients (n = 21) categorized as having proven/putative invasive pulmonary aspergillosis or *Aspergillus* colonization, according to the Blot algorithm [16]

	All (n = 21)	Proven/putative aspergillosis (n = 13)	*Aspergillus* colonization (n = 8)	p value[a]
Pulmonary infiltrates	21 (100)	13 (100)	8 (100)	>0.99
Alveolar consolidation	19 (90)	11 (85)	8 (100)	0.11
Lung nodules	15 (71)	8 (61)	7 (87)	0.33
Ground-glass opacities	14 (67)	10 (77)	4 (50)	0.34
Cavitation	3 (14)	1 (8)	2 (25)	0.53
Halo sign	3 (14)	2 (15)	1 (12)	>0.99
Pleural effusion	12 (57)	8 (61)	4 (50)	0.67

[a] p value comes from the Fisher exact test; categorical variables are shown as n (%)

patient with proven IPA, 10 over 16 patients with putative IPA and 4 over 18 patients with *Aspergillus* respiratory tract colonization.

The association between *Aspergillus* status, as categorized with the Blot et al. algorithm, and in-ICU mortality was assessed by logistic regression analysis. Both in univariable analysis [OR = 7.98 (1.80–35.36), $p = 0.006$] and after adjusting for covariates significantly associated with ICU mortality, putative/proven IPA was strongly associated with in-ICU mortality [aOR = 9.58 (1.97–46.52), $p = 0.005$], while *Aspergillus* colonization was not [aOR = 0.64 (0.21–1.99), $p = 0.44$] (Table 6). Of note, within the putative/proven IPA subgroup (n = 17), 10/12 immunocompromised and 5/5 non-immunocompromised patients died in the ICU.

Discussion

We herein report *Aspergillus*-positive lower respiratory tract specimen culture in an 8 % prevalence of patients with ARDS, half of whom had putative or proven IPA. Immunosuppression and pneumonia were more frequent among patients having at least one positive sample for *Aspergillus*. Immunocompromised ARDS patients were more frequently categorized as having putative or proven IPA, while non-immunocompromised patients were more likely categorized as having *Aspergillus* respiratory tract colonization. Importantly, patients with one

or more positive respiratory tract sample for *Aspergillus* had a worse outcome than others only when categorized as having putative/proven IPA according to the Blot algorithm.

The current series is, to the best of our knowledge, the largest one to focus on *Aspergillus*-positive respiratory tract samples in ARDS patients. The 8 % prevalence of patients having at least one positive sample for *Aspergillus*, in our population with ARDS, is significantly higher than the 1 % rate prospectively reported by Bassetti et al. in unselected mechanically ventilated patients, suggesting ARDS is a risk factor for *Aspergillus* respiratory colonization and/or infection [14]. Four percent of our ARDS patients (n = 17/423) were eventually classified as having proven or putative IPA, which is less than the 13 % prevalence of proven IPA that was previously reported in an autopsy study of 64 patients with ARDS [15], likely due to differences in case-mix and methods between this study and ours. Such figures are consistent with the fact that the Blot et al. algorithm was previously shown to have 61 % specificity and positive predictive value and 92 % sensitivity and negative predictive value, implying that its ability to exclude IPA might be better than in diagnosing it [16, 26]. Strikingly, the median delay between the first respiratory sample positive for *Aspergillus* spp. and mechanical ventilation initiation was 3 days, consistent with a previous study in mechanically ventilated

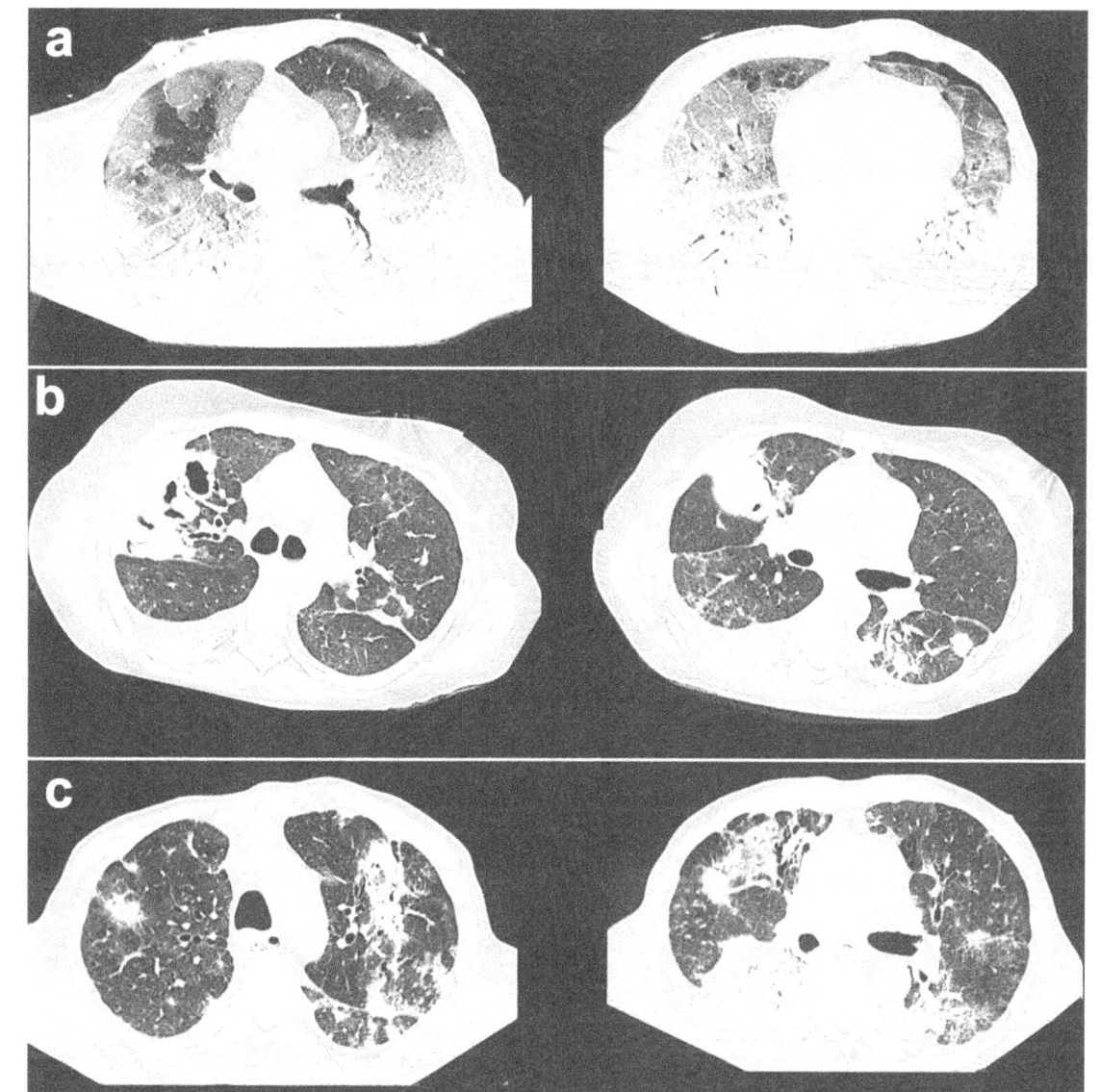

Fig. 2 Chest CT scan images in patients with ARDS and one or more respiratory tract culture positive for *Aspergillus* spp., categorized as having putative invasive pulmonary aspergillosis (IPA) or *Aspergillus* colonization [16]. CT scan slices depicted **a** ARDS-typical bilateral basal consolidations, together with ground-glass opacities (*left panel*) and left anterior pneumothorax (*right panel*) in a patient categorized as having putative IPA; **b** *right upper* lobe cavitation (*left panel*), together with nodular lesions (*right panel*) in a patient with necrotizing group A *Streptococcus*, categorized as having *Aspergillus* respiratory tract colonization; and **c** nodular lesions with ground-glass opacities (*left panel*) and alveolar consolidations (*right panel*) in a patient categorized as having putative IPA

non-ARDS patients [11], suggesting that respiratory tract colonization by *Aspergillus* spores had occurred prior to ARDS onset. The combination of ARDS-associated alveolar damage and associated local immune dysregulation [27], together with sepsis-induced immunosuppression [28], might, through alterations in innate immunity and antigen presentation processes [29], account for the development of IPA in previously colonized patients. Other previously described conditions at risk of IPA in

critically ill non-immunosuppressed patients include COPD, present in only 11 % of our Aspergillus[+] group, as compared to 31 % in a large series and, to a lesser extent, cirrhosis and corticosteroids, observed in less than 10 % of cases [6]. Surprisingly, however, corticosteroid administration was not associated with mortality in a recent series of mechanically ventilated patients with proven or putative Aspergillosis [6]. Although we found a trend toward more high-dose steroids administration in the

Table 5 Management and outcomes of ARDS patients with (*Aspergillus*+) or without (*Aspergillus*−) one or more respiratory tract sample positive for *Aspergillus* spp.

	All (n = 423)	*Aspergillus*− (n = 388)	*Aspergillus*+ (n = 35)	p value
Microbiological examinations				
Number of endobronchial samples	4.0 (2.0–7.0)	3.5 (2.0–7.0)	4.5 (2.7–9.2)	0.019
Including BAL	211 (48)	181 (45)	30 (86)	<0.0001
Duration of ICU stay (days)	12 (6–22)	12 (6–22)	14 (7–35)	0.14
Ventilator-free days at day 28 (days)	0 (0–17)	0 (0–22)	0 (0–16)	0.19
Ventilator-acquired pneumonia	146 (35)	135 (35)	11 (31)	0.85
Treatment				
Prone position	169 (40)	153 (40)	16 (46)	0.48
Nitric oxide inhalation	117 (28)	108 (28)	9 (26)	0.85
Paralyzing agents	380 (92)	348 (92)	32 (91)	>0.99
ECMO	21 (5)	18 (5)	3 (9)	0.40
Shock	350 (83)	321 (83)	29 (83)	>0.99
Renal replacement therapy	122 (29)	105 (27)	17 (49)	0.011
Corticosteroids				
"Stress-dose" steroids[a]	144 (34)	134 (34)	10 (29)	0.58
"High-dose" steroids[b]	96 (23)	84 (22)	12 (34)	0.094
In-ICU mortality	209 (50)	188 (48)	21 (60)	0.22

ECMO extracorporeal membrane oxygenation, *BAL* bronchoalveolar lavage

[a] Hydrocortisone 200 mg/day

[b] Prednisone equivalent >1 mg/kg/day; continuous variables are shown as median (interquartile range 25–75); categorical variables are shown as n (%)

Table 6 Univariable and multivariable logistic regression analyses of factors associated with ICU mortality in ARDS patients

	n	Death n (%)	Univariable analysis OR (95 % CI)	p	Multivariable analysis aOR (95 % CI)	p
Age (years)	–	–	1.02 (1.01–1.03)	<0.0001	1.02 (1.00–1.03)	0.029
Year of inclusion	–	–	0.89 (0.82–0.95)	<0.001	–	–
Liver cirrhosis						
Yes	44	31 (70.5)	2.69 (1.37–5.31)	0.004	2.62 (1.24–5.54)	0.012
No	379	178 (47.0)	1		1	
Immunosuppression						
Yes	100	58 (58.0)	1.57 (1.00–2.47)	0.050	1.83 (1.08–3.11)	0.024
No	323	151 (46.7)	1		1	
PaO_2/FiO_2 ratio (mmHg)	–	–	0.99 (0.99–0.99)	<0.0001	0.99 (0.99–0.99)	<0.0001
SAPS II	–	–	1.03 (1.02–1.04)	<0.0001	1.02 (1.00–1.03)	0.018
LODS	–	–	1.19 (1.13–1.25)	<0.0001	1.12 (1.05–1.20)	<0.001
Antifungal treatment[a]						
Yes	17	12 (70.6)	2.55 (0.88–7.36)	0.084	–	–
No	406	197 (48.5)	1			
Blot et al. algorithm[16]						
No *Aspergillus* spp. colonization	388	188 (48.5)	1	–	1	–
Aspergillus spp. colonization	18	6 (33.3)	0.53 (0.20–1.45)	0.22	0.64 (0.21–1.99)	0.44
Putative or proven IPA	17	15 (88.2)	7.98 (1.80–35.36)	0.006	9.58 (1.97–46.52)	0.005

IPA invasive pulmonary aspergillosis

[a] As prescribed for a suspicion of invasive pulmonary aspergillosis; the Hosmer–Lemeshow goodness of fit test showed good calibration of the model ($p = 0.28$); the area under the curve of the model is 0.78 (0.73–0.82); OR (95 % CI), odds ratio (95 % confidence interval); aOR, adjusted odds ratio

Aspergillus$^+$ group, their relationship with subsequent IPA and death could not be assessed in our study due to its limited statistical power.

The recent clinical algorithm proposed by Blot et al. for discriminating between ICU patients with *Aspergillus* respiratory tract colonization and those with IPA, allows for categorizing non-immunocompromised patients as having putative IPA, provided semiquantitative culture of BAL fluid is positive for *Aspergillus*, together with a positive cytological smear showing branching hyphae [16]. This criterion (4b) becomes indeed crucial in non-immunocompromised ARDS patients who all meet, by definition, the radiological criterion of the Blot algorithm (criterion 3), while both the relevance and reproducibility of several of the clinical criteria (e.g., dyspnea, pleuritic chest pain, pleuritic rub) can be questioned in critically ill mechanically ventilated patients. Nevertheless, and as expected, immunosuppression was strongly associated with proven/putative IPA in our series; however, it is noteworthy that non-immunocompromised patients accounted for one-third of patients classified as having probable infection, all of whom ($n = 5/5$) eventually died, suggesting putative IPA portends a dismal prognosis even in non-immunocompromised patients.

Although the purpose of our study was not to evaluate the performance value of GM antigen measurement, our results suggest that its detection is more efficient in BAL fluid than in plasma to discriminate between proven/putative IPA and *Aspergillus* colonization, in line with a previous prospective study conducted in non-ARDS critically ill patients [30]. In the context of ARDS patients with a positive culture for *Aspergillus,* a positive GM test in BAL fluid may be a helpful tool to reinforce the diagnostic suspicion of IPA and may thus incite clinicians to start antifungal therapy.

While the number of chest CT scans available in the current study was limited, our results suggest that, in the particular context of ARDS, its diagnostic yield to discriminate between putative aspergillosis and *Aspergillus* colonization is limited, most patients exhibiting non-specific findings such as alveolar consolidations.

In our series, the overall positivity of one or more respiratory sample for *Aspergillus* was not significantly associated with higher in-ICU mortality. Still, the risk of in-ICU mortality was significantly higher in ARDS patients with proven/putative IPA, as opposed to those with *Aspergillus* colonization, and as compared to those having no positive respiratory tract culture for *Aspergillus*, even after adjusting on significantly associated covariables. The benefit/risk ratio of antifungal therapy has not been assessed in ICU patients when categorized as having proven/putative IPA according to the recently proposed algorithm [16]. Our findings of a higher in-ICU

mortality among a cohort of ARDS patients suggest that the initiation of such treatment should be considered in this specific subgroup, including non-immunocompromised patients, who also exhibited a strikingly high ICU mortality ($n = 5/5$ died). Of note, a previous observational study in critically ill COPD patients having putative IPA reported no improvement in ICU and long-term mortality in patients receiving antifungal treatment as compared to others, suggesting the severity of the underlying diseases was a key prognostic factor [7]. Strikingly, in the current series, six patients of the putative IPA subgroup ($n = 16$) did not receive an antifungal treatment, reflecting the fact that the criteria on which such treatment should be initiated in patients having *Aspergillus* spp.-positive respiratory tract samples are not standardized yet.

Our study has a number of limitations. First, due to its monocentric design, our results may not be applicable to other centers, thereby limiting their generalizability, since risk exposure to *Aspergillus*, prevalence of colonization and subsequent IPA may vary between centers. Moreover, the number and the type of respiratory tract samples performed were not standardized over the study period, potentially hampering the isolation of *Aspergillus* spp. in patients having had limited microbiological investigations. Second, this was a retrospective study with possible associated errors in data abstraction. However, due to the relatively low frequency of IPA, prospective studies in the specific subgroup of ARDS patients would be hardly feasible due to the low rate of *Aspergillus* colonization [8]. Third, our patients were admitted over a 10-year period, with inherently associated selection bias related to variations in coding habits between years. Moreover, during this relatively long time period, exposure to *Aspergillus* spores might have varied due to environmental factors. However, we found no association between the year of ICU admission and the risk of having one or more respiratory tract sample positive for *Aspergillus* spp. Fourth, several known prognostic factors for ARDS, including pulmonary artery pressure level or right ventricular dysfunction [31], were not available due to the retrospective nature of the study. Last, due to the limited number of patients having had a chest CT scan performed ($n = 21/35$), our study does not allow for drawing definite conclusions regarding the performance of chest CT scan in discriminating between putative aspergillosis and *Aspergillus* colonization in the context of ARDS.

Conclusions

We report a prevalence of 8 % of *Aspergillus*-positive lower respiratory tract specimen culture and 4 % of proven or putative IPA during ARDS. Immunocompromised ARDS patients were more likely to be categorized as having a putative or proven IPA, while non-immuno-compromised patients were more frequently classified as having *Aspergillus* respiratory tract colonization. Immunosuppression and pneumonia were associated with having at least one positive sample for *Aspergillus*. In this cohort of ARDS patients, having one or more positive sample for *Aspergillus* had no impact on outcome when classified as a mere respiratory tract colonization. In contrast, patients classified as having putative/proven IPA had a higher risk of in-ICU mortality, suggesting antifungal treatment should be assessed in this subgroup.

Abbreviations
ARDS: acute respiratory distress syndrome; ICU: intensive care unit; IPA: invasive pulmonary aspergillosis.

Authors' contributions
NDP, MD, JR, FS, FF, FB and AG collected the data; NDP, MD and DC analyzed the data and wrote the manuscript; and KR, GC, FF, FB, AMD and CBB revised the manuscript. NDP is the guarantor of the article. All authors read and approved the final manuscript.

Author details
[1] Groupe Henri Mondor-Albert Chenevier, Centre Hospitalier Universitaire Henri Mondor, DHU A-TVB, Service de Réanimation Médicale, Assistance Publique-Hôpitaux de Paris, 51, Avenue du Maréchal de Lattre de Tassigny, 94010 Créteil Cedex, France. [2] Groupe de Recherche CARMAS, Faculté de Médecine de Créteil, Université Paris Est Créteil, 94010 Créteil, France. [3] Centre Hospitalier Universitaire Henri Mondor, DHU A-TVB, Antenne de Pneumologie, Assistance Publique-Hôpitaux de Paris, 94010 Créteil, France. [4] Unité de Mycologie, Département de Biologie-Pathologie, Centre Hospitalier Universitaire Henri Mondor, DHU VIC, Assistance Publique-Hôpitaux de Paris, 94010 Créteil, France.

Competing interests
The authors declare they have no competing interests.

Funding
This study did not receive funding from external or internal sources.

References
1. De Pauw B, Walsh TJ, Donnelly JP, Stevens DA, Edwards JE, Calandra T, Pappas PG, Maertens J, Lortholary O, Kauffman CA, et al. Revised definitions of invasive fungal disease from the European Organization for Research and Treatment of Cancer/Invasive Fungal Infections Cooperative Group and the National Institute of Allergy and Infectious Diseases Mycoses Study Group (EORTC/MSG) Consensus Group. Clin Infect Dis. 2008;46:1813–21.
2. Koulenti D, Garnacho-Montero J, Blot S. Approach to invasive pulmonary aspergillosis in critically ill patients. Curr Opin Infect Dis. 2014;27:174–83.
3. Dimopoulos G, Piagnerelli M, Berre J, Eddafali B, Salmon I, Vincent JL. Disseminated aspergillosis in intensive care unit patients: an autopsy study. J Chemother. 2003;15:71–5.
4. Meersseman W, Vandecasteele SJ, Wilmer A, Verbeken E, Peetermans WE, Van Wijngaerden E. Invasive aspergillosis in critically ill patients without malignancy. Am J Respir Crit Care Med. 2004;170:621–5.
5. Wauters J, Baar I, Meersseman P, Meersseman W, Dams K, De Paep R, Lagrou K, Wilmer A, Jorens P, Hermans G. Invasive pulmonary aspergillosis is a frequent complication of critically ill H1N1 patients: a retrospective study. Intensive Care Med. 2012;38:1761–8.
6. Taccone FS, Van den Abeele AM, Bulpa P, Misset B, Meersseman W, Cardoso T, Paiva JA, Blasco-Navalpotro M, De Laere E, Dimopoulos G, et al. Epidemiology of invasive aspergillosis in critically ill patients: clinical presentation, underlying conditions, and outcomes. Crit Care. 2015;19:7.
7. Delsuc C, Cottereau A, Frealle E, Bienvenu AL, Dessein R, Jarraud S, Dumitrescu O, Le Marechal M, Wallet F, Friggeri A, et al. Putative invasive pulmonary aspergillosis in critically ill patients with chronic obstructive pulmonary disease: a matched cohort study. Crit Care. 2015;19:421.
8. Bassetti M, Mikulska M, Repetto E, Bernardini C, Soro O, Molinari MP, Mussap M, Pallavicini FM, Viscoli C. Invasive pulmonary aspergillosis in intensive care units: Is it a real problem? J Hosp Infect. 2009;74:186–7.
9. Garnacho-Montero J, Amaya-Villar R, Ortiz-Leyba C, Leon C, Alvarez-Lerma F, Nolla-Salas J, Iruretagoyena JR, Barcenilla F. Isolation of *Aspergillus* spp. from the respiratory tract in critically ill patients: risk factors, clinical presentation and outcome. Crit Care. 2005;9:R191–9.
10. Vandewoude K, Blot S, Benoit D, Depuydt P, Vogelaers D, Colardyn F. Invasive aspergillosis in critically ill patients: analysis of risk factors for acquisition and mortality. Acta Clin Belg. 2004;59:251–7.
11. Vandewoude KH, Blot SI, Depuydt P, Benoit D, Temmerman W, Colardyn F, Vogelaers D. Clinical relevance of *Aspergillus* isolation from respiratory tract samples in critically ill patients. Crit Care. 2006;10:R31.
12. Ranieri VM, Rubenfeld GD, Thompson BT, Ferguson ND, Caldwell E, Fan E, Camporota L, Slutsky AS. Acute respiratory distress syndrome: the Berlin definition. JAMA. 2012;307:2526–33.
13. Bellani G, Laffey JG, Pham T, Fan E, Brochard L, Esteban A, Gattinoni L, van Haren F, Larsson A, McAuley DF, et al. Epidemiology, patterns of care, and mortality for patients with acute respiratory distress syndrome in intensive care units in 50 countries. JAMA. 2016;315:788–800.
14. Lugosi M, Alberti C, Zahar JR, Garrouste M, Lemiale V, Descorps-Desclere A, Ricard JD, Goldgran-Toledano D, Cohen Y, Schwebel C, et al. Aspergillus in the lower respiratory tract of immunocompetent critically ill patients. J Infect. 2014;69:284–92.
15. de Hemptinne Q, Remmelink M, Brimioulle S, Salmon I, Vincent JL. ARDS: a clinicopathological confrontation. Chest. 2009;135:944–9.
16. Blot SI, Taccone FS, Van den Abeele AM, Bulpa P, Meersseman W, Brusselaers N, Dimopoulos G, Paiva JA, Misset B, Rello J, et al. A clinical algorithm to diagnose invasive pulmonary aspergillosis in critically ill patients. Am J Respir Crit Care Med. 2012;186:56–64.
17. Antachopoulos C. Invasive fungal infections in congenital immunodeficiencies. Clin Microbiol Infect. 2010;16:1335–42.
18. Lortholary O, Meyohas MC, Dupont B, Cadranel J, Salmon-Ceron D, Peyramond D, Simonin D. Invasive aspergillosis in patients with acquired immunodeficiency syndrome: report of 33 cases. French Cooperative Study Group on Aspergillosis in AIDS. Am J Med. 1993;95:177–87.
19. Le Gall JR, Lemeshow S, Saulnier F. A new Simplified Acute Physiology Score (SAPS II) based on a European/North American multicenter study. JAMA. 1993;270:2957–63.
20. Le Gall JR, Klar J, Lemeshow S, Saulnier F, Alberti C, Artigas A, Teres D. The Logistic Organ Dysfunction system. A new way to assess organ dysfunction in the intensive care unit. ICU Scoring Group. JAMA. 1996;276:802–10.
21. The Acute Respiratory Distress Syndrome Network. Ventilation with lower tidal volumes as compared with traditional tidal volumes for acute lung injury and the acute respiratory distress syndrome. N Engl J Med. 2000;342:1301–8.
22. Mercat A, Richard JC, Vielle B, Jaber S, Osman D, Diehl JL, Lefrant JY, Prat G, Richecoeur J, Nieszkowska A, et al. Positive end-expiratory pressure setting in adults with acute lung injury and acute respiratory distress syndrome: a randomized controlled trial. JAMA. 2008;299:646–55.
23. Papazian L, Forel JM, Gacouin A, Penot-Ragon C, Perrin G, Loundou A, Jaber S, Arnal JM, Perez D, Seghboyan JM, et al. Neuromuscular blockers in early acute respiratory distress syndrome. N Engl J Med. 2010;363:1107–16.
24. Guerin C, Reignier J, Richard JC, Beuret P, Gacouin A, Boulain T, Mercier E, Badet M, Mercat A, Baudin O, et al. Prone positioning in severe acute respiratory distress syndrome. N Engl J Med. 2013;368:2159–68.
25. Ferguson ND, Fan E, Camporota L, Antonelli M, Anzueto A, Beale R, Brochard L, Brower R, Esteban A, Gattinoni L, et al. The Berlin definition of ARDS: an expanded rationale, justification, and supplementary material. Intensive Care Med. 2012;38:1573–82.

26. Azoulay E, Afessa B. Diagnostic criteria for invasive pulmonary aspergillosis in critically ill patients. Am J Respir Crit Care Med. 2012;186:8–10.

27. Boomer JS, To K, Chang KC, Takasu O, Osborne DF, Walton AH, Bricker TL, Jarman SD 2nd, Kreisel D, Krupnick AS, et al. Immunosuppression in patients who die of sepsis and multiple organ failure. JAMA. 2011;306:2594–605.

28. Hotchkiss RS, Monneret G, Payen D. Sepsis-induced immunosuppression: from cellular dysfunctions to immunotherapy. Nat Rev Immunol. 2013;13:862–74.

29. Camargo JF, Husain S. Immune correlates of protection in human invasive aspergillosis. Clin Infect Dis. 2014;59:569–77.

30. Meersseman W, Lagrou K, Maertens J, Wilmer A, Hermans G, Vanderschueren S, Spriet I, Verbeken E, Van Wijngaerden E. Galactomannan in bronchoalveolar lavage fluid: a tool for diagnosing aspergillosis in intensive care unit patients. Am J Respir Crit Care Med. 2008;177:27–34.

31. MekontsoDessap A, Boissier F, Charron C, Begot E, Repesse X, Legras A, Brun-Buisson C, Vignon P, Vieillard-Baron A. Acute cor pulmonale during protective ventilation for acute respiratory distress syndrome: prevalence, predictors, and clinical impact. Intensive Care Med. 2016;42:862–70.

3

Assessment and predictors of physical functioning post-hospital discharge in survivors of critical illness

Kevin J. Solverson[1], Christopher Grant[1,2] and Christopher J. Doig[1,3]*

Abstract

Background: Prior studies of physical functioning after critical illness have been mostly limited to survivors of acute respiratory distress syndrome. The purpose of this study was to objectively assess muscle strength and physical functioning in survivors of critical illness from a general ICU and the associations of these measures to health-related quality of life (HRQL), mental health and critical illness variables.

Methods: This was a prospective cohort study of 56 patients admitted to a medical ICU (length of stay ≥4 days) from April 1, 2009, and March 31, 2010. Patients were assessed in clinic at 3 months post-hospital discharge. Muscle strength and physical functioning were measured using hand-held dynamometry and the 6-min walk test. HRQL was assessed using the short-form 36 (SF-36) and EuroQol-5D (EQ-5D) questionnaires.

Results: Three months post-hospital discharge, median age- and sex-matched muscle strength was reduced across all muscle groups. The median 6-min walk distance was 72 % of predicted. Physical functioning was associated with reductions in self-reported HRQL (SF-36, EQ-5D) and increased anxiety. Univariate regression modeling showed that reduced muscle strength and 6-min walk distance were associated with sepsis but not ICU length of stay. Multivariate regression modeling showed that sepsis and corticosteroid use were associated with a reduced 6-min walk distance, but again ICU length of stay was not.

Conclusions: Survivors of critical illness have reduced strength in multiple muscle groups and impaired exercise tolerance impacting both HRQL and mental health. These outcomes were worsened by sepsis and corticosteroid use in the ICU but not ICU length of stay. Interventions to minimizing the burden of sepsis in critically ill patients may improve long-term outcomes.

Keywords: Critical care, Muscle weakness, Muscle strength dynamometer, Sepsis, Recovery of function, Adult

Background

As more patients are surviving critical illness, examining longer-term outcomes becomes increasingly important. There is increasing evidence that critical illness survivors have impaired physical functioning, increased prevalence of mental health disorders and reduced health-related quality of life (HRQL) [1–6].

*Correspondence: cdoig@ucalgary.ca
[1] Department of Critical Care Medicine, Cumming School of Medicine, University of Calgary, 3134 Hospital Drive NW, Calgary, AB T2N 2T9, Canada
Full list of author information is available at the end of the article

Critically ill patients have been shown to develop multifactorial weakness termed ICU-acquired weakness (ICUAW), and these patients are at risk of prolonged ICU lengths of stay, increased mechanical ventilation time, prolonged weakness and poor hospital outcomes [7–13]. Muscle biopsies taken during critical illness have shown wasting of the muscle fibers and increased catabolic metabolism [14–17]. Risk factors for ICUAW include prolonged immobility, mechanical ventilation, corticosteroid and neuromuscular blockade administration and cytokine-related injury from systemic inflammation [5, 7, 9, 10, 17–24]. However, the duration of physical impairment after hospital discharge secondary to critical illness and the predictors of severity remain unclear.

Studies that have objectively examined long-term physical function have primarily focused on survivors of acute respiratory distress syndrome (ARDS) and not the general ICU survivor population. Long-term physical function of ARDS survivors was first objectively described by Herridge et al. [5] landmark paper using the 6-min walk test (6MWT). Recent post-ICU studies have used manual muscle testing (MMT) for the assessment of muscle strength in addition to the 6MWT; however, MMT has limitations including a ceiling effect in less severe muscle weakness [25, 26]. Isokinetic muscle strength testing using hand-held dynamometry has been shown to be a more sensitive and objective method of strength testing compared to MMT [25, 27–30]. However, to date hand-held dynamometry has not been used in the ICU survivor population, despite its common use in other patient populations [31–34].

The goal of our study was to objectively examine muscle strength and physical functioning using hand-held dynamometry and the 6MWT in critical illness survivors 3 months after hospital discharge. Additionally, we sought to determine whether muscle strength or physical functioning was associated with HRQL, mental health or critical illness variables such as severity and type of illness and ICU length of stay.

Methods

Design

This was a prospective longitudinal cohort study of patients who were admitted to a 25-bed multidisciplinary tertiary referral ICU, which also served as the trauma center for southern Alberta [35]. Enrollment occurred between April 1, 2009, and March 31, 2010. At the time of study enrollment, there were two full-time equivalent physiotherapists; however, no patients were mobilized while intubated in the ICU. The initiation of physiotherapy was up to the discretion of the attending physician.

Patients assessed in the ICU follow-up clinic were adult patients (≥18 years), admitted to the ICU with a minimum 4-day length of ICU stay. Patients were excluded if they had traumatic brain injuries, spinal cord injuries, pre-existing neurocognitive or neuromuscular disorders, acute strokes or lived outside of the immediate municipality of Calgary. Patients in the ICU were screened for eligibility during the initial 48 h and approached for follow-up once they had been admitted to the ICU for a minimum of 4 days. Due to limited capacity in the ICU follow-up clinic, patients were enrolled consecutively until clinical capacity was met at which point screening would be temporally suspended. Patients enrolled in the ICU were assessed at 3 months after hospital discharge.

A total of 61 patients met inclusion criteria, 4 patients declined follow-up, and 1 patient was lost to follow-up. Attendance at the clinic was presented as a natural continuation of care following hospitalization, which individuals had the option to refuse. We sought permission from these patients to include their clinical data in our study. This study was approved by the University of Calgary Human Research Ethics Board (ID# E-22574), and written informed consent was obtained from all patients.

Instruments/questionnaires

A single trained individual (author KS) assessed peripheral muscle strength using hand-held dynamometry. The JAMAR (5030J1) hydraulic hand dynamometer and the Chatillon dynamometer (K-MSC-200) were used for all muscle strength assessments. All measurements were taken in kilograms to the nearest hundredth of a kilogram. Each muscle group (handgrip, triceps, biceps, ankle dorsiflexors, hamstrings and quadriceps) was measured according to previously validated protocols [36]. For each muscle group, patients were asked to exert a maximal effort for 3–4 s against the dynamometer, which was in a fixed position. Three measurements were collected for each muscle group, alternating between patient sides between measurements. For each muscle group, the highest force generated on the patient's dominant side was used for analysis. The National Isometric Muscle Strength Database Consortium [36] was used for age- and sex-standardized normative values. The 6MWT was used to assess overall physical functioning. Previously published guidelines and procedures were followed [37], and age and sex normative values were obtained from Enright et al. [38].

The assessment of HRQL was done using short-form 36 (SF-36) and EuroQol-5D (EQ-5D) surveys [39]. The SF-36 survey was reported as each domain ranging from 0 to 100 (higher scores indicate better HRQL), and the physical and mental composite scores (PCS, MCS) were standardized to Canadian population norms (score of 50 represents the average normative value) [40]. The Hospital Anxiety and Depression Scale (HADS) was used to assess anxiety and depression, scores ranging from 0 to 21 [41]. A score >7 on either the anxiety or depression section indicates severe symptoms. All questionnaires were administered at the time of the patient's clinical visit.

Statistical analysis

All clinical data were entered into a study-specific database. These data were merged with clinical and outcome data from an ICU-specific longitudinal database, details described elsewhere [42]. All data analysis was performed using Stata 11.0 (Stata Corp, College Station,

TX). Descriptive statistics were used to report patient demographics, hand-held dynamometry testing and the 6MWT.

Multiple linear regression models were used to assess the association between the strength of each muscle group (independent variable), 6MWT, EQ-5D and the SF-36 (dependent variables). The EQ-5D domains were modeled as a dichotomous variable (0 = no problems, 1 = reporting any problems). Multiple univariate and a single multivariate linear regression analysis assessed the association of the following ICU risk factors (dependent variables) to patient's predicted peripheral muscle strength or 6MWT (independent variables): (1) ICU length of stay (LOS), (2) hospital LOS, (3) severity of illness as measured by the mean Acute Physiology and Chronic Health Evaluation (APACHE) II score, (4) degree of organ failure measure by the Sequential Organ Failure Assessment (SOFA) score, (5) presence of sepsis (defined using the 2001 American College of Chest Physicians guideline [43]), (6) presence of ARDS (defined as a PaO2:FiO2 ratio of 200 or less while mechanically ventilated with evidence of airspace disease in all four quadrants on chest radiograph), (7) any corticosteroid use, (8) any neuromuscular blocker use (9), duration of ventilation and (10) Functional Comorbidity Index score. For the multivariate linear regression, all ICU risk factors were analyzed in the model and variables that had a p value <0.05 were carried forward in the analysis to create the final model.

Results

During the study period, 56 patients were seen in the ICU follow-up clinic. The median (IQR) age was 61 years (41, 68), and 54 % were males (Table 1). Prior to ICU admission, 57 % of patients had one or more pre-existing comorbidity and 100 % were living independently at home. The median (IQR) first APACHE II score and maximum SOFA scores were 19 (16, 24) and 11 (9, 14), respectively. Only 18 % of patients received corticosteroids, and 21 % received neuromuscular blockers anytime while in the ICU. No patient with ARDS received corticosteroids. The median (IQR) days of mechanical ventilation and ICU and hospital LOS were 8 days (4, 11), 11 days (6, 15) and 12 days (8, 12), respectively. The median (IQR) time to follow-up was 72 days (54, 92) after hospital discharge.

Patient's median dynamometry-measured muscle strength was reduced across all muscle groups when compared to age- and sex-matched data (Table 2). The median (IQR) percent-predicted strength of the handgrips 61 % (25, 108), quadriceps 59 % (35, 88) and the ankle dorsiflexors 62 % (42, 92) all showed the greatest impairment 3 months after critical illness. For all the

Table 1 Baseline patient characteristics

Variable	All patients (n = 56)[a]
Baseline characteristics prior to admission	
Age (year)	61 (41, 68)
Male [n (%)]	30 (54)
Pre-existing comorbidity [n (%)]	32 (57)
Charlson comorbidity index score	3 (1, 4)
Functional Comorbidity Index score	1 (0, 2)
Living independently at home [n (%)]	56 (100)
Body mass index (kg/m^2)	26 (22, 33)
ICU characteristics	
Diagnosis at ICU admission [n (%)]	
Respiratory failure	37 (66)
Intra-abdominal infection	7 (13)
Urologic infection	3 (5)
Poly-trauma	4 (7)
Other	5 (9)
Sepsis present during admission [n (%)]	39 (70)
ARDS present during admission [n (%)]	13 (23 %)
Any corticosteroid use [n (%)]	10 (18)
Daily dose corticosteroids if received any, mg (prednisone equivalent)	57 (35, 82)
Any neuromuscular blocker use [n (%)]	12 (21)
APACHE II score	19 (16, 24)
SOFA score maximum value	11 (9, 14)
Length of mechanical ventilation (day)	8 (4, 11)
Length of ICU stay (day)	11 (6, 15)
Length of hospital stay (day)	12 (8, 21)
Time to follow-up after hospital discharge (day)	72 (54, 92)

ARDS acute respiratory distress syndrome, *APACHE II* Acute Physiology and Chronic Health Evaluation, *SOFA* Sequential Organ Failure Assessment, *ICU* intensive care unit

[a] Reported as median (interquartile range) unless specified

muscle groups, over 50 % of the patients did not achieve 80 % of their age- and sex-matched predicted strength. The median (IQR) distance walked in 6 min and percent predicted were 382 m (291, 480) and 70 % (53, 88), respectively. In total, 55 % of patients did not achieve at least 80 % of their age- and sex-matched predicted 6MWT distance. The maximum strength results of each muscle group statistically correlated with the 6MWT distance.

Table 3 outlines individual regression analyses evaluating the associations of physical functioning to HRQL and mental health. Reporting problems in the domains mobility (p = 0.003), usual activities (p = 0.006), pain and discomfort (p = 0.031) of the EQ-5D were each associated with reduced predicted 6MWT distance. Patient's overall impression of their global health using the EQ-5D VAS was also associated with performance on the 6MWT (p = 0.025). Among the muscle groups strength tested,

Table 2 Muscle strength and physical functioning of critical illness survivors at 3 months after hospital discharge measured using hand-held dynamometry and the 6-min walk test

Variable (n = 56)	Measurement (median, IQR)	% predicted (median, IQR)	% of patients < 80% predicted strength	Correlation with the 6MWT (R^2, p value)
Maximum muscle strength (kg)[a]				
Grip	20.4 (9.1, 30.6)	61 % (25, 108)	60	0.28 (<0.001)
Triceps	12.3 (8.7, 16.7)	71 % (45, 126)	52	0.31 (<0.001)
Biceps	14.5 (11.7, 19.0)	72 % (45, 126)	52	0.28 (<0.001)
Hamstrings	13.2 (10.3, 17.6)	77 % (47, 114)	53	0.30 (<0.001)
Quadriceps	20.3 (16.4, 25.6)	59 % (35, 88)	69	0.14 (0.013)
Ankle dorsiflexors	13.7 (10.6, 17.2)	62 % (42, 92)	57	0.13 (<0.001)

6MWT 6-min walk test

[a] Strength results reported as the maximum force generated on the dominant body side

Table 3 Associations of physical functioning and health-related quality of life at 3 months after hospital discharge

Variable n = 50[a]	6-Minute walk test	Grip	Triceps	Biceps	Hamstrings	Quadriceps	Ankle dorsiflexors
EuroQol-5D[b]							
Mobility	−0.211 (0.003)	−0.297 (0.030)	−0.223 (0.144)	−0.228 (0.097)	−0.283 (0.021)	−0.252 (0.019)	−0.140 (0.125)
Self-care	−0.177 (0.067)	−0.132 (0.435)	−0.170 (0.372)	0.165 (0.336)	−0.198 (0.190)	−0.177 (0.197)	−0.142 (0.212)
Usual activities	−0.177 (0.006)	−0.166 (0.153)	−0.044 (0.736)	−0.061 (0.606)	−0.103 (0.335)	−0.070 (0.446)	−0.127 (0.105)
Pain/discomfort	−0.125 (0.031)	−0.020 (0.855)	−0.011 (0.929)	−0.105 (0.345)	−0.096 (0.359)	−0.072 (0.412)	−0.031 (0.688)
Anxiety/depression	−0.123 (0.079)	−0.099 (0.476)	−0.120 (0.421)	−0.065 (0.630)	−0.021 (0.866)	−0.001 (0.994)	−0.007 (0.941)
Visual analog scale[c]	0.050 (0.025)	0.324 (0.428)	0.028 (0.534)	0.018 (0.662)	0.026 (0.480)	−0.010 (0.759)	−0.009 (0.746)
Short-from 36							
Physical functioning[d]	0.005 (0.001)	0.006 (0.019)	0.004 (0.178)	0.004 (0.112)	0.005 (0.026)	0.004 (0.062)	0.003 (0.063)
Physical composite score[e]	0.010 (0.001)	0.008 (0.185)	0.000 (0.997)	0.007 (0.266)	0.009 (0.105)	0.008 (0.113)	0.004 (0.320)
Mental composite score[e]	0.005 (0.118)	0.010 (0.128)	0.003 (0.712)	0.006 (0.409)	0.005 (0.416)	0.005 (0.308)	0.004 (0.453)
HADS[f]							
Anxiety	−0.029 (0.001)	−0.023 (0.176)	−0.025 (0.179)	−0.025 (0.130)	−0.023 (0.123)	−0.018 (0.16)	−0.014 (0.251)
Depression	−0.016 (0.098)	−0.033 (0.080)	−0.008 (0.718)	−0.023 (0.214)	−0.012 (0.174)	−0.027 (0.067)	0.010 (0.450)

ICU intensive care unit, *LOS* length of stay, *APACHE* Acute Physiology and Chronic Health Evaluation, *SOFA* Sequential Organ Failure Assessment, *6MWT* 6-min walk test

[a] β-Coefficients (p value) modeled as univariate regression analyses. 6MWT and muscle strength modeled as percent predicted. β-Coefficients represent the percent change in the physical functioning variable per unit change in exposure variable

[b] Each domain of the EuroQol-5D questionnaire modeled as 0 "no problems" and 1 "any problems"

[c] Visual analog scale of the EQ-5D scores ranges from 0 to 10 based on patients perspective of current overall health

[d] The physical function domain is standardized to a 0–100 scale, and higher scores indicate better health-related quality of life

[e] Physical and mental composite scores of the short-form 36 survey, standardized to Canadian norms. Scores can range from 0 to 100 and are standardized to 50, which represents the average Canadian's health-related quality of life

[f] Hospital Anxiety and Depression Scale (HADS), scores range from 0 to 21, significant symptoms of anxiety/depression defined as scores ≥8

grip (p = 0.030), hamstring (p = 0.021) and quadriceps (p = 0.019) weakness were associated with increasing impairment on the mobility domain of the EQ-5D.

The physical function domain of the SF-36 was associated with the percent-predicted 6MWT distance (p < 0.001), grip strength (p = 0.019) and hamstring strength (p = 0.026). The 6MWT percent-predicted distance was associated with the physical composite score of the SF-36 (p = 0.003) and the anxiety score of the Hospital and Anxiety Depression Scale. Patient's percent-predicted 6MWT and muscle strength for all muscle groups, except triceps, were statistically associated with reported values in the general health domain (patient's perspective of overall health) of the SF-36. Additionally, patients predicted grip strength and 6MWT were associated with the vitality, social functioning and role emotional domains, with the 6MWT also associated with the physical role and emotional role domains (data not shown).

Univariate regression analysis showed that ICU LOS (p = 0.002), number of days mechanically ventilated (p = 0.002), the presence of sepsis (p = 0.044) and corticosteroid use in the ICU (p = 0.019) were independently associated with patient's percent-predicted 6MWT distance (Table 4). Sepsis was the only ICU risk factor associated with a reduction in the 6MWT by an estimated 17 % and reductions in strength of all muscle groups (except quadriceps). Muscle strength did not correlate with patient's ICU or hospital LOS. Both the 6MWT and peripheral muscle strength did not show an association with the Functional Comorbidity Index, APACHE II or SOFA scores. There were no associations found between neuromuscular medication use or the presence of ARDS in the ICU and the 6MWT, peripheral muscle strength or self-reported physical functioning (SF-36, EQ-5D) (data not shown).

The multivariate linear regression analysis assessing predictors of 6MWT distance included the ICU risk factors that were statistically significant in the univariate regression, with the exception of mechanical ventilation duration as it is highly correlated with ICU LOS. The presence of sepsis ($\beta = -0.159$, p = 0.030) and any corticosteroid use ($\beta = -0.188$, p = 0.037) in the ICU were associated with patient's age- and sex-matched 6MWT distance ($R^2 = 0.24$), and ICU LOS ($\beta = -0.002$, p = 0.233) was no longer statistically significant. Additionally, total cumulative steroid dose and average daily corticosteroid dose were analyzed in regression model and there was no association with physical function or muscle strength (data not shown).

Discussion

This is the first study to report the use of hand-held dynamometry assessment of multiple muscle groups in the general ICU survivor population. We demonstrated that approximately 3 months after hospital discharge the majority of ICU survivors experienced persistent muscle weakness across all muscle groups. The quadriceps were the weakest muscle group measured, with the median percent-predicted strength achieved at 59 %. Fan et al. [23] described grip strength in ARDS survivors, in keeping with our results, reporting a range of 50–70 % percent-predicted strength 3–12 months after ICU discharge. Global muscle weakness in ARDS survivors, measured using MMT, has a reported prevalence between 8 and 22 % during the first year after discharge [23, 24]. However, we found that over 50 % of patients did not achieve 80 % of their age- and sex-matched predicted hand-held dynamometry-measured muscle strength. These differences may be due to the limited sensitivity of MMT to detect less severe weakness [24], or that our study included all ICU patients versus only ARDS patients.

A reduction in percent-predicted 6MWT distance and grip strength was associated with a decrease in the physical functioning domain on the SF-36 survey, similar to results found in prior studies [22–24]. We found that poor 6MWT performance was also associated with reduced HRQL in nearly all of the domains of the EQ-5D and SF-36, including the physical composite score, suggesting there is a strong link between patients overall physical functioning and HRQL. Further supporting this finding, the muscle strength of patient's was independently associated with the patient's perception of their mobility and general health on the SF-36. Poor 6MWT performance was associated with increased symptoms of anxiety, showing the connection between physical functioning and mental health [6]. It is important to note there was an expected association between muscle strength and the 6MWT; however, the 6MWT was

Table 4 Summary of predictors of muscle strength and physical functioning at 3 months after hospital discharge

Variable n = 50[a]	6-Minute walk test	Grip	Triceps	Biceps	Hamstrings	Quadriceps	Ankle dorsiflexors
ICU LOS, days	−0.003 (0.041)	−0.002 (0.85)	−0.010 (0.305)	−0.005 (0.537)	−0.001 (0.806)	0.000 (0.922)	−0.001 (0.685)
Hospital LOS, days	−0.003 (0.079)	−0.001 (0.965)	0.002 (0.727)	0.003 (0.498)	0.000 (0.969)	0.003 (0.274)	0.001 (0.755)
Mechanical ventilation, days	−0.004 (0.045)	−0.001 (0.905)	−0.009 (0.378)	−0.004 (0.610)	−0.001 (0.899)	0.001 (0.809)	−0.001 (0.742)
Presence of sepsis	−0.168 (0.029)	−0.389 (0.009)	−0.328 (0.045)	−0.315 (0.033)	−0.328 (0.016)	−0.134 (0.262)	−0.197 (0.049)
APACHE II score	−0.003 (0.642)	−0.002 (0.868)	−0.008 (0.515)	0.003 (0.802)	0.003 (0.755)	0.011 (0.212)	0.006 (0.397)
SOFA score	0.011 (0.257)	0.022 (0.229)	0.021 (0.325)	0.027 (0.167)	0.020 (0.219)	0.019 (0.174)	0.017 (0.154)
Functional Comorbidity Index	−0.019 (0.593)	−0.070 (0.247)	−0.111 (0.114)	−0.050 (0.437)	−0.000 (0.998)	0.013 (0.803)	−0.044 (0.274)
Any corticosteroid use[b]	−0.215 (0.019)	−0.304 (0.092)	−0.382 (0.062)	−0.359 (0.052)	−0.320 (0.047)	−0.222 (0.137)	−0.221 (0.058)

ICU intensive care unit, *LOS* length of stay, *APACHE* Acute Physiology and Chronic Health Evaluation, *SOFA* Sequential Organ Failure Assessment, *6MWT* 6-min walk test

[a] β-Coefficients (p value) modeled as univariate regression analyses. 6MWT and muscle strength modeled as percent predicted. β-Coefficients represent the percent change in the physical functioning variable per unit change in exposure variable

[b] Also analyzed using cumulative ICU and average daily corticosteroid dose with no significance found

associated with more domains of HRQL than muscle strength alone. This finding highlights that the 6MWT accounts for more than just physical functioning or muscle strength, and is a composite assessment that may also be influenced by cardiopulmonary status, mental health, motivation, neurological status and bodily pain [24, 44, 45].

ICU LOS is thought to be a surrogate marker for immobility [23]. This is a well-described risk factor for muscle wasting and weakness in both healthy controls and patients in ICU [10, 46]. However, in our multivariate regression analysis ICU LOS was not found to be a predictor of muscle strength or 6MWT. The model included both corticosteroid use and the presence of sepsis, suggesting that ICU LOS, an indicator of immobility, may be confounded or collinearly correlated by these variables. Therefore, interventions to reduce immobility in the ICU may not decrease the prevalence of long-term impaired muscle strength or physical functioning. However, the benefits of interventions such as early mobilization still need to be examined in long-term randomized controlled trials using the appropriate physical outcome measures [47–50].

The presence of sepsis during critical illness was significantly associated with both impaired physical functioning and muscle weakness in nearly all muscle groups (the most of any ICU risk factor) as part of the univariate and multivariate linear regression analysis. Systemic inflammation and cytokine release have been shown to induce muscle injury and increase the incidence of ICUAW detected in the ICU [7, 51–53]. Our findings support a premise that inflammation during critical illness can result in long-term detectable impairment of muscle function [3]. Our study suggests sepsis, as a mechanism possibly related to the acute systemic inflammatory process, may be more important than ICU LOS or immobility in long-term physical impairment.

Our analysis showed that any exposure to corticosteroid use during critical illness was associated with reduced physical functioning. This supports the findings of prior studies in ARDS survivors and recommendations to avoid corticosteroid use in the ICU in order to lessen the degree of patient's long-term functional disability [5, 10, 24]. We did not see any effect on physical functioning when analyzing average daily corticosteroid dose or cumulative dose, similar to other studies [10]. Prior studies examining the effects of corticosteroids were limited to patients who had ARDS, but surprisingly none of our patients who had ARDS (23 %) received any corticosteroids. This highlights the variability of clinical practice across institutions and the importance of studying long-term physical functioning outcomes across the general ICU population.

The limitations of this study include that it is a single-center study with a relatively small sample size. Additionally, patient recruitment was limited due to the small capacity of the follow-up clinic. Patients who may have met inclusion criteria were not screened, potentially creating selection bias. However, patient selection was random and we had a relatively few number of patients decline enrollment or who were lost to follow-up.

Conclusion
We found that in survivors of critical illness approximately 3 months after hospital discharge patients had significant impairment in muscle strength and physical functioning measured using hand-held dynamometry and the 6MWT. Patients with impaired physical functioning and muscle weakness were found to have reduced HRQL. Sepsis and corticosteroid use were found to be an important risk factor for reduced long-term physical function, whereas ICU length of stay (a surrogate for immobility) was not.

Abbreviations
ARDS: acute respiratory distress syndrome; APACHE II: Acute Physiology and Chronic Health Evaluation II; ESS: Epworth Sleepiness Scale; EQ-5D: EuroQol-5D; HADS: Hospital Anxiety and Depression Scale; ICU: intensive care unit; ICUAW: intensive care unit-acquired weakness; IQR: interquartile range; LOS: length of stay; MCS: mental composite summary; MMT: manual muscle testing; PCS: physical composite summary; PQSI: Pittsburgh Sleep Quality Index; PSG: polysomnography; SF-36: short-form 36; SOFA: Sequential Organ Failure Assessment; 6MWT: 6-min walk test.

Authors' contributions
KS designed the study, performed data collection and analyses and wrote the manuscript. CG interpreted the data and edited the manuscript. CD designed the study, performed data collection and analyses and edited the manuscript. All authors read and approved the final manuscript.

Author details
[1] Department of Critical Care Medicine, Cumming School of Medicine, University of Calgary, 3134 Hospital Drive NW, Calgary, AB T2N 2T9, Canada. [2] Division of Physical Medicine and Rehabilitation, Cumming School of Medicine, University of Calgary, 3134 Hospital Drive NW, Calgary, AB T2N 2T9, Canada. [3] Department of Community Health Sciences, Cumming School of Medicine, University of Calgary, 3134 Hospital Drive NW, Calgary, AB T2N 2T9, Canada.

Funding
This work was funded as part of a grant from Alberta Innovates Health Solutions

Competing interests
The authors declare that they have no competing interests.

References
1. Dowdy DW, Eid MP, Dennison CR, Mendez-Tellez PA, Herridge MS, Guallar E, et al. Quality of life after acute respiratory distress syndrome: a meta-analysis. Intensive Care Med. 2006;32(8):1115–24.

2. Barnato AE, Albert SM, Angus DC, Lave JR, Degenholtz HB. Disability among elderly survivors of mechanical ventilation. Am J Respir Crit Care Med. 2011;183(8):1037–42.

3. Iwashyna TJ, Ely EW, Smith DM, Langa KM. Long-term cognitive impairment and functional disability among survivors of severe sepsis. JAMA. 2010;304(16):1787–94.

4. Jackson JC, Mitchell N, Hopkins RO. Cognitive functioning, mental health, and quality of life in ICU survivors: an overview. Crit Care Clin. 2009;25(3):615–28.

5. Herridge MS, Cheung AM, Tansey CM, Matte-Martyn A, Diaz-Granados N, Al-Saidi F, et al. One-year outcomes in survivors of the acute respiratory distress syndrome. N Engl J Med. 2003;348(8):683–93.

6. Bienvenu OJ, Colantuoni E, Mendez-Tellez PA, Dinglas VD, Shanholtz C, Husain N, et al. Depressive symptoms and impaired physical function after acute lung injury: a 2-year longitudinal study. Am J Respir Crit Care Med. 2012;185(5):517–24.

7. De Jonghe B, Lacherade JC, Durand MC, Sharshar T. Critical illness neuromuscular syndromes. Crit Care Clin. 2007;23(1):55–69.

8. Ginz HF, Iaizzo PA, Girard T, Urwyler A, Pargger H. Decreased isometric skeletal muscle force in critically ill patients. Swiss Med Wkly. 2005;135(37–38):555–61.

9. Stevens RD, Dowdy DW, Michaels RK, Mendez-Tellez PA, Pronovost PJ, Needham DM. Neuromuscular dysfunction acquired in critical illness: a systematic review. Intensive Care Med. 2007;33(11):1876–91.

10. De Jonghe B, Sharshar T, Lefaucheur JP, Authier FJ, Durand-Zaleski I, Boussarsar M, et al. Paresis acquired in the intensive care unit: a prospective multicenter study. JAMA. 2002;288(22):2859–67.

11. Bierbrauer J, Koch S, Olbricht C, Hamati J, Lodka D, Schneider J, et al. Early type II fiber atrophy in intensive care unit patients with nonexcitable muscle membrane. Crit Care Med. 2012;40(2):647–50.

12. Ali NA, O'Brien JM Jr, Hoffmann SP, Phillips G, Garland A, Finley JC, et al. Acquired weakness, handgrip strength, and mortality in critically ill patients. Am J Respir Crit Care Med. 2008;178(3):261–8.

13. Hough CL, Steinberg KP, Thompson BT, Rubenfeld GD, Hudson LD. Intensive care unit-acquired neuromyopathy and corticosteroids in survivors of persistent ARDS. Intensive Care Med. 2009;35(1):63–8.

14. Levine S, Nguyen T, Taylor N, Friscia ME, Budak MT, Rothenberg P, et al. Rapid disuse atrophy of diaphragm fibers in mechanically ventilated humans. N Engl J Med. 2008;358(13):1327–35.

15. Wollersheim T, Woehlecke J, Krebs M, Hamati J, Lodka D, Luther-Schroeder A, et al. Dynamics of myosin degradation in intensive care unit-acquired weakness during severe critical illness. Intensive Care Med. 2014;40(4):528–38.

16. Hermans G, Casaer MP, Clerckx B, Guiza F, Vanhullebusch T, Derde S, et al. Effect of tolerating macronutrient deficit on the development of intensive-care unit acquired weakness: a subanalysis of the EPaNIC trial. Lancet Respir Med. 2013;1(8):621–9.

17. Puthucheary ZA, Rawal J, McPhail M, Connolly B, Ratnayake G, Chan P, et al. Acute skeletal muscle wasting in critical illness. JAMA. 2013;310(15):1591–600.

18. Schefold JC, Bierbrauer J, Weber-Carstens S. Intensive care unit-acquired weakness (ICUAW) and muscle wasting in critically ill patients with severe sepsis and septic shock. J Cachex Sarcopenia Muscle. 2010;1(2):147–57.

19. Herridge MS, Batt J, Hopkins RO. The pathophysiology of long-term neuromuscular and cognitive outcomes following critical illness. Crit Care Clin. 2008;24(1):179–99.

20. van der Schaaf M, Dettling DS, Beelen A, Lucas C, Dongelmans DA, Nollet F. Poor functional status immediately after discharge from an intensive care unit. Disabil Rehabil. 2008;30(23):1812–8.

21. Semmler A, Okulla T, Kaiser M, Seifert B, Heneka MT. Long-term neuromuscular sequelae of critical illness. J Neurol. 2013;260(1):151–7.

22. Herridge MS, Tansey CM, Matte A, Tomlinson G, Diaz-Granados N, Cooper A, et al. Functional disability 5 years after acute respiratory distress syndrome. N Engl J Med. 2011;364(14):1293–304.

23. Fan E, Dowdy DW, Colantuoni E, Mendez-Tellez PA, Sevransky JE, Shanholtz C, et al. Physical complications in acute lung injury survivors: a two-year longitudinal prospective study. Crit Care Med. 2014;42(4):849–59.

24. Needham DM, Wozniak AW, Hough CL, Morris PE, Dinglas VD, Jackson JC, et al. Risk factors for physical impairment after acute lung injury in a national, multicenter study. Am J Respir Crit Care Med. 2014;189(10):1214–24.

25. Bohannon RW. Manual muscle testing: does it meet the standards of an adequate screening test? Clin Rehabil. 2005;19(6):662–7.

26. Bohannon RW. Quantitative testing of muscle strength: issues and practical options for the geriatric population. Top Geriatr Rehabil. 2002;18(2):1–17.

27. Noreau L, Vachon J. Comparison of three methods to assess muscular strength in individuals with spinal cord injury. Spinal Cord. 1998;36(10):716–23.

28. Elliott D, Denehy L, Berney S, Alison JA. Assessing physical function and activity for survivors of a critical illness: a review of instruments. Aust Crit Care. 2011;24(3):155–66.

29. Visser J, Mans E, de Visser M, van den Berg-Vos RM, Franssen H, de Jong JM, et al. Comparison of maximal voluntary isometric contraction and hand-held dynamometry in measuring muscle strength of patients with progressive lower motor neuron syndrome. Neuromuscul Disord. 2003;13(9):744–50.

30. van der Ploeg RJ, Oosterhuis HJ, Reuvekamp J. Measuring muscle strength. J Neurol. 1984;231(4):200–3.

31. Robles PG, Mathur S, Janaudis-Fereira T, Dolmage TE, Goldstein RS, Brooks D. Measurement of peripheral muscle strength in individuals with chronic obstructive pulmonary disease: a systematic review. J Cardiopulm Rehabil Prev. 2011;31(1):11–24.

32. Baldwin CE, Paratz JD, Bersten AD. Muscle strength assessment in critically ill patients with handheld dynamometry: an investigation of reliability, minimal detectable change, and time to peak force generation. J Crit Care. 2013;28(1):77–86.

33. Vanpee G, Hermans G, Segers J, Gosselink R. Assessment of limb muscle strength in critically ill patients: a systematic review. Crit Care Med. 2014;42(3):701–11.

34. Vanpee G, Segers J, Van Mechelen H, Wouters P, Van den Berghe G, Hermans G, et al. The interobserver agreement of handheld dynamometry for muscle strength assessment in critically ill patients. Crit Care Med. 2011;39(8):1929–34.

35. Laupland KB, Zygun DA, Davies HD, Church DL, Louie TJ, Doig CJ. Population-based assessment of intensive care unit-acquired bloodstream infections in adults: Incidence, risk factors, and associated mortality rate. Crit Care Med. 2002;30(11):2462–7.

36. The National Isometric Muscle Strength (NIMS) Database Consortium. Muscular weakness assessment: use of normal isometric strength data. Arch Phys Med Rehabil. 1996;77(12):1251–5.

37. ATS Committee on Proficiency Standards for Clinical Pulmonary Function Laboratories. ATS statement: guidelines for the six-minute walk test. Am J Respir Crit Care Med. 2002;166(1):111–7.

38. Enright PL, Sherrill DL. Reference equations for the six-minute walk in healthy adults. Am J Respir Crit Care Med. 1998;158(5 Pt 1):1384–7.

39. Hayes JA, Black NA, Jenkinson C, Young JD, Rowan KM, Daly K, et al. Outcome measures for adult critical care: a systematic review. Health Technol Assess. 2000;4(24):1–111.

40. Hopman WM, Towheed T, Anastassiades T, Tenenhouse A, Poliquin S, Berger C, Canadian Multicentre Osteoporosis Study Research Group, et al. Canadian normative data for the SF-36 health survey. CMAJ. 2000;163(3):265–71.

41. Zigmond AS, Snaith RP. The hospital anxiety and depression scale. Acta Psychiatr Scand. 1983;67(6):361–70.

42. Doig CJ, Zygun DA, Fick GH, Laupland KB, Boiteau PJ, Shahpori R, et al. Study of clinical course of organ dysfunction in intensive care. Crit Care Med. 2004;32(2):384–90.

43. Levy MM, Fink MP, Marshall JC, Abraham E, Angus D, Cook D, et al. 2001 SCCM/ESICM/ACCP/ATS/SIS international sepsis definitions conference. Crit Care Med. 2003;31(4):1250–6.

44. Benington S, McWilliams D, Eddleston J, Atkinson D. Exercise testing in survivors of intensive care—is there a role for cardiopulmonary exercise testing? J Crit Care. 2012;27(1):89–94.

45. Solway S, Brooks D, Lacasse Y, Thomas S. A qualitative systematic overview of the measurement properties of functional walk tests used in the cardiorespiratory domain. Chest. 2001;119(1):256–70.

46. Brower RG. Consequences of bed rest. Crit Care Med. 2009;37(10 Suppl):S422–8.

47. Morris PE, Goad A, Thompson C, Taylor K, Harry B, Passmore L, et al. Early intensive care unit mobility therapy in the treatment of acute respiratory failure. Crit Care Med. 2008;36(8):2238–43.

48. Schweickert WD, Pohlman MC, Pohlman AS, Nigos C, Pawlik AJ, Esbrook CL, et al. Early physical and occupational therapy in mechanically ventilated, critically ill patients: a randomised controlled trial. Lancet. 2009;373(9678):1874–82.
49. Kayambu G, Boots RJ, Paratz JD. Early rehabilitation in sepsis: a prospective randomised controlled trial investigating functional and physiological outcomes: the i-PERFORM Trial (Protocol Article). BMC Anesthesiol. 2011;11:21.
50. Hermans G, De Jonghe B, Bruyninckx F, Van den Berghe G. Interventions for preventing critical illness polyneuropathy and critical illness myopathy. Cochrane Database Syst Rev. 2009;1:006832.
51. Baracos V, Rodemann HP, Dinarello CA, Goldberg AL. Stimulation of muscle protein degradation and prostaglandin E2 release by leukocytic pyrogen (interleukin-1). A mechanism for the increased degradation of muscle proteins during fever. N Engl J Med. 1983;308(10):553–8.
52. Wagenmakers AJ. Muscle function in critically ill patients. Clin Nutr. 2001;20(5):451–4.
53. Klaude M, Mori M, Tjader I, Gustafsson T, Wernerman J, Rooyackers O. Protein metabolism and gene expression in skeletal muscle of critically ill patients with sepsis. Clin Sci. 2012;122(3):133–42.

4

Efficiency of an electronic device in controlling tracheal cuff pressure in critically ill patients

Anahita Rouzé[1], Julien De Jonckheere[2], Farid Zerimech[3], Julien Labreuche[4], Erika Parmentier-Decrucq[1], Benoit Voisin[1], Emmanuelle Jaillette[1], Patrice Maboudou[3], Malika Balduyck[3,5] and Saad Nseir[1,6]*

Abstract

Background: Despite intermittent control of tracheal cuff pressure (P_{cuff}) using a manual manometer, cuff under-inflation (<20 cmH$_2$O) and overinflation (>30 cmH$_2$O) frequently occur in intubated critically ill patients, resulting in increased risk of microaspiration and tracheal ischemic lesions. The primary objective of our study was to determine the efficiency of an electronic device in continuously controlling P_{cuff}. The secondary objective was to determine the impact of this device on the occurrence of microaspiration of gastric or oropharyngeal secretions.

Methods: Eighteen patients requiring mechanical ventilation were included in this prospective randomized controlled crossover study. They randomly received either continuous control of P_{cuff} with Mallinckrodt® device for 24 h, followed by discontinuous control with a manual manometer for 24 h, or the reverse sequence. During the 48 h after randomization, P_{cuff} was continuously recorded, and pepsin and alpha amylase were quantitatively measured in tracheal aspirates. P_{cuff} target was 25 cmH$_2$O.

Results: Clinical characteristics were similar during the two study periods, as well as mean airway pressure. Percentage of time spent with cuff overinflation or underinflation was significantly lower during continuous control compared with routine care period [median (IQR) 0.8 (0.1, 2) vs 20.9 (3.1, 40.1), $p = 0.0009$]. No significant difference was found in pepsin [median (IQR) 230 (151, 300) vs 259 (134, 368), $p = 0.95$] or in alpha amylase level [median (IQR) 1475 (528, 10,333) vs 2400 (1342, 15,391), $p = 0.19$] between continuous control and routine care periods, respectively.

Conclusions: The electronic device is efficient in controlling P_{cuff}, compared with routine care using a manometer. Further studies are needed to evaluate the impact of this device on intubation-related complications.

Trial registration ClinicalTrials.gov Identifier: NCT01965821

Keywords: Tracheal cuff, Intubation, Mechanical ventilation, Complications, Microaspiration

Background

In spite of the increased use of noninvasive ventilation and high-flow nasal oxygen [1–3], intubation is still frequently performed in up to 85 % of critically ill patients requiring mechanical ventilation [4]. This invasive procedure is associated with several potential complications, such as microaspiration of contaminated oropharyngeal and gastric secretions, ventilator-associated pneumonia, and tracheal ischemic lesions [5–10]. These intubation-related complications occur when tracheal cuff is inadequately inflated [11].

Current recommendations are to keep cuff pressure (P_{cuff}) between 20 and 30 cmH$_2$O, using a manometer [12]. Unfortunately, these recommendations are not followed in a high percentage of ICUs [13]. Even

*Correspondence: s-nseir@chru-lille.fr
[1] Centre de Réanimation, CHU Lille, 59000 Lille, France
Full list of author information is available at the end of the article

when tracheal cuff is routinely monitored and adjusted by nurses, patients spend a large amount of time up to 30–50 % outside the targeted range [14–18]. Moreover, P_{cuff} drops under 20 cmH$_2$O each time the manometer is connected [19]. Several new devices are available to continuously control P_{cuff} and prevent complications related to underinflation or overinflation of tracheal cuff [20–22]. Although many devices are available on the market, few of them were evaluated and validated by well-conducted clinical studies. These devices could be classified into mechanical and electronic. The advantages in using an electronic device are its easy use and the lower cost, compared with a pneumatic device.

The efficiency of the electronic device was evaluated in one in vitro study [23]. However, to our knowledge no clinical randomized controlled study has evaluated the efficiency of the electronic device in critically ill patients receiving mechanical ventilation for more than 48 h. Therefore, we conducted this randomized controlled trial to determine the efficiency of the electronic device in continuously controlling P_{cuff}. The secondary objective of this study was to evaluate the impact of continuous control of P_{cuff}, using the electronic device, on microaspiration of gastric contents in intubated critically ill patients.

Methods

This prospective randomized controlled crossover study was performed during a 1-year period, in a 10-bed ICU at the university hospital of Lille (France), in accordance with the Helsinki Declaration.

Inclusion and exclusion criteria

Inclusion criteria were: age >18 years and mechanical ventilation through a tracheal tube for a predicted duration of at least 48 h. Exclusion criteria were: mechanical ventilation through a tracheostomy, enrollment in another study that might interfere with the current study results, pregnancy, and contraindication for enteral nutrition.

Randomization

Patients were randomly assigned to receive continuous control of P_{cuff} with the electronic device (Mallinckrodt electronic cuff pressure controller®, VBM Medizintechnik GmbH, Sulz am Neckar, Germany) for 24 h, followed by discontinuous control (every 8 h) with a manual manometer (Hi-Lo Hand Pressure Gauge®, Mallinckrodt, Medtronic TM) for 24 h (Fig. 1), or the reverse sequence (Fig. 2). The target of P_{cuff} was 25 cmH$_2$O during the two periods. Randomization was performed using a computer-generated random assignment list in balanced blocs of six. Treatment assignments were contained in sealed opaque envelopes sequentially numbered.

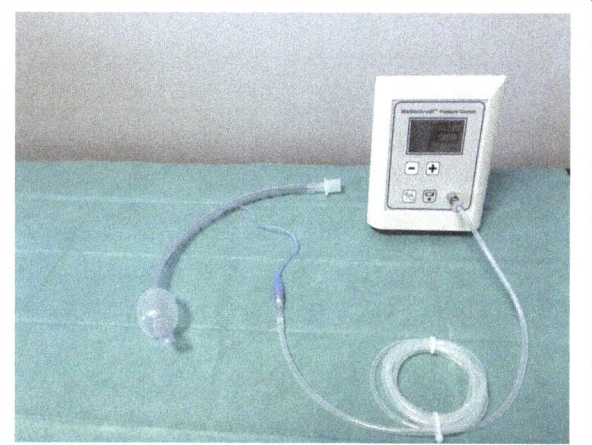

Fig. 1 Electronic device connected to a tracheal tube

Study objectives and outcome measurement

The primary objective was to determine the efficiency of the electronic device in reducing percentage of time spent with underinflation or overinflation of tracheal cuff, compared with routine care using a manometer. The secondary objectives included the impact of the electronic device on percentage of patients with underinflation or overinflation of tracheal cuff, percentage of time spent with underinflation of tracheal cuff, percentage of time spent with overinflation of tracheal cuff, percentage of time spent with normal (20–30 cmH$_2$O) tracheal cuff, P_{cuff}, and coefficient of variation of P_{cuff}, compared with routine care, and its impact on microaspiration of gastric and oropharyngeal secretions.

P_{cuff} and airway pressure were continuously recorded at a digitizing frequency of 100 Hz for 48 h (Physiotrace®; Estaris, Lille, France) [24], including 24 h of continuous control of P_{cuff} using the mechanical device and 24 h of manual control of P_{cuff} using the manometer (Fig. 3). Pepsin and alpha amylase were quantitatively measured in all tracheal aspirates during the two study periods [25, 26]. In order to avoid interference between the two periods regarding pepsin and alpha amylase levels, tracheal aspirate performed during the first 2 h of each study period was not analyzed. The engineer who analyzed the data (JDJ) and the physicians who measured pepsin and alpha amylase (FZ, PM, and MB) were blinded to study group assignment.

Study population

All patients were intubated with a high-volume low-pressure PVC standard-cuffed tracheal tube. Tracheal tube size was 8 and 7.5 in men and women, respectively. During the manometer period, nurses adjusted P_{cuff} every 8 h. Tracheal suctioning was performed, using open suction system, 6 times a day, or more frequently if clinically indicated.

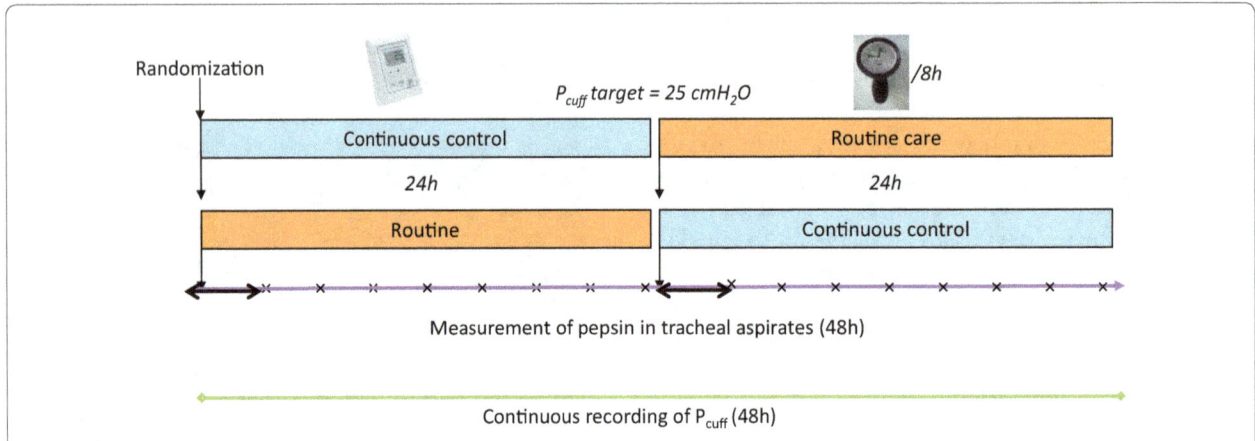

Fig. 2 Study design. *Red arrows* indicate washout periods for pepsin and amylase measurement, and *times symbol* indicates each tracheal aspirate performed for pepsin and amylase measurement

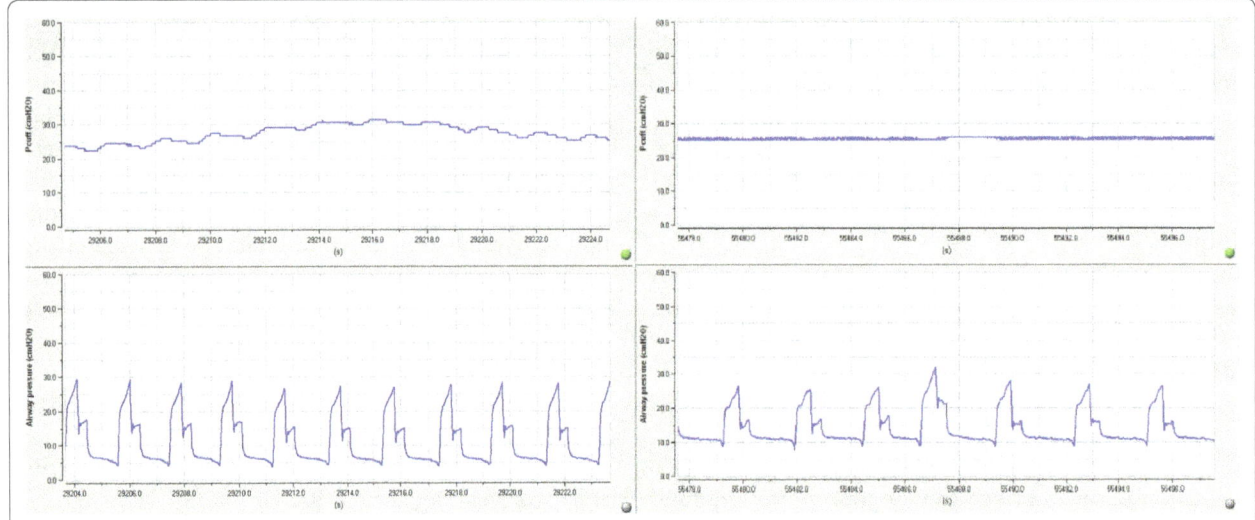

Fig. 3 An example of cuff and airway pressure recording. At *left*, cuff pressure (*above*), and airway pressure (*below*), during routine care. At *right*, cuff pressure (*above*) and airway pressure (*below*) during continuous control of cuff pressure

Semi-recumbent position was used during mechanical ventilation. During routine care period, P_{cuff} was adjusted, using the manometer, before turning and oral care.

Definitions

The primary outcome was the percentage of time spent with underinflation or with overinflation of tracheal cuff. Secondary outcomes included mean P_{cuff}, coefficient of variation of P_{cuff}, percentage of patients with underinflation of tracheal cuff, percentage of patients with overinflation of tracheal cuff, percentage of time spent with normal (20–30 cmH$_2$O) cuff pressure, percentage of time spent with underinflation of tracheal cuff, percentage of time spent with overinflation of tracheal cuff, mean

pepsin and alpha amylase level, percentage of tracheal aspirates positive for pepsin, and percentage of tracheal aspirates positive for alpha amylase.

Underinflation of tracheal cuff was defined as P_{cuff} <20 cmH$_2$O for >5 min over the 24-h period of recording. Overinflation of tracheal cuff was defined as P_{cuff} >30 cmH$_2$O for >5 min over the 24-h period of recording [14]. The coefficient of variation of P_{cuff} was calculated as standard deviation/mean P_{cuff} × 100.

Microaspiration of gastric contents was defined by the presence of pepsin at significant level (>200 ng/mL) in tracheal aspirate. Microaspiration of oropharyngeal secretions was defined by the presence of alpha amylase at significant level (>1685 UI/L) in tracheal aspirate [26].

Statistical analyses

Sample size calculation

Based on previous results [14, 15], the mean percentage of time spent with underinflation or overinflation of tracheal cuff was 30 % [standard deviation (SD) = 20 %] in patients intubated with a PVC-cuffed tracheal tube receiving routine care of P_{cuff} using a manual manometer. The expected mean percentage of time with underinflation or overinflation of tracheal cuff using the mechanical device was 10 % (expected difference of 20 %). In a parallel-group design, $n = 22$ patients per group will be required to detect this difference with a two-sided test, a power of 90 %, an alpha risk of 5 %, and a SD of 20 %. In a crossover design, the sample size determination is based on SD within subject difference, which can be derived from SD of measure and coefficient correlation (r) between the two measures on the same subject [27]. The sample size can therefore be derived from the number of patients to be included in parallel-group design, as follows: $n * (1 - r)$. Thus, assuming a conservative value of 0.2 for r, the number of patients to include is 18.

Result analysis

All analyses were performed in an intention-to-treat manner. Distribution of quantitative variables was tested using Shapiro–Wilk test. Normally and non-normally distributed variables were expressed as mean ± SD and median (25th, 75th interquartile), respectively. The statistical significance was set at $p < 0.05$.

The primary outcome was compared using a mixed linear model, adjusting for the period effect. Interaction between study period and assigned treatment, i.e., continuous control of P_{cuff} or routine care, was tested. Qualitative and quantitative patient characteristics and secondary outcomes were compared between the two 24-h periods using McNemar and Wilcoxon tests, respectively.

Results

During the study period, 23 patients were eligible. Five patients were excluded for different reasons, and 18 patients were included and were all analyzed (Fig. 4).

Patient characteristics

Patient characteristics are presented in Table 1.

No significant difference was found between the two study periods regarding ventilator mode and settings, sedation, Ramsay score, or neuromuscular blocking agent use. Prone position was not used in included patients, during the two study periods. All other characteristics were also similar during the two periods (Table 2).

No significant difference was found in duration of P_{cuff} and airway pressure recording [median (IQR) 23 (23, 23.3 vs 23.5 h (23, 24), $p = 0.066$], or in mean airway pressure [13.2 (10.7, 15.5) vs 13.1 cmH$_2$O (10.8, 15.6)] between continuous control and routine care periods, respectively.

Primary outcome

The percentage of time spent with underinflation, or with overinflation, was significantly lower during continuous control of P_{cuff} compared with routine care [median (IQR) 0.8 (0.1, 2) vs 20.9 (3.1, 40.1), $p = 0.0009$]. No significant interaction was found between study period and the assigned treatment ($p = 0.91$).

Secondary outcomes

Mean P_{cuff} and percentage of time spent with P_{cuff} 20–30 cmH$_2$O were significantly higher during continuous control of P_{cuff} compared with routine care. Percentage of patients with underinflation, percentage of time spent with underinflation, percentage of time spent with overinflation, and coefficient of variation of P_{cuff} were significantly lower during continuous control compared with routine care of tracheal cuff. Percentage of patients with overinflation was similar during the two study periods (Table 3).

No significant difference was found in pepsin level, in percentage of tracheal aspirates positive for pepsin, in alpha amylase level, or in percentage of tracheal aspirates positive for alpha amylase between the two study periods (Table 3).

Discussion

Our results suggest that the electronic device is efficient in controlling P_{cuff}. However, no significant impact of continuous control of P_{cuff} was found on microaspiration of gastric or oropharyngeal secretions.

To our knowledge, our study is the first clinical randomized controlled study to evaluate the efficiency of the electronic device in continuously controlling P_{cuff} in critically ill patients. A previous in vitro study found similar results [23]. In addition, Lorente et al. [28] conducted a prospective observational study to determine the impact of continuous control of P_{cuff}, using the same electronic device, on the incidence of VAP. The authors reported significantly lower rate of P_{cuff} determinations <20 cmH$_2$O (mean ± SD 0 vs 9 ± 8, $p < 0.001$), P_{cuff} determinations >30 cmH$_2$O (mean ± SD 0 vs 4 ± 5, $p < 0.001$), and substantial decrease (51 %) in VAP incidence in patients who received continuous control of P_{cuff}, compared with those received routine care. However, the efficiency of the electronic device in continuously controlling P_{cuff} was not the primary objective of the study. In addition, P_{cuff} was not continuously recorded, and the study was not randomized.

The percentage of time spent with underinflation (median 9.1 %) and with overinflation (median 2.4 %)

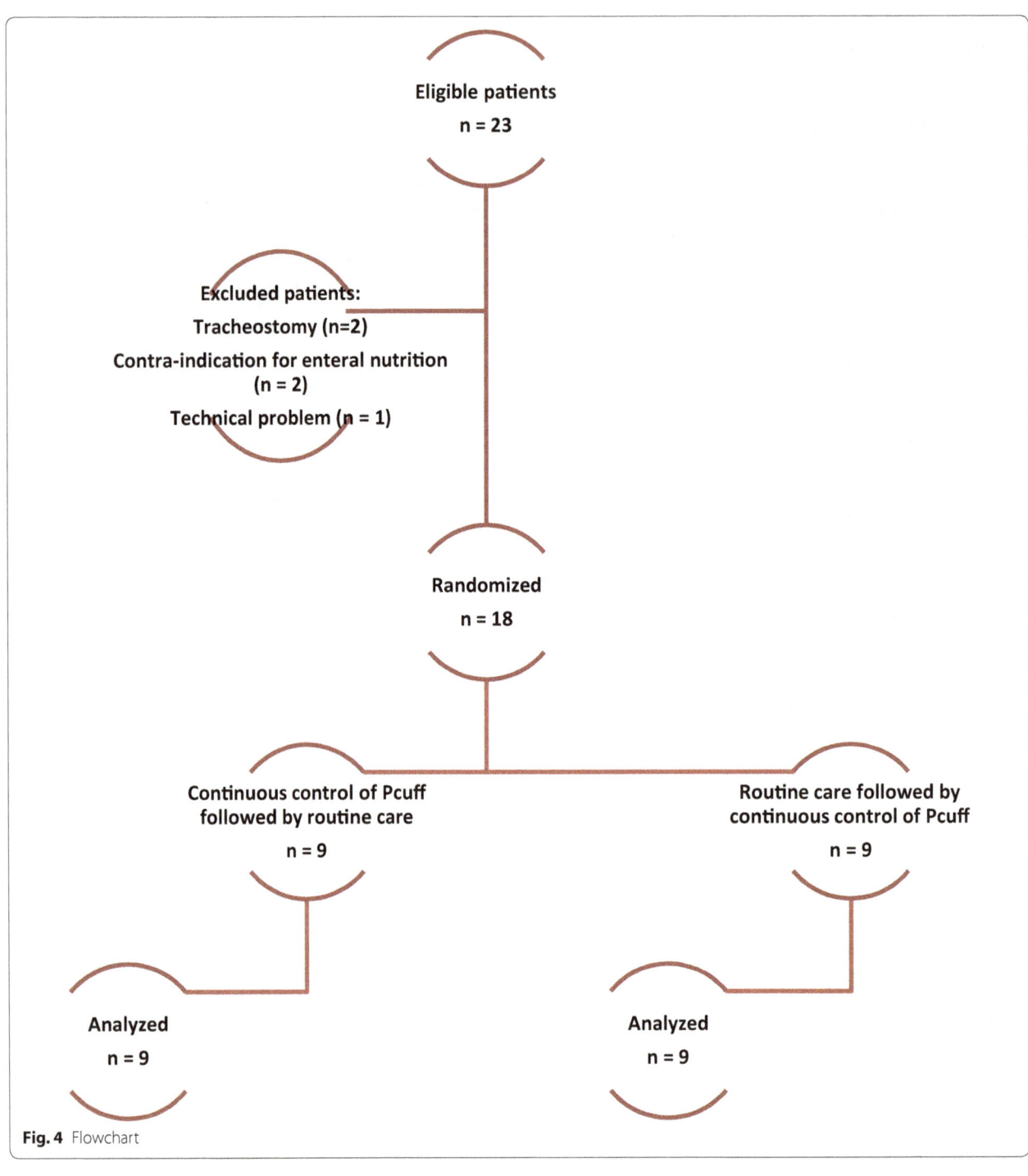

Fig. 4 Flowchart

during routine care was lower than previously reported [14, 15]. The small number of patients included in the current study ($n = 18$) could explain this difference. Duration of prior intubation was identified as an independent risk factor for underinflation of tracheal cuff [14]. However, duration of prior intubation was quite similar in the current study (median 4 days) compared with previous studies

(2 and 5 days, respectively) [14, 15]. Another explanation could be the different patient characteristics between the current study and previous ones. The percentage of non-sedated patients was lower in the current study (22 %) compared with the two previous ones (35 and 53 %, respectively). The absence of sedation was identified as an independent risk factor for underinflation of tracheal cuff [14].

Table 1 Patient characteristics

Number of included patients	18
Age (years), mean ± SD	54 ± 18
Male gender, n (%)	13 (72)
Weight (kg), median (IQR)	72 (66, 81)
SAPS II, mean ± SD	43 ± 16
LOD score, mean ± SD	6 ± 3
Cause for ICU admission, n 5 %	
Neurologic failure	7 (38)
Respiratory failure	6 (33)
Shock	5 (27)
Duration of mechanical ventilation before inclusion (days), median (IQR)	4 (2, 6)
Total duration of mechanical ventilation (days), median (IQR)	12 (7, 25)
Length of ICU stay (days), median (IQR)	21 (11, 30)
Ventilator-associated pneumonia, n (%)	3 (15)
ICU mortality, n (%)	10 (55)

SAPS Simplified Acute Physiology Score, LOD logistic organ dysfunction, IQR interquartile range

No significant impact of continuous control of P_{cuff} was found on microaspiration of gastric and oropharyngeal secretions. Several explanations could be suggested for this finding. Microaspiration of gastric contents was a secondary outcome, and our study was probably underpowered to detect such an effect. The higher, but not significant, level of alpha amylase during continuous control, compared with routine care periods, is in keeping with this hypothesis. Although this secondary outcome was negative, the results could be helpful for future studies, aiming at evaluating the impact of continuous control of P_{cuff} on microaspiration. In addition, the duration of tracheal aspirate collection (24 h) during the two study periods was probably too short to evaluate this effect. Further, the above-mentioned in vitro study reported that the electronic device might interfere with self-expanding properties of some PVC-cuffed tracheal tubes [23]. Therefore, the rapid correction of overinflation of P_{cuff} during cough could result in short sudden drop of P_{cuff} and microaspiration of gastric contents. Further studies are needed to confirm this hypothesis. The short washout period (2 h) used in this study might have resulted in overlap in pepsin and alpha amylase results between the two periods. Whilst pepsin half-life is relatively short [29], alpha amylase half-life is unknown. This might have influenced the impact of continuous control of P_{cuff} on microaspiration of gastric and oropharyngeal secretions.

Table 2 Patient characteristics during the 48 h following randomization

Variables	Continuous control of P_{cuff} n = 18	Routine care n = 18	p
Ventilatory mode[a]			>0.99
ACV	13 (72)	13 (72)	
PSV	9 (50)	10 (56)	
Mean P_{peak} (cmH$_2$O)	31 (21, 35)	30 (24, 34)	0.64
Mean PEEP (cmH$_2$O)	7 (5, 9)	6 (5, 8)	0.73
Mean FiO$_2$	0.45 (0.40, 0.50)	0.40 (0.40, 0.50)	0.41
Number of tracheal suctions	6 (5, 7)	6 (6, 7)	>0.99
Sedation	12 (67)	14 (78)	0.50
Ramsay score	5 (3, 6)	4 (3, 6)	0.86
Neuromuscular blocking agent use	1 (6)	0 (0)	>0.99
Head-of-bed position <30°	4 (22)	6 (33)	0.50
Fiberoptic bronchoscopy	2 (11)	2 (11)	>0.99
Transport outside the ICU	0 (0)	1 (6)	>0.99
Aerosolized medication	2 (11)	2 (11)	>0.99
¡NO	2 (11)	1 (6)	>0.99
Quantity of enteral nutrition (mL/day)	1000 (500, 1500)	1000 (875, 1125)	0.31
Gastric residual volume (mL)	0 (0, 61)	0 (0, 100)	0.52
Vomiting	2 (11)	2 (11)	>0.99
Prokinetic drugs	1 (6)	1 (6)	>0.99
Stress ulcer prophylaxis or treatment	16 (89)	16 (89)	>0.99

Data are number of patients (%) or median (Interquartile range)

P_{cuff} cuff pressure, ACV assist–control ventilation, PSV pressure support ventilation, P_{peak} peak pressure, PEEP positive end-expiratory pressure, FiO$_2$ fraction of inspired oxygen, ¡NO inhaled nitric oxide

[a] Some patients received two ventilator modes during continuous control of P_{cuff}, or during routine care

Table 3 Secondary outcomes

Variables	Continuous control $n = 18$	Routine care $n = 18$	p
Mean P_{cuff} (cmH$_2$O)	25.9 (25.5, 26.4)	22.7 (21.6, 24.8)	0.001
Coefficient of P_{cuff} variation (%)	4.1 (1.5, 6.1)	7.7 (4.4, 11.5)	<0.001
P_{cuff} 20–30 cmH$_2$O			
Yes	18 (100)	18 (100)	>0.99
% of recording time	99.1 (97.9, 99.9)	73.5 (54.4–96.8)	<0.001
P_{cuff} <20 cmH$_2$O			
Yes	0 (0)	13 (72)	<0.001
% of recording time	0.0 (0, 0)	9.1 (0.0–36.1)	0.001
P_{cuff} >30 cmH$_2$O			
Yes	11 (61)	14 (78)	0.25
% of recording time	0.8 (0.1, 2.1)	2.4 (0.7, 9.4)	<0.001
Pepsin (ng/mL)	230 (151, 300)	259 (134, 369)	0.95
% of tracheal aspirates positive for pepsin	67 (0, 100)	71 (0, 100)	0.83
Alpha amylase (ng/mL)	1475 (528, 10,333)	2400 (1342–15,391)	0.19
% of tracheal aspirates positive for alpha amylase	40 (0, 100)	33 (0, 100)	0.92

Data are number of patients (%) or median (interquartile range)

P_{cuff} cuff pressure

Yes indicates that a patient had the variable at least once

Given the efficiency of the electronic device, the absence of potential harm, and the reduction in nurse workload, one could argue that use of such a device could be recommended in every intubated critically ill patient. However, the level of evidence on the clinical benefit of using continuous control of P_{cuff} is still low [30]. In addition, cost-effectiveness of this preventive measure of VAP was not evaluated. Therefore, further randomized controlled trials aiming at evaluating the impact of continuous control of P_{cuff} on VAP incidence are required to evaluate the efficiency of this preventive measure.

Some limitations of our study should be acknowledged. First, this was a single-center study. Therefore, our results could not be generalized to patients hospitalized in other ICUs. We did not evaluate the impact of continuous control of P_{cuff} using the electronic device on ventilator-associated pneumonia or tracheal ischemic lesions. However, our study design did not allow such an evaluation, because each patient was his own control. This design is probably the best first step to evaluate the efficiency of the electronic device, because of potential patient-related confounders, such as tracheal size, shape, respiratory resistance, and airway pressure. Further, the study was not blinded. However, investigators who assessed continuous P_{cuff} recording and pepsin were blinded to study group assignment.

Conclusions

The electronic device evaluated in this study is efficient in continuously controlling P_{cuff} in critically ill patients. Further randomized controlled studies are needed to determine the impact of continuous control of P_{cuff}, using the electronic device, on intubation-related complications, such as microaspiration, VAP, and tracheal ischemia.

Abbreviations
P_{cuff}: cuff pressure; SAPS: Simplified Acute Physiology Score; LOD: logistic organ dysfunction.

Authors' contributions
AR, JDJ, MB, FZ, and SN designed the study. AR, JDJ, EP, BV, EJ, FZ, and PM collected data. JL and SN performed statistical analysis. AR and SN wrote the manuscript. All authors participated in the final revision of the manuscript and approved the submitted version. All authors read and approved the final manuscript.

Author details
[1] Centre de Réanimation, CHU Lille, 59000 Lille, France. [2] Centre d'Investigation Clinique, CHU Lille, 59000 Lille, France. [3] Centre de Biologie et de Pathologie, CHU Lille, 59000 Lille, France. [4] EA 2694 - Santé publique : épidémiologie et qualité des soins, CHU Lille, 59000 Lille, France. [5] Faculté de Pharmacie, Université Lille, 59000 Lille, France. [6] Faculté de Médecine, Université Lille, 59000 Lille, France.

Acknowledgements
None.

Competing interests
SN received fees from Medtronic for lecture, and from Ciel Medical for advisory board. AR, JDJ, FZ, JL, EP, BV, EJ, PM and MB: none.

References

1. Papazian L, Corley A, Hess D, Fraser JF, Frat J-P, et al. Use of high-flow nasal cannula oxygenation in ICU adults: a narrative review. Intensive Care Med. 2016;42:1336–49

2. Cabrini L, Landoni G, Oriani A, Plumari VP, Nobile L, et al. Noninvasive ventilation and survival in acute care settings: a comprehensive systematic review and metaanalysis of randomized controlled trials. Crit Care Med. 2015;43:880–8.

3. Martinez-Urbistondo D, Alegre F, Carmona-Torre F, Huerta A, Fernandez-Ros N, et al. Mortality prediction in patients undergoing non-invasive ventilation in intermediate care. PLoS One. 2015;10:e0139702.

4. Esteban A, Frutos-Vivar F, Muriel A, Ferguson ND, Peñuelas O, et al. Evolution of mortality over time in patients receiving mechanical ventilation. Am J Respir Crit Care Med. 2013;188:220–30.

5. Nseir S, Zerimech F, Jaillette E, Artru F, Balduyck M. Microaspiration in intubated critically ill patients: diagnosis and prevention. Infect Disord Drug Targets. 2011;11:413–23.

6. Touat L, Fournier C, Ramon P, Salleron J, Durocher A, et al. Intubation-related tracheal ischemic lesions: incidence, risk factors, and outcome. Intensive Care Med. 2013;39:575–82.

7. Blot SI, Poelaert J, Kollef M. How to avoid microaspiration? A key element for the prevention of ventilator-associated pneumonia in intubated ICU patients. BMC Infect Dis. 2014;14:119.

8. Branson RD, Gomaa D, Rodriquez D. Management of the artificial airway. Respir Care. 2014;59:974–89 **(discussion 989–990)**.

9. Carter EL, Duguid A, Ercole A, Matta B, Burnstein RM, et al. Strategies to prevent ventilation-associated pneumonia: the effect of cuff pressure monitoring techniques and tracheal tube type on aspiration of subglottic secretions: an in vitro study. Eur J Anaesthesiol. 2014;31:166–71.

10. Blot SI, Rello J, Koulenti D. The value of polyurethane-cuffed endotracheal tubes to reduce microaspiration and intubation-related pneumonia: a systematic review of laboratory and clinical studies. Crit Care. 2016;20:203.

11. Jaillette E, Martin-Loeches I, Artigas A, Nseir S. Optimal care and design of the tracheal cuff in the critically ill patient. Ann Intensive Care. 2014;4:7.

12. American Thoracic Society, Infectious Diseases Society of America. Guidelines for the management of adults with hospital-acquired, ventilator-associated, and healthcare-associated pneumonia. Am J Respir Crit Care Med 2005;171:388–16.

13. Talekar CR, Udy AA, Boots RJ, Lipman J, Cook D. Tracheal cuff pressure monitoring in the ICU: a literature review and survey of current practice in Queensland. Anaesth Intensive Care. 2014;42:761–70.

14. Nseir S, Brisson H, Marquette C-H, Chaud P, Di Pompeo C, et al. Variations in endotracheal cuff pressure in intubated critically ill patients: prevalence and risk factors. Eur J Anaesthesiol. 2009;26:229–34.

15. Nseir S, Zerimech F, De Jonckheere J, Alves I, Balduyck M, et al. Impact of polyurethane on variations in tracheal cuff pressure in critically ill patients: a prospective observational study. Intensive Care Med. 2010;36:1156–63.

16. Lizy C, Swinnen W, Labeau S, Poelaert J, Vogelaers D, et al. Cuff pressure of endotracheal tubes after changes in body position in critically ill patients treated with mechanical ventilation. Am J Crit Care. 2014;23:e1–8.

17. Geng G, Hu J, Huang S. The effect of endotracheal tube cuff pressure change during gynecological laparoscopic surgery on postoperative sore throat: a control study. J Clin Monit Comput. 2015;29:141–4.

18. Lou Sole M, Su X, Talbert S, Penoyer DA, Kalita S, et al. Evaluation of an intervention to maintain endotracheal tube cuff pressure within therapeutic range. Am J Crit Care. 2011;20:109–18.

19. Farré R, Rotger M, Ferrer M, Torres A, Navajas D. Automatic regulation of the cuff pressure in endotracheally-intubated patients. Eur Respir J. 2002;20:1010–3.

20. Duguet A, D'Amico L, Biondi G, Prodanovic H, Gonzalez-Bermejo J, et al. Control of tracheal cuff pressure: a pilot study using a pneumatic device. Intensive Care Med. 2007;33:128–32.

21. Nseir S, Rodriguez A, Saludes P, De Jonckheere J, Valles J, et al. Efficiency of a mechanical device in controlling tracheal cuff pressure in intubated critically ill patients: a randomized controlled study. Ann Intensive Care. 2015;5:54.

22. Chenelle CT, Oto J, Sulemanji D, Fisher DF, Kacmarek RM. Evaluation of an automated endotracheal tube cuff controller during simulated mechanical ventilation. Respir Care. 2015;60:183–90.

23. Weiss M, Doell C, Koepfer N, Madjdpour C, Woitzek K, et al. Rapid pressure compensation by automated cuff pressure controllers worsens sealing in tracheal tubes. Br J Anaesth. 2009;102:273–8.

24. De Jonckheere J, Logier R, Dassonneville a, Delmar G, Vasseur C. PhysioTrace: an efficient toolkit for biomedical signal processing. In: Conference proceedings of the IEEE engineering in medicine and biology, vol. 7; 2005. p. 6739–41.

25. Nseir S, Zerimech F, Fournier C, Lubret R, Ramon P, et al. Continuous control of tracheal cuff pressure and microaspiration of gastric contents in critically ill patients. Am J Respir Crit Care Med. 2011;184:1041–7.

26. Dewavrin F, Zerimech F, Boyer A, Maboudou P, Balduyck M, et al. Accuracy of alpha amylase in diagnosing microaspiration in intubated critically-ill patients. PLoS One. 2014;9:e90851.

27. Julious SA. Sample sizes for clinical trials with normal data. Stat Med. 2004;23:1921–86.

28. Lorente L, Lecuona M, Jiménez A, Lorenzo L, Roca I, et al. Continuous endotracheal tube cuff pressure control system protects against ventilator-associated pneumonia. Crit Care. 2014;18:R77.

29. Metheny NA, Dahms TE, Chang Y-H, Stewart BJ, Frank PA, et al. Detection of pepsin in tracheal secretions after forced small-volume aspirations of gastric juice. JPEN J Parenter Enter Nutr. 2004;28:79–84.

30. Nseir S, Lorente L, Ferrer M, Rouzé A, Gonzalez O, et al. Continuous control of tracheal cuff pressure for VAP prevention: a collaborative meta-analysis of individual participant data. Ann Intensive Care. 2015;5:43.

5

Invasive fungal tracheobronchitis in mechanically ventilated critically ill patients: underlying conditions, diagnosis, and outcomes

Chun-Yu Lin[1,3†], Wei-Lun Liu[4,5,6†], Che-Chia Chang[7], Hou-Tai Chang[8], Han-Chung Hu[2,3], Kuo-chin Kao[2,3], Ning-Hung Chen[2,3], Ying-Jen Chen[1,3], Cheng-Ta Yang[2,3], Chung-Chi Huang[2,3*] and George Dimopoulos[9]

Abstract

Background: Invasive fungal tracheobronchitis (IFT) is a severe form of pulmonary fungal infection that is not limited to immunocompromised patients. Although respiratory failure is a crucial predictor of death, information regarding IFT in critically ill patients is limited.

Methods: In this retrospective, multicenter, observational study, we enrolled adults diagnosed as having IFT who had been admitted to the intensive care unit between January 2007 and December 2015. Their demographics, clinical imaging data, bronchoscopic and histopathological findings, and outcomes were recorded.

Results: This study included 31 patients who had been diagnosed as having IFT, comprising 24 men and 7 women with a mean age of 64.7 ± 13.7 years. All patients developed respiratory failure and received mechanical ventilation before diagnosis. Eighteen (58.1%) patients had diabetes mellitus, and 12 (38.7%) had chronic lung disease. Four (12.9%) patients had hematologic disease, and none of the patients had neutropenia. Twenty-five (80.6%) patients were diagnosed as having proven IFT, and the remaining patients had probable IFT. *Aspergillus* spp. (61.3%) were the most common pathogenic species, followed by Mucorales (25.8%) and *Candida* spp. (6.5%). The diagnoses in six (19.4%) patients were confirmed only through bronchial biopsy and histopathological examination, whereas their cultures of bronchoalveolar lavage fluid were negative for fungi. The overall in-hospital mortality rate was 93.5%.

Conclusions: IFT in critically ill patients results in a high mortality rate. Diabetes mellitus is the most prevalent underlying disease, followed by chronic lung disease. In addition to *Aspergillus* spp., Mucorales is another crucial pathogenic species. Bronchial lesion biopsy is the key diagnostic strategy.

Keywords: Invasive fungal tracheobronchitis, Aspergillosis, Mucormycosis, Critical care, Outcome

Background

Invasive fungal disease is a life-threatening disease that mostly occurs in immunocompromised patients. The incidence of pulmonary fungal infection has dramatically increased in recent years [1]. *Aspergillus* spp. is the most common pathogenic species among pulmonary fungal infection [2, 3]. The overall mortality rate of invasive aspergillosis is approximately 50% [4–6]. Moreover, the

*Correspondence: cch4848@cloud.cgmh.org.tw
†Chun-Yu Lin and Wei-Lun Liu contributed equally to the work
[2] Department of Pulmonary and Critical Care Medicine, Chang Gung Memorial Hospital at Linkou, Taoyuan, Taiwan
Full list of author information is available at the end of the article

frequency of invasive fungal infections caused by non-*Aspergillus* filamentous fungi is also increasing, and these infections are associated with devastating outcomes similar to that of invasive aspergillosis [5]. In addition to patients with conventional risk factors including neutropenia and those who have undergone stem cell transplantations, patients with chronic obstructive pulmonary disease, chronic renal failure, and liver cirrhosis may develop invasive fungal infections [2, 7, 8]. Critically ill patients who are admitted to intensive care units (ICUs) have been increasingly recognized as a population at a particularly high risk of pulmonary fungal infection [2]. Moreover, invasive aspergillosis in critically ill patients without malignancy who receive mechanical ventilation results in very poor outcomes and a mortality rate of 90% [9].

Invasive fungal tracheobronchitis (IFT) is a rare but severe form of pulmonary fungal infection that has been increasingly observed in critically ill patients [2, 10]. Diagnosing IFT is considerably difficult because of the nonspecific clinical manifestations and the low yields in microbiological tests [2, 11, 12]. The mortality rate of IFT caused by different fungi varies from 20 to 80% [11, 13–16]. Patients with *Aspergillus* tracheobronchitis who have developed acute respiratory failure exhibit substantially poorer outcomes than those without respiratory distress do (mortality rate 69.2–93.8 vs. 25–32.8%) [11, 15, 16]. Moreover, ICU admission is a strong predictor of death in patients with non-*Aspergillus* mold invasive infections [5]. However, information regarding IFT in critically ill patients is limited.

The aim of the current study is to evaluate the diagnostic approach and the outcomes of IFT in critically ill patients.

Methods
Study design and subjects
In this retrospective, multicenter, observational study, we included critically ill adult patients with IFT who had been admitted to medical ICUs between January 2007 and December 2015 at the Linkou and Chiayi branches of Chang Gung Memorial Hospital, Far Eastern Memorial Hospital, and the Liouying branch of Chi Mei Medical Center. This study was approved by the institutional review boards of Chang Gung Memorial Hospital (CGMH 104-7452B). The patients were classified as having proven or probable IFT by using the revised definitions for invasive fungal infections from the European Organization for the Research and Treatment of Cancer/Mycosis Study Group (EORTC/MSG) [17]. Histopathology was used to diagnose proven IFT. Probable IFT refers to the presence of positive cultures for fungal species from bronchoalveolar lavage (BAL) specimens accompanied by tracheobronchitis. All patients underwent fiberoptic bronchoscopy. From the bronchoscopic findings, IFT was classified into pseudomembranous, ulcerative, or obstructive forms according to Denning's classification [18]. The patients' demographic data; underlying diseases; clinical presentation; disease severity; laboratory parameters; bronchoscopic, microbiological, and histopathological findings; medications; and outcomes were recorded.

Overall in-hospital mortality was assessed. If the study patients were alive, survival was recorded until the date they were lost to follow-up or the date the study concluded. Because of the retrospective, observational

nature of this study and the lack of any modification in the general management of the patients, the need for informed consent was waived.

Statistical analyses
All statistical analyses were performed using GraphPad Prism statistical software (GraphPad Prism, version 5.01). The categorical variables are presented as counts (percentages), and the continuous variables are presented as the means ± standard deviations.

Results
This study included 31 critically ill patients who had been diagnosed as having IFT, comprising 24 men and 7 women with a mean age of 64.7 ± 13.7 years. Table 1 summarizes the demographics and underlying conditions of the patients who were hospitalized in the medical ICU for IFT. Thirty (96.8%) patients had underlying diseases. Only one patient, who was a light smoker, had no medical history. Diabetes mellitus (DM; 18 patients, [58.1%]) was the most predominant underlying condition in the IFT patients. The median HbA1c level was 8.1% (5.4–13%). Five patients were newly diagnosed as having DM. Nine patients were taking oral anti-diabetic agents. Four patients had received insulin therapy. Three of these DM patients had proteinuria and chronic renal disease. Chronic lung disease (12 patients [38.7%]) was the second most predominant underlying disease. Four patients (12.9%) had solid organ tumors, and four (12.9%) had hematologic disease. None of these IFT patients had chronic renal failure or neutropenia, and none had undergone solid organ transplantations. Moreover, 17 patients (54.8%) had received systemic steroid treatment before diagnosis. Three patients (9.7%) developed IFT after being diagnosed as having H1N1 pneumonia. The overall in-hospital mortality rate was 93.5% (29 patients). The median time spent in the ICU before diagnosis was 5 days (0–19 days). The median length of ICU stay was 14 days (2–85 days). The median survival time after diagnosis was 10 days (0–85 days). Table 2 summarizes the clinical manifestations of the critically ill patients with IFT. The mean Acute Physiology and Chronic Health Evaluation II (APACHE II) score on ICU admission was 23.1 ± 10.4. Because of respiratory failure, all patients received mechanical ventilation before diagnosis. Furthermore, 21 patients (67.7%) underwent computed tomography (CT). Consolidation was the most frequent finding (19 patients [61.3%]). Only one patient exhibited the air crescent sign on CT, and none of the patients had the halo sign. All patients underwent bronchoscopies and BAL. Moreover, 27 and 12 patients (87.1 and 38.7%) had the pseudomembranous and ulcerative forms of IFT, respectively. The obstructive form (4 patients [12.9%]) was the least frequent form of IFT (Table 2). Bronchial biopsy was performed in 27

Table 1 Demographics and underlying conditions of 31 patients with invasive fungal tracheobronchitis

Variable	No. of patients (%)
Age, years (mean ± SD)	64.7 ± 13.7
Gender, male	24 (77.4)
Current/ex-smoker	15 (48.4)
Underlying disease	30 (96.8)
DM	18 (58.1)
Chronic lung disease	12 (38.7)
COPD/asthma	8 (25.8)
Old TB	2 (6.5)
Bronchiectasis	2 (6.5)
Solid organ cancer	4 (12.9)
Hematologic disease	4 (12.9)
Liver cirrhosis	3 (9.7)
Systemic steroids before diagnosis	17 (54.8)
Duration of steroids before ICU admission, day, median (IQR)	49 (14–90)
Daily dosage of steroids, mg, median (IQR)	50 (29–71)
Inhaled corticosteroids before diagnosis	3 (9.7)
H1N1 infection before diagnosis	3 (9.7)

SD standard deviation, DM diabetes mellitus, COPD chronic obstructive pulmonary disease, TB tuberculosis, ICU intensive care unit, IQR interquartile range

patients (87%). Biopsy was not performed in the remaining four patients (12.9%) because of the extremely low platelet count (<5000 per mm^3) or severe hypoxemia under ventilator support (fraction of inspired oxygen 100%). None of the patients had developed massive hemoptysis or hypoxemia after the bronchial biopsy. Figure 1 illustrates the distinct histological images and indistinguishable bronchoscopic and radiographic findings of IFT caused by different fungal species. The mortality rate did not differ significantly between the patients with proven and probable IFT (96% [24 of 25] vs. 83.3% [5 of 6]; $p = 0.35$).

In this study, *Aspergillus* spp. was found to be the most common pathogenic species of IFT (19 patients [61.3%]), followed by Mucorales (8 patients [25.8%]). *Candida* spp. was the causative pathogen of IFT in two patients (6.5%). A further two patients were infected by undifferentiated mold (Table 2). The galactomannan antigen levels were evaluated in 16 of the 19 patients with *Aspergillus* tracheobronchitis and in 4 of the 12 patients with non-*Aspergillus*-related fungal tracheobronchitis. In patients with *Aspergillus* tracheobronchitis, the galactomannan antigen levels in the serum and BAL were 3.44 ± 2.8 and 4.87 ± 2.6, respectively. In patients with non-*Aspergillus*-related fungal tracheobronchitis, the galactomannan antigen levels were less than 0.5. The two survivors were infected by *Aspergillus* spp. and undifferentiated mold. The mortality rate did

Table 2 Clinical manifestations of 31 patients with invasive fungal tracheobronchitis

Variable	No. of patients (%)
APACHE II score on ICU admission, mean ± SD	23.1 ± 10.4
AKI requiring RRT	14 (45.2)
RF before diagnosis reached	31 (100)
Time in the ICU before diagnosis, days (IQR)	5 (1.8–8)
Length of ICU stay, days (IQR)	14 (8–27)
Concurrent bacterial sepsis	18 (58.1)
Parenchymal involvement	31 (100)
CT scan	21 (67.7)
Consolidation	19 (61.3)
Cavitation	4 (12.9)
Air crescent sign	1 (3.2)
Bronchoscopic classification	
Pseudomembranous	27 (87.1)
Ulcerative	12 (38.7)
Obstructive	4 (12.9)
Diagnosis of IFT	
Proven	25 (80.6)
Probable	6 (19.4)
Pathogen	
Aspergillus spp.	19 (61.3)
Aspergillus fumigatus	11 (35.4)
Aspergillus flavus	2 (6.5)
Aspergillus terrus	1 (3.2)
Undifferentiated *Aspergillus* species	5 (16.1)
Mucorales	8 (25.8)
Candida spp.	2 (6.5)
Undifferentiated mold	2 (6.5)
BAL fungal culture	
Positive	25 (80.6)
Negative	6 (19.4)
Galactomannan level in *Aspergillus* tracheobronchitis	
Serum (index)	3.44 ± 2.8
BAL (index)	4.87 ± 2.6
Antifungal therapy	29 (93.5)
Voriconazole	15 (48.4)
Echinocandin	19 (61.3)
Combination therapy	8 (25.8)

APACHE II Acute Physiology and Chronic Health Evaluation II, ICU intensive care unit, SD standard deviation, AKI acute kidney injury, RRT renal replacement therapy, RF respiratory failure, IQR interquartile range, CT computed tomography, IFT invasive fungal tracheobronchitis, BAL bronchoalveolar lavage

not differ among patients with IFT caused by different fungal species. Only nine patients (29%) had positive fungal culture results for lower respiratory tract specimens before bronchoscopy. Six patients (19.4%) had negative fungal culture results for BAL fluid after bronchoscopy. They were diagnosed through histopathology of bronchial biopsy specimens.

Invasive fungal tracheobronchitis in mechanically ventilated critically ill patients: underlying...

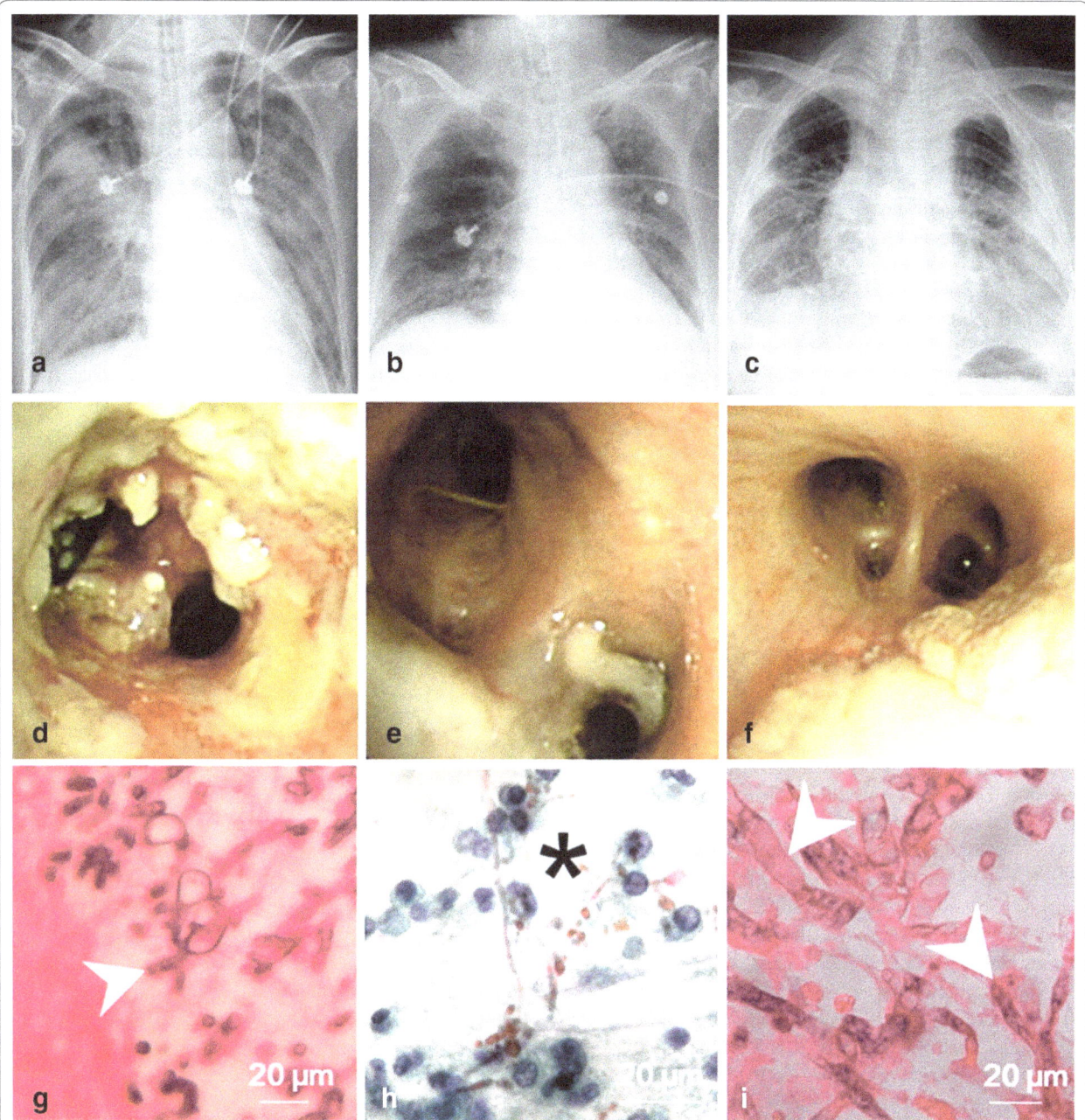

Fig. 1 Chest radiograph and bronchoscopic and histological examinations of IFT. **a** Invasive Aspergillus tracheobronchitis. **b** Invasive Candida tracheobronchitis. **c** Mucorales-related invasive tracheobronchitis. **d** Bronchoscopic view of invasive Aspergillus tracheobronchitis. **e** Bronchoscopic view of invasive Candida tracheobronchitis. **f** Bronchoscopic view of Mucorales-related invasive tracheobronchitis. **g** Histopathological examination revealed septate fungal hyphae branching at a 45° angle (*arrowhead*), which is characteristic of *Aspergillus* spp. (magnification: 400×). **h** Histopathological examination revealed yeast cells and pseudohyphae (*star*), which are characteristic of *Candida* spp. (magnification: 400×). **i** Histopathological examination revealed broad, thin-walled, non-septate hyphae, which are characteristic of Mucormycete (*left arrowhead*) and the other septate fungal hyphae branching at a sharp angle, which are characteristic of *Aspergillus* spp. (*right arrowhead*) (magnification: 400×)

Discussion

To the best of our knowledge, this study was the largest series of IFT in mechanically ventilated critically ill patients. The main findings of our study are as follows.

First, 80.6% of the patients had proven IFT, whereas the remaining patients (19.4%) had probable IFT. Second, DM was the most frequent predominant underlying condition in our IFT patients (58.1%), followed by chronic lung disease (38.7%). Third, less than 15% of the patients had a hematologic disease. Fourth, none of the patients had neutropenia or had undergone solid organ transplantations. Fifth, the mortality rate was 93.5%. All patients developed acute respiratory failure before diagnosis and were admitted to the ICU with high APACHE II scores (23.1 ± 10.4).

Invasive fungal infection was reported to mainly affect immunocompromised patients, particularly those with hematologic malignancy [17]. However, *Aspergillus* spp. has recently been shown to cause invasive fungal disease in patients with chronic lung disease and critically ill patients with liver cirrhosis [7, 19–24]. This is mainly attributed to the administration of broad spectrum antibiotics, corticosteroids, and immunoparalysis related to sepsis [2, 22, 25–27]. In a cohort study of 156 patients with *Aspergillus* tracheobronchitis, Fernández-Ruiz et al. [15] reported that 6.5% of them had DM, 23.7% received mechanical ventilation because of respiratory failure, most patients were immunocompromised, and the mortality rate was 39.1%. Karnak et al. [13] reviewed 228 patients with endobronchial fungal disease and found that 54% of them were immunocompromised, and 11% had DM; the mortality rate was 52% in patients with endobronchial mucormycosis. In our cohort, DM was the most prevalent underlying condition (58.1%), whereas only four patients (12.9%) had hematologic disease, and none of the patients were neutropenic. Numerous studies have reported that acute respiratory failure and ICU admission are crucial prognostic factors for invasive fungal disease [5, 15, 27–30]. In the current study, we found that patients with IFT who developed respiratory failure exhibited high mortality. He et al. [14] reported that patients with *Aspergillus* tracheobronchitis and the involvement in parenchyma demonstrated higher mortality, suggesting that *Aspergillus* tracheobronchitis is an early stage of invasive pulmonary aspergillosis. By contrast, Patterson and Strek [2] argued that tracheobronchitis is a form of invasive pulmonary aspergillosis and is associated with poor outcomes because of delayed diagnosis. Furthermore, Karnak et al. [13] also found that 7–20% of patients with invasive pulmonary aspergillosis simultaneously manifested fatal tracheobronchial involvement. The overall mortality of invasive fungal infection is approximately 50% [5, 6], and the mortalities of endobronchial fungal disease caused by different fungi range widely from 20 to 80% [11, 13–16]. In our cohort, the overall in-hospital mortality rate was 93.5% even though none of the patients had neutropenia or immunosuppression. Cornillet et al. suggested that among non-neutropenic patients with invasive aspergillosis, the nonspecific symptoms and the difficulty in diagnosis lead to suboptimal management and the late administration of treatment. This delayed administration of treatment results in a higher mortality in non-neutropenic patients than in neutropenic patients (89 vs. 60%) and may explain the high mortality observed in our cohort [24, 31].

Diagnosing IFT is considerably difficult because of the nonspecific clinical manifestations and the lack of a diagnostic tool to distinguish colonization from infection [2, 12, 32, 33]. Radiological findings are usually nonspecific in patients with aspergillosis. The typical halo and air crescent signs on CT images of the lungs are associated with low sensitivity for invasive fungal infection and are rarely observed in non-neutropenic patients [12, 21]. In the current study, the air crescent sign was detected on the CT scan of only one patient. The galactomannan antigen levels in BAL fluid are useful for diagnosing invasive pulmonary aspergillosis [34]. However, in addition to *Aspergillus spp.*, other fungi may cause invasive tracheobronchitis without affecting the galactomannan antigen levels [13]. Invasive aspergillosis is the most frequent invasive fungal infection among hematologic patients (59.2–74.3%), followed by invasive fungal infections caused by Mucorales (7.2–13.9%) [35, 36]. Karnak et al. [13] also found that *Aspergillus* spp. is the most common pathogenic species of endobronchial fungal disease (53%), and Mucorales accounted for only 13.4%. In the current study, *Aspergillus* spp. was the most common pathogenic species (61.3%), followed by Mucorales (25.8%).

Considering the increasing incidence of invasive aspergillosis in critically ill patients and the strict host criteria in the revised definitions for invasive fungal disease from the EORTC/MSG [17], Blot et al. [37] validated a clinical algorithm to diagnose invasive pulmonary aspergillosis in the ICU. They proposed *Aspergillus*-positive lower respiratory tract specimen culture as the entry criterion and that physicians should increasingly consider the possibility of invasive pulmonary aspergillosis [20, 22, 37]. However, the rate of positive fungal culture results for BAL fluid is only 25–77% and can further decrease after antifungal therapy [13, 31, 32]. In our patients, less than 30% had positive cultures for fungi before bronchoscopy, and 20% had negative BAL fluid cultures after bronchoscopy. The incidence of IFT may be underestimated if the diagnosis is based only on positive cultures. Hence, we believe that bronchoscopy should be the main diagnostic approach for IFT.

In 1995, Denning proposed three forms of *Aspergillus* tracheobronchitis, pseudomembranous, obstructive, and ulcerative [18]. Thereafter, Karnak et al. [13] demonstrated that endobronchial fungal disease can be caused by six different fungi. The origins of invasive fungal diseases are difficult to differentiate on the basis of radiographic or bronchoscopic findings (Fig. 1). Direct microscopy of tracheobronchial specimens is essential for observing fungal morphology, enabling a presumptive diagnosis of IFT and earlier administration of antifungal treatment [12]. Transbronchial lung biopsy or bronchial aspiration is relatively risky in patients with angioinvasive fungal infection, particularly in patients with coagulopathy or thrombocytopenia [26, 38]. By contrast, the biopsy of bronchial lesions is less invasive and relatively safe; biopsy exhibits a higher sensitivity than BAL fluid culture alone [14, 16]. In our study, all patients underwent bronchoscopy and BAL cultures and 25 underwent bronchial biopsy. None of the patients developed massive hemoptysis or hypoxemia after the procedure.

The present study had some limitations. First, this study was retrospective. Second, this study included only cases with proven and probable IFT; thus, some of the possible cases may have been overlooked, and the outcomes may have been underestimated.

Conclusion

IFT in mechanically ventilated critically ill patients is a devastating disease irrespective of the host's immune status. DM is the most prevalent underlying disease, followed by chronic lung disease. The mortality rate is very high in IFT patients who develop respiratory failure. In addition to *Aspergillus* spp. (61.3%), Mucorales is another crucial pathogenic species (25.8%). Early diagnosis of IFT is based on bronchoscopy. Bronchoscopy with the biopsy of bronchial lesions should be the preferred diagnostic strategy. Large, prospective studies are urgently required to improve the outcome of IFT in critically ill patients.

Abbreviations
IFT: invasive fungal tracheobronchitis; ICU: intensive care unit; BAL: bronchoalveolar lavage; COPD: chronic obstructive pulmonary disease; APACHE II: Acute Physiology and Chronic Health Evaluation II; CT: computed tomography.

Authors' contributions
CYL and WLL had full access to all of the data in the study and take responsibility for the integrity of the data and the accuracy of the data analysis. CYL was involved in the study design and contributed to the data collection and writing, review, and revision of the manuscript. WLL was involved in the study design and contributed to the data collection and writing, review, and revision of the manuscript. CCC contributed to the data collection and review of the manuscript. HTC contributed to the data collection and review of the manuscript. HCH contributed to data interpretation and commented on the manuscript. KK contributed to data collection and commented on the manuscript. NHC supervised data collection and commented on the manuscript. YJC was involved in the study design, supervised statistical analysis, and data interpretation. CTY contributed to data interpretation and commented on the manuscript. GD contributed to data interpretation and commented on the manuscript. CCH provided substantial support to the study design, data analysis, patient recruitment, and manuscript revision. All authors read and approved the final manuscript.

Author details
[1] Department of General Medicine and Geriatrics, Chang Gung Memorial Hospital at Linkou, Taoyuan, Taiwan. [2] Department of Pulmonary and Critical Care Medicine, Chang Gung Memorial Hospital at Linkou, Taoyuan, Taiwan. [3] College of Medicine, Chang Gung University, Taoyuan, Taiwan. [4] Department of Intensive Care Medicine, Chi Mei Medical Center, Liouying, Tainan, Taiwan. [5] College of Health Sciences, Graduate Institute of Medical Sciences, Chang Jung Christian University, Tainan, Taiwan. [6] College of Medicine, Fu Jen Catholic University, New Taipei, Taiwan. [7] Department of Pulmonary and Critical Care Medicine, Chang Gung Memorial Hospital at Chiayi, Chiayi, Taiwan. [8] Department of Critical Care Medicine, Far Eastern Memorial Hospital, New Taipei City, Taiwan. [9] Department of Critical Care, ATTIKON University Hospital, University of Athens, Medical School, Athens, Greece.

Acknowledgements
We thank all of the investigators and members of the Division of Pulmonary and Critical Care Medicine and the Department of Internal Medicine at Chang Gung Memorial Hospital for their efforts.

Competing interests
The authors declare that they have no competing interests.

References
1. Limper AH, Knox KS, Sarosi GA, et al. An official American Thoracic Society statement: treatment of fungal infections in adult pulmonary and critical care patients. Am J Respir Crit Care Med. 2011;183:96–128. doi:10.1164/rccm.2008-740ST.
2. Patterson KC, Strek ME. Diagnosis and treatment of pulmonary aspergillosis syndromes. Chest. 2014;146:1358–68. doi:10.1378/chest.14-0917.
3. Chamilos G, Marom EM, Lewis RE, et al. Predictors of pulmonary zygomycosis versus invasive pulmonary aspergillosis in patients with cancer. Clin Infect Dis. 2005;41:60–6. doi:10.1086/430710.
4. Segal BH. Aspergillosis. N Engl J Med. 2009;360:1870–84. doi:10.1056/NEJMra0808853.
5. Slavin M, van Hal S, Sorrell TC et al. Invasive infections due to filamentous fungi other than Aspergillus: epidemiology and determinants of mortality. Clin Microbiol Infect. 2015;21: 490 e491–490 e410. doi:10.1016/j.cmi.2014.12.021.
6. Nivoix Y, Velten M, Letscher-Bru V, et al. Factors associated with overall and attributable mortality in invasive aspergillosis. Clin Infect Dis. 2008;47:1176–84. doi:10.1086/592255.
7. Meersseman W, Lagrou K, Maertens J, Van Wijngaerden E. Invasive aspergillosis in the intensive care unit. Clin Infect Dis. 2007;45:205–16. doi:10.1086/518852.
8. Muskett H, Shahin J, Eyres G, et al. Risk factors for invasive fungal disease in critically ill adult patients: a systematic review. Crit Care. 2011;15:R287. doi:10.1186/cc10574.
9. Meersseman W, Vandecasteele SJ, Wilmer A, et al. Invasive aspergillosis in critically ill patients without malignancy. Am J Respir Crit Care Med. 2004;170:621–5. doi:10.1164/rccm.200401-093OC.
10. Ferrell BA, Tolle JJ. Invasive endobronchial mucormycosis. Am J Respir Crit Care Med. 2014;190:e28. doi:10.1164/rccm.201312-2229IM.
11. He H, Ding L, Li F, Zhan Q. Clinical features of invasive bronchial-pulmonary aspergillosis in critically ill patients with chronic obstructive respiratory diseases: a prospective study. Crit Care. 2011;15:R5. doi:10.1186/cc9402.
12. Bassetti M, Righi E, De Pascale G, et al. How to manage aspergillosis in non-neutropenic intensive care unit patients. Crit Care. 2014;18:458. doi:10.1186/s13054-014-0458-4.
13. Karnak D, Avery RK, Gildea TR, et al. Endobronchial fungal disease: an under-recognized entity. Respiration. 2007;74:88–104. doi:10.1159/000094708.
14. He H, Jiang S, Zhang L, et al. Aspergillus tracheobronchitis in critically ill patients with chronic obstructive pulmonary diseases. Mycoses. 2014;57:473–82. doi:10.1111/myc.12185.
15. Fernandez-Ruiz M, Silva JT, San-Juan R, et al. Aspergillus tracheobronchitis report of 8 cases and review of the literature. Medicine. 2012;91:261–73. doi:10.1097/MD.0b013e31826c2ccf.

16. Tasci S, Glasmacher A, Lentini S, et al. Pseudomembranous and obstructive Aspergillus tracheobronchitis—optimal diagnostic strategy and outcome. Mycoses. 2006;49:37–42. doi:10.1111/j.1439-0507.2005.01180.x.

17. De Pauw B, Walsh TJ, Donnelly JP, et al. Revised definitions of invasive fungal disease from the European Organization for Research and Treatment of Cancer/Invasive Fungal Infections Cooperative Group and the National Institute of Allergy and Infectious Diseases Mycoses Study Group (EORTC/MSG) Consensus Group. Clin Infect Dis. 2008;46:1813–21. doi:10.1086/588660.

18. Denning DW. Commentary: unusual manifestations of aspergillosis. Thorax. 1995;50:812–3. doi:10.1136/thx.50.7.812.

19. Leav BA, Fanburg B, Hadley S. Invasive pulmonary aspergillosis associated with high-dose inhaled fluticasone. N Engl J Med. 2000;343:586. doi:10.1056/NEJM200008243430818.

20. Garbino J, Fluckiger U, Elzi L, et al. Survey of aspergillosis in non-neutropenic patients in Swiss teaching hospitals. Clin Microbiol Infect. 2011;17:1366–71. doi:10.1111/j.1469-0691.2010.03402.x.

21. Guinea J, Torres-Narbona M, Gijon P, et al. Pulmonary aspergillosis in patients with chronic obstructive pulmonary disease: incidence, risk factors, and outcome. Clin Microbiol Infect. 2010;16:870–7. doi:10.1111/j.1469-0691.2009.03015.x.

22. Dimopoulos G, Frantzeskaki F, Poulakou G, Armaganidis A. Invasive aspergillosis in the intensive care unit. Ann N Y Acad Sci. 2012;1272:31–9. doi:10.1111/j.1749-6632.2012.06805.x.

23. Delsuc C, Cottereau A, Frealle E, et al. Putative invasive pulmonary aspergillosis in critically ill patients with chronic obstructive pulmonary disease: a matched cohort study. Crit Care. 2015;19:421. doi:10.1186/s13054-015-1140-1.

24. Cornillet A, Camus C, Nimubona S, et al. Comparison of epidemiological, clinical, and biological features of invasive aspergillosis in neutropenic and nonneutropenic patients: a 6-year survey. Clin Infect Dis. 2006;43:577–84. doi:10.1086/505870.

25. Hotchkiss RS, Monneret G, Payen D. Immunosuppression in sepsis: a novel understanding of the disorder and a new therapeutic approach. Lancet Infect Dis. 2013;13:260–8. doi:10.1016/S1473-3099(13)70001-X.

26. Kosmidis C, Denning DW. The clinical spectrum of pulmonary aspergillosis. Thorax. 2015;70:270–7. doi:10.1136/thoraxjnl-2014-206291.

27. Taccone FS, Van den Abeele AM, Bulpa P, et al. Epidemiology of invasive aspergillosis in critically ill patients: clinical presentation, underlying conditions, and outcomes. Crit Care. 2015;19:7. doi:10.1186/s13054-014-0722-7.

28. Kennedy KJ, Daveson K, Slavin MA, et al. Mucormycosis in Australia: contemporary epidemiology and outcomes. Clin Microbiol Infect. 2016;. doi:10.1016/j.cmi.2016.01.005.

29. Spellberg B, Kontoyiannis DP, Fredricks D, et al. Risk factors for mortality in patients with mucormycosis. Med Mycol. 2012;50:611–8. doi:10.3109/13693786.2012.669502.

30. Vandewoude K, Blot S, Benoit D, et al. Invasive aspergillosis in critically ill patients: analysis of risk factors for acquisition and mortality. Acta Clin Belg. 2004;59(5):251–7.

31. Bulpa P, Dive A, Sibille Y. Invasive pulmonary aspergillosis in patients with chronic obstructive pulmonary disease. Eur Respir J. 2007;30:782–800. doi:10.1183/09031936.00062206.

32. Panigrahi MK, Manju R, Kumar SV, Toi PC. Pulmonary mucormycosis presenting as nonresolving pneumonia in a patient with diabetes mellitus. Respir Care. 2014;59:e201–5. doi:10.4187/respcare.03205.

33. Wang XM, Guo LC, Xue SL, Chen YB. Pulmonary mucormycosis: a case report and review of the literature. Oncol Lett. 2016;11:3049–53. doi:10.3892/ol.2016.4370

34. Meersseman W, Lagrou K, Maertens J, et al. Galactomannan in bronchoalveolar lavage fluid: a tool for diagnosing aspergillosis in intensive care unit patients. Am J Respir Crit Care Med. 2008;177:27–34. doi:10.1164/rccm.200704-606OC.

35. Klingspor L, Saaedi B, Ljungman P, Szakos A. Epidemiology and outcomes of patients with invasive mould infections: a retrospective observational study from a single centre (2005–2009). Mycoses. 2015;58:470–7. doi:10.1111/myc.12344.

36. Neofytos D, Horn D, Anaissie E, et al. Epidemiology and outcome of invasive fungal infection in adult hematopoietic stem cell transplant recipients: analysis of Multicenter Prospective Antifungal Therapy (PATH) Alliance registry. Clin Infect Dis. 2009;48:265–73. doi:10.1086/595846.

37. Blot SI, Taccone FS, Van den Abeele AM, et al. A clinical algorithm to diagnose invasive pulmonary aspergillosis in critically ill patients. Am J Respir Crit Care Med. 2012;186:56–64. doi:10.1164/rccm.201111-1978OC.

38. Di Carlo P, Cabibi D, La Rocca AM, et al. Post-bronchoscopy fatal endobronchial hemorrhage in a woman with bronchopulmonary mucormycosis: a case report. J Med Case Rep. 2010;4:398. doi:10.1186/1752-1947-4-398.

6

Hemodynamic effects of short-term hyperoxia after coronary artery bypass grafting

Hendrik J. F. Helmerhorst[1,2,3]*, Rob B. P. de Wilde[1], Dae Hyun Lee[4], Meindert Palmen[5], Jos R. C. Jansen[1], David J. van Westerloo[1] and Evert de Jonge[1]

Abstract

Background: Although oxygen is generally administered in a liberal manner in the perioperative setting, the effects of oxygen administration on dynamic cardiovascular parameters, filling status and cerebral perfusion have not been fully unraveled. Our aim was to study the acute hemodynamic and microcirculatory changes before, during and after arterial hyperoxia in mechanically ventilated patients after coronary artery bypass grafting (CABG) surgery.

Methods: This was a single-center physiological study in a tertiary care ICU in the Netherlands. Twenty-two patients scheduled for ICU admission after elective CABG were enrolled in the study between September 2014 and September 2015.

In the ICU, patients were exposed to a fraction of inspired oxygen (FiO_2) of 90% allowing a 15-min wash-in period. Various hemodynamic parameters were measured using direct pressure signals and continuous arterial waveform analysis at three sequential time points: before, during and after hyperoxia.

Results: During a 15-min exposure to a fraction of inspired oxygen (FiO_2) of 90%, the partial pressure of arterial oxygen (PaO_2) and arterial oxygen saturation (SaO_2) were significantly higher. The systemic resistance increased ($P < 0.0001$), without altering the heart rate. Stroke volume variation and pulse pressure variation decreased slightly. The cardiac output did not significantly decrease ($P = 0.08$). Mean systemic filling pressure and arterial critical closing pressure increased ($P < 0.01$), whereas the percentage of perfused microcirculatory vessels decreased ($P < 0.01$). Other microcirculatory parameters and cerebral blood flow velocity showed only slight changes.

Conclusions: We found that short-term hyperoxia affects hemodynamics in ICU patients after CABG. This was translated in several changes in central circulatory variables, but had only slight effects on cardiac output, cerebral blood flow and the microcirculation.

Keywords: Hyperoxia, Arterial oxygenation, Hemodynamics, Microcirculation, Cerebral blood flow velocity, Intensive care unit, Thoracic surgery

Background

During and after coronary artery bypass grafting (CABG), patients are supported with mechanical ventilation and supplemental oxygen. Despite its lifesaving characteristics and key role in the treatment of vasodilatory shock, oxygen therapy may harbor considerable risks given the relationship between prolonged hyperoxia, lung injury and adverse outcome [1–5]. The effects of supplemental oxygen may be even more pertinent during cardiovascular events considering the direct effects of high arterial oxygen concentrations on the vascular tone [6, 7]. Arterial hyperoxia has the potential to alter hemodynamics and has been associated with adverse outcomes and mortality after cardiac arrest, myocardial infarction, stroke, brain injury and during mechanical ventilation [8–14], yet not during cardiopulmonary bypass [15, 16]. It is well established that high oxygen concentrations

*Correspondence: H.J.F.Helmerhorst@lumc.nl
[1] Department of Intensive Care Medicine, Leiden University Medical Center, Post Box 9600, Leiden 2300 RC, The Netherlands
Full list of author information is available at the end of the article

induce vasoconstriction and increase the resistance of the systemic circulation. However, the effects on vital parameters may be diverse and the venous and arterial aspects of the circulation have not been clearly distinguished in previous studies. Furthermore, the microcirculation may react differently than systemic hemodynamics [17].

Achieving hemodynamic stabilization is an important clinical prerequisite for early extubation and dismissal from the intensive care unit (ICU) after cardiothoracic surgery. Any intervention that influences hemodynamics and blood flow to the bypassed myocardial territories may impact functional recovery and requires optimal fine-tuning to achieve the best outcome. Although oxygen is generally administered in a liberal manner in the perioperative setting, the unraveling of the effects of oxygen administration on dynamic cardiovascular parameters, filling status and cerebral perfusion may provide novel insights in the pathophysiological mechanisms involved in hyperoxic exposure. Our aim was to study the acute hemodynamic and microcirculatory changes during increased oxygen supply in mechanically ventilated ICU patients after CABG surgery.

Methods

Participants

Adult patients with symptomatic coronary artery disease without recent myocardial infarction scheduled for ICU admission after coronary artery bypass surgery were screened for eligibility. Patients with congestive heart failure, severe arrhythmias, intracardiac shunts, extensive peripheral arterial occlusive disease, symptomatic pulmonary disease, aortic aneurysm and/or significant valvular disease were not considered for inclusion. Patients with signs of severe hemodynamic instability (e.g., rapid changes in vascular resistance, use of inotropic agents) during ICU admission were excluded. Study approval was granted by the local medical ethics committee (LUMC P14.046), and all patients signed informed consent. The study was registered with the Netherlands Trial Register, number NTR5064, registration date February 2015.

Measurements

Anesthesia during surgery was maintained with propofol and sufentanil. Ventilation was adjusted to achieve normocapnia. FiO_2 was 0.4, and a positive end-expiratory pressure of 5 cm H_2O was applied. Directly after surgery, patients were admitted to the ICU and received standard postoperative care. Continuous infusion of propofol and sufentanil was maintained for all patients, and no bolus medications (fluids, vasoactive or sedative agents) were administered.

Mean arterial blood pressure (MAP) was measured via a 20-G radial arterial catheter inserted by Seldinger technique. Central venous pressure (CVP) was measured with a central venous catheter inserted in the right internal jugular vein (MultiCath venous catheter, Vigon GmbH & Co, Aachen, Germany). Pressure transducers (PX600F, Edwards Lifesciences) for the arterial and central venous signals were referenced to the intersection of the anterior axillary line and the fifth intercostal space. The airway pressure was measured at the entrance of the endotracheal tube and balanced at zero level against ambient air. Standard electrocardiogram leads were used to monitor heart rate. Body temperature was measured using a rectal temperature probe.

Beat-to-beat values of cardiac output (CO), stroke volume, stroke volume variation (SVV), pulse pressure variation (PPV) and heart rate (HR) were obtained by Modelflow using continuous arterial waveform analysis as previously described [18, 19]. Hemodynamics were also monitored by the LiDCO*plus* monitor (LiDCO Group Plc., London, UK).

Before starting the protocol, the mechanical ventilation in volume-controlled mode was switched to airway pressure release ventilation (APRV), with settings adjusted to achieve the same minute ventilation, which allows for external control of the ventilator (Evita 4, Dräger AG, Lübeck, Germany). A computer program was used to control the ventilator as described previously [20]. During the study interval, all patients were hemodynamically stable and ventilator settings, sedation and vasoactive therapy remained unchanged.

At least three videos of ten sequences (40 frames each) visualizing different sites of the sublingual microcirculation were recorded per patient per time point by the same dedicated researcher using sidestream dark field (SDF) imaging with the MicroScan Video Microscope (MicroVision Medical BV, Amsterdam, The Netherlands). The three best quality videos from representative multiple site imaging were analyzed, and calculated parameters were averaged. Previously suggested key points for optimal image acquisition were considered, and maximal efforts were undertaken to avoid pressure artifacts and eliminate secretions [21]. SDF imaging data were recorded and analyzed using real-time quality feedback on adequate focus, contrast and stability with GlycoCheck (GlycoCheck BV, Maastricht, The Netherlands), as described previously [22]. The GlycoCheck software automatically calculates the perfused boundary region (PBR), which is a previously validated dimension of the permeable part of the endothelial glycocalyx that does allow red blood cell penetration [23, 24]. The red blood cell (RBC) filling percentage is calculated an estimate for microvascular perfusion. Recorded videos were also imported for offline analysis in Automated Vascular Analysis (AVA) software 4.1 (MicroVision Medical BV). The software automatically separates outcome parameters for large (mostly venules) or small (mostly capillaries) vessels using a diameter cut-off value of 20 μm. Total vessel density (TVD), perfused vessel density (PVD), valid vessel density (VVD) and De Backer Score were calculated as measures of microvascular vessel density; the percentage of perfused vessels (%PV) was calculated as the number of vessels continuously perfused divided by the total number of vessels of the same type. The heterogeneity index was defined as the difference between maximal and minimal proportions of perfused vessels evaluated at each visualized area divided by the mean value of the areas [25].

Blood flow velocity (BFV) in the right middle cerebral artery (MCA) was measured at an insonation depth of 50–52 mm by transcranial Doppler (TCD) monitoring using a Pioneer TC 4040. When the optimal TCD signal was achieved, a 2-MHz TCD transducer probe was fixed over the temporal window using an adjustable headset (Marc 500, Spencer Technologies, Nicolet Biomedical).

Experimental procedure

Approximately one hour after ICU admission the experimental procedures were initiated. All measurements were performed with patients in supine position at three sequential time points: pre-intervention, during intervention and post-intervention. Before the intervention (T1), FiO_2 was titrated to a level targeting a partial pressure of arterial oxygen (PaO_2) between 67.5 mmHg (9 kPa) and 82.5 mmHg (11 kPa) and a complete set of hemodynamic measurements was performed. The intervention (T2) commenced by increasing the FiO_2 to 0.9, and after a 15-min wash-in period, all hemodynamic measurements were repeated. Thereafter (T3), the FiO_2 was decreased by targeting baseline PaO_2 levels, and after 15-min wash-out period, the final control measurements were completed. Before, during and after the intervention, arterial blood gas samples were analyzed to determine arterial oxygenation.

Four 12-second inspiratory hold maneuvers were applied using ventilator plateau pressures of 5, 15, 25 and 35 cm H_2O as previously reported [20]. Each successive inspiratory hold was performed when the initial hemodynamic steady state was reestablished. When the plateau pressure increases, CVP increases concomitantly, whereas CO and MAP decrease with a short delay, reaching a steady state at 7–10 s after inflation. From these steady state measurements, a venous return curve was constructed by fitting a linear regression line through four values of CVP and CO. The extrapolated value at zero flow is the mean systemic filling pressure (P_{msf}). Similarly, the ventricular output curve was fitted through the values of MAP and CO, where the regression line crosses the zero flow intercept at the critical closing pressure (P_{cc}) [19].

The resistance of the systemic circulation (R_{sys}) was calculated as the ratio of the pressure difference between MAP and mean CVP, and CO. The resistance at the arterial and venous side of the circulation was also separately calculated as resistance for ventricular output $R_{vo} = (MAP - P_{cc})/CO$ and resistance for venous return $R_{vr} = (P_{msf} - CVP)/CO$ [26].

Statistical analysis

As this was an exploratory physiological intervention study studying multiple hemodynamic parameters, we did not specifically rely on sample size calculation for one single outcome.

The intervention (T2, *hyperoxia*) and post-intervention measurements (T3, *normoxia*) were compared to baseline (T1, *normoxia*) measurements, using a paired *t* tests or Wilcoxon signed-rank test, depending on the underlying distribution.

Multivariate linear mixed models with random effects per patient were used to compare the exposure (T2) with the non-exposure (T1 and T3) measurements, to account for within-subject correlation and were adjusted for age, temperature, the administered dose of propofol and norepinephrine, and the achieved levels of arterial carbon dioxide ($PaCO_2$) and hemoglobin (Hb).

To account for multiple testing, the indicated levels of statistical significance were lowered to 0.01. All statistical analyses were conducted using R version 3.2.1 (R Foundation for Statistical Computing, Vienna, Austria).

Results

Patients were screened for eligibility from September 2014 until September 2015. Four patients were excluded due to severe postoperative hemodynamic or respiratory instability in the ICU. Baseline characteristics of the twenty-two included patients are listed in Table 1. All participating patients were free of surgical complications, fully recovered from anesthesia within 8 h after surgery and were discharged from the ICU on the first postoperative day. During the experimental procedure, all patients received a glucose 2.5% in 0.45% saline solution at 84 ml/h, propofol (range 200–400 mg h^{-1}) and sufentanil (range 5–25 μg h^{-1}). Two patients additionally received norepinephrine (0.02 and 0.04 μg kg^{-1} min^{-1}) at a constant rate in order to keep the blood pressure in a similar range (MAP higher than 65 mmHg) as the other included patients during the experimental procedure. This was accounted for in the multivariate linear mixed model, and excluding these patients did not materially change the magnitude or direction of our univariate findings.

Table 1 Patient characteristics

Characteristics	All patients ($n = 22$)
Descriptive characteristics	
Age (year)	63 (59–66)
Male/female (n)	17/5
BMI (kg/m^2)	26 (25–29)
Body temperature (°C)	37 (36–37)
APACHE IV	40 (33–61)
SAPS II	28 (24–32)
Surgical characteristics	
Perfusion time (min)	105 (91–121)
Clamp time (min)	73 (63–82)
ICU ventilator settings	
P_{insp} (cm H$_2$O)	18 (16–19)
V_T (ml)	585 (484–650)
PEEP (cm H$_2$O)	5 (5–5)
Respiratory rate (breaths min^{-1})	12 (12–14)
ICU medication	
Propofol (mg h^{-1})	250 (200–288)
Sufentanil (mg h^{-1})	10 (6–10)
Norepinephrine (µg kg^{-1} min^{-1})	0 (0–0), range 0–0.04

Data are medians (interquartile range), unless stated otherwise

BMI body mass index, *APACHE* Acute Physiology and Chronic Health Evaluation Score, *SAPS* Simplified Acute Physiology Score, P_{insp} inspiratory pressure, V_T tidal volume, *PEEP* positive end-expiratory pressure

Table 2 Variables of arterial blood gas analyses during different time periods

Variable	T1	T2	T3
	Pre	Hyperoxia	Post
FiO$_2$ (%)	25 (21–30)	90 (90–90)	21 (21–25)
Arterial blood gas analyses[a]			
SaO$_2$ (%)	94.9 (1.9)	99.0 (0.3)***	95.7 (1.8)
PaO$_2$ (mmHg)	83.5 (12.2)	390.2 (93.2)***	87.8 (21.5)
PaCO$_2$ (mmHg)	39.8 (8.1)	36.0 (7.9)**	34.5 (8.7)***
Hb (mmol L^{-1})	7.2 (0.8)	7.4 (0.7)	7.4 (0.8)
Ht (L L^{-1})	0.34 (0.04)	0.35 (0.03)	0.35 (0.04)
Glucose (mmol L^{-1})	7.5 (1.6)	7.4 (1.7)	7.7 (1.8)
Lactate (mmol L^{-1})	1.25 (0.38)	1.20 (0.40)	1.25 (0.34)

Data are means (SD). For FiO$_2$, medians (interquartile range) are provided

FiO$_2$ fraction of inspired oxygen, *SaO$_2$* arterial oxygen saturation, *PaO$_2$* partial pressure of arterial oxygen, *PaCO$_2$* partial pressure of arterial carbon dioxide, *Hb* hemoglobin, *Ht* hematocrit

* $P < 0.01$; ** $P < 0.001$; *** $P < 0.0001$ for paired comparison between indicated outcome and baseline (T1)

[a] Arterial blood gas samples analyzed prior to the start of hemodynamic measurement

Arterial blood gas parameters

Arterial blood gas values at the three different time points are shown in Table 2. PaO$_2$ levels pre- and post-hyperoxia matched well with the targeted levels. Also, pre- and post-hyperoxia arterial oxygen saturation (SaO$_2$) was similar. During hyperoxia PaO$_2$ and SaO$_2$ were significantly higher.

PaCO$_2$ decreased over time, whereas hemoglobin, hematocrit, glucose and lactate levels did not change.

Hemodynamic parameters

Hemodynamic values at the three different time points are shown in Table 3. After starting the intervention with 90% oxygen supply, R_{sys} increased ($P < 0.0001$), without altering the heart rate. SVV and PPV decreased slightly. CO did not significantly decrease ($P = 0.08$).

During the hyperoxia period P_{msf} and the slope of the venous return curve (Slope$_{vrc}$) increased (Fig. 1). P_{cc} increased, whereas the slope of the left ventricular output curve (Slope$_{voc}$) did not change. R_{sys} and R_{vr} increased because of the higher MAP and P_{msf} at constant CO. R_{vo} did not change because MAP and P_{cc} increased similarly.

We did not find any reduction in cerebral blood flow and only slight shifts in microcirculatory scores were noted. The percentage of perfused vessels decreased during hyperoxia ($P = 0.01$). No changes in vascular density were detected for either large or small vessels.

The results were virtually unchanged when multivariate mixed models were used (Table 3).

Discussion

In this single-center physiological intervention study, we found that a 15-min exposure to hyperoxia affects hemodynamics in ICU patients after CABG. This was translated in several changes in central circulatory variables and in the percentage of perfused microcirculatory vessels, but showed no alterations in cardiac output and cerebral blood flow.

The circulation of blood can be described by either the CO or the venous return. As only blood returning to the heart can be pumped out in the systemic circulation, venous return should always equal CO. Major determinants of CO are preload, contractility and afterload. During hyperoxia, left ventricular afterload clearly increased. The absence of a measurable decrease in CO may be explained by a concomitant increase in preload. Indeed, we found higher CVP during hyperoxia. The alternative explanation, i.e., increased contractility, is unlikely as we found no increase in the slope of the cardiac output curve during hyperoxia.

The circulation can also be described by the venous return to the heart, which is driven by P_{msf} − CVP. During hyperoxia P_{msf} increased more than CVP. However, this did not lead to an increase of venous return due to the simultaneous increase in venous resistance.

Table 3 Crude hemodynamic measurements during different time periods and adjusted change in estimate with hyperoxic ventilation

Hemodynamic variables	T1 Pre	T2 Hyperoxia	T3 Post	Hyperoxia vs. normoxia Adjusted change in estimate (95% CI)	P value
Central circulatory variables[a]					
MAP (mmHg)	77 (11)	85 (11)***	78 (11)	6.76 (3.88; 9.63)	<0.0001
CVP (mmHg)	9.1 (1.7)	9.6 (1.7)	9.3 (1.6)	0.35 (0.11; 0.60)	0.01
HR (beats min^{-1})	84 (14)	82 (14)	83 (15)	−0.55 (−3.05; 2.06)	0.68
Calculated variables					
CO Modelflow (L min^{-1})[b]	5.12 (1.04)	4.97 (1.13)	4.98 (1.18)	−0.08 (−0.27; 0.11)	0.41
SVV (%)[b]	13.6 (9.3)	13.2 (6.9)	15.3 (7.4)	−1.76 (−3.38; −0.03)	0.05
PPV (%)[b]	15.6 (10.3)	15.1 (7.6)	16.6 (4.9)	−1.30 (−2.99; 0.49)	0.16
CO LiDCOplus (L min^{-1})[c]	4.80 (1.10)	4.62 (1.10)	4.79 (1.27)	−0.12 (−0.40; 0.08)	0.21
Derived parameters[d]					
R_{sys} (mmHg min L^{-1})	13.4 (4.9)	15.3 (5.9)***	13.6 (5.1)	1.82 (0.96; 2.67)	<0.001
P_{vr} (mmHg)	11.7 (3.3)	13.5 (3.5)*	12.1 (2.8)	1.47 (0.61; 2.37)	<0.01
R_{vr} (mmHg min L^{-1})	2.4 (0.8)	2.8 (1.0)**	2.5 (0.8)	0.39 (0.21; 0.58)	<0.001
$Slope_{vrc}$ (L min^{-1} mmHg^{-1})	−0.46 (0.16)	−0.38 (0.13)**	−0.44 (0.15)	0.07 (0.03; 0.10)	<0.001
P_{msf} (mmHg)	20.8 (3.5)	23.1 (4.0)*	21.4 (2.9)	1.90 (0.95; 2.93)	<0.001
R_{vo} (mmHg min L^{-1})	7.9 (3.2)	7.9 (4.3)	7.7 (1.9)	−0.09 (−1.17; 1.03)	0.87
$Slope_{voc}$ (L min^{-1} mmHg^{-1})	0.13 (0.05)	0.15 (0.11)	0.14 (0.04)	0.01 (−0.03; 0.05)	0.62
P_{cc} (mmHg)	38.8 (9.8)	47.9 (15.1)*	40.9 (8.9)	8.55 (4.13; 12.68)	<0.001
Cerebral blood flow[e]					
BFV_{mca} (cm s^{-1})	34.6 (10.6)	32.3 (10.3)	33.6 (11.5)	−1.42 (−3.80; 1.01)	0.26
Pulsatility index	0.95	0.96	1.0	−0.03 (−0.07; 0.01)	0.17
Resistance index	0.57	0.57	0.58	0 (−0.01; 0.01)	0.66
Microcirculation[f]					
RBC filling (%)	72.3 (4.4)	71.1 (5.0)	72.9 (5.1)	−1.87 (−3.29; −0.34)	0.02
PBR (μm)	2.1 (0.2)	2.2 (0.2)	2.1 (0.2)	0.05 (−0.03; 0.12)	0.21
TVD (mm/mm^2)	12.2 (3.5)	12.7 (3.5)	12.0 (3.4)	0.35 (−0.96; 2.08)	0.66
PVD (mm/mm^2)	12.0 (3.7)	12.1 (2.9)	12.0 (3.1)	−0.03 (−1.50; 1.70)	0.97
VVD (μm/mm^2)	712 (117)	672 (130)	699 (93)	−37.29 (−80.97; 8.01)	0.11
De Backer Score (n/mm)	14.2 (1.2)	15.1 (1.6)	14.4 (1.6)	0.86 (0.23; 1.51)	0.01
PV (%)	99.6 (1.3)	93.2 (8.3)*	97.4 (6.1)	−4.72 (−7.64; −2.00)	<0.01
	100 (IQR 99–100)	98 (IQR 85–100)	100 (IQR 99–100)	–	–
Heterogeneity index (%)	13 [9–14]	22 [21–23]***	21 [15–21]***	–	–

Change in estimate (95% CI) with intervention (hyperoxia) in reference to normoxia periods from linear mixed model adjusted for age, temperature, Hb, PaCO$_2$, norepinephrine dose and propofol dose. P value calculated using t tests with Satterthwaite approximations to degrees of freedom

Data are means (SD). For PV (%), medians (interquartile range) are provided

MAP mean arterial pressure, CVP central venous pressure, HR heart rate, CO cardiac output, SVV stroke volume variation, PPV pulse pressure variation, R_{sys} resistance of the systemic circulation, P_{vr} pressure difference between P_{msf} and P_{cv}, R_{vr} resistance for venous return, $Slope_{vrc}$ slope of venous return curve, P_{msf} mean systemic filling pressure, R_{vo} resistance for ventricular output, $Slope_{voc}$ slope of ventricular output curve, P_{cc} critical closing pressure, BFV_{mca} blood flow velocity in middle cerebral artery, RBC red blood cell, PBR perfused boundary region, TVD total vascular density, PVD perfused vascular density, VVD valid vascular density, PV perfused vessels

* $P < 0.01$; ** $P < 0.001$; *** $P < 0.0001$ for paired comparison between indicated outcome and baseline (T1)

[a] Directly measured from radial artery and central venous catheters

[b] Calculated beat-to-beat by pulse contour analysis from Modelflow and averaged over indicated time period

[c] Calculated by pulse contour analysis from LiDCOplus 15 min after starting the exposure at indicated time period

[d] Secondarily derived from Modelflow calculated variables

[e] Directly measured using transcranial Doppler on middle cerebral artery

[f] Calculated from sublingual sidestream dark field imaging analyses

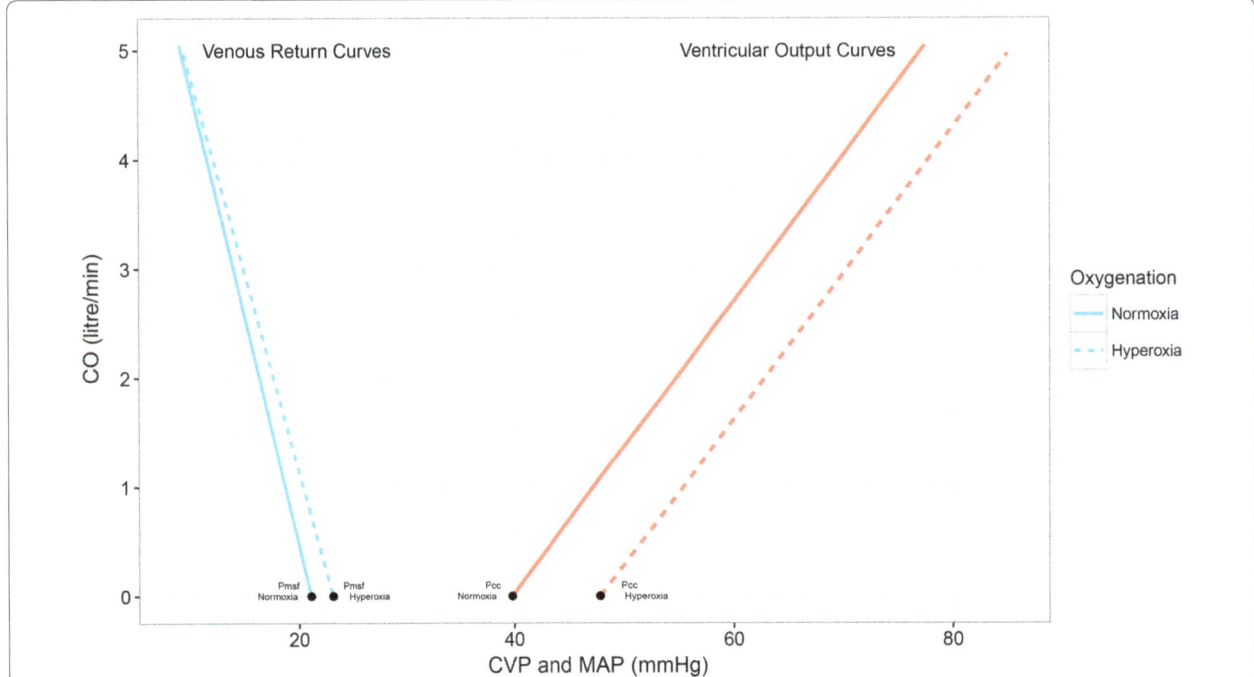

Fig. 1 Venous return and ventricular output curves by arterial oxygenation status. Relationship between cardiac output (CO) and central venous pressure (CVP) in a venous return curve and between CO and mean arterial blood pressure (MAP) in a ventricular output curve for the averaged patient (Table 3). At zero blood flow mean systemic filling pressure (P_{msf}) and critical closing pressure (P_{cc}) are indicated. Venous return curves and ventricular output curves for arterial normoxia and hyperoxia are given

Vasoconstriction may be the key driver of most if not all effects of hyperoxia on hemodynamics. Not only does it increase blood pressure, afterload and venous resistance, it also leads to a shift of blood from unstressed to stressed volume, as indicated by increases in P_{msf} and CVP. We also observed an increase in P_{cc} by hyperoxia. P_{cc} is a theoretical pressure defined by dynamic pressure flow-relations and represents the arterial pressure, below which conceptually no flow will be possible. It is a combined estimate representing all vascular circuits. Theoretically, P_{cc} is the sum of arterial wall tension and the pressure surrounding the blood vessel. P_{cc} may differ importantly between different vessels, and measured P_{cc} is an average value for the complete vasculature. An increase in P_{cc} may be especially relevant in certain disease states such as increased intracranial pressure and abdominal compartment syndrome with high pressures surrounding the vessels. In both situations, P_{cc} is markedly elevated. For example, intracerebral blood flow will decrease to zero when arterial blood pressure is lower than the critical closing pressure of the brain and beyond the limits of cerebral autoregulation. In such states, vasoconstriction, by either vasoactive drugs or hyperoxia, may have either beneficial effects by increasing blood pressure or harmful effects by increasing arterial wall tone and thereby P_{cc}.

In our study, we could not show a reduction in perfusion of the brain by hyperoxia. Similarly, in a previous report perfusion changes at all oxygen levels were relatively small [27, 28]. It should be noted that all these studies were performed in situations with normal intracranial pressure. In situations with intracranial hypertension, such as in traumatic brain injury, we cannot rule out that a further increase of P_{cc} by hyperoxia will decrease the pressure difference between P_a and P_{cc} which can lead to a lower perfusion and possible ischemia of the brain.

Comparing our findings with earlier studies on the effects of hyperoxia on hemodynamics, the cardiac output fall was less than in healthy volunteers [29] and the decrease in the percentage of perfused vessels of the microcirculation was also in a different order of magnitude than previously observed [30]. Recognizing the perfused boundary region of microcirculatory vessels as a surrogate measure for the dimension of the glycocalyx, we could not detect any hyperoxia-induced alterations. Considering the effects on the venous system, more pronounced effects are to be expected in the smaller vessels compared to larger vessels. As a limited number of arterioles are present in the sublingual mucosa, where capillaries and venules are more abundant, only slight changes were anticipated in the analyzed microcirculation when high oxygen levels are applied.

Study differences may be largely explained by the use of anesthesia and mechanical ventilation as both affect hemodynamics and anesthesia also induces a considerable decrease in stressed volume. Furthermore, even in the presence of healthy lungs, both mechanical ventilation and bypass surgery may inflict an inflammatory response which can modify the effects of hyperoxic ventilation on the circulation in comparison with healthy subjects. Remaining differences may be clarified by the short exposure time in our procedures, although no further increase in PaO_2 was to be expected from a longer exposure and therefore a steady state in hemodynamics was assumed.

The increase in stressed volume and P_{msf} by hyperoxia mimics the effects of administering a fluid bolus, yet without increasing the R_{vr}. It is well known that the effects of extra fluids on CO are most pronounced in situations with underfilling of the vasculature explaining the relative conservation of cardiac output during hyperoxia in our postoperative, sedated patients, compared to healthy subjects. The effects of hyperoxia closely resemble the effects of norepinephrine and are in contrast to the effects of propofol [31, 32]. We earlier showed that intravenous administration of norepinephrine resulted in increases in R_{sys}, R_{vr} and P_{msf}. Interestingly, CO increased in some but not all patients after norepinephrine [32]. An increase in CO was associated with a higher SVV. Thus, it appears likely that the effects of a shift from unstressed to stressed volume by vasoconstriction, with an increase in P_{msf}, is mostly found in patients with vasoplegia and/or a decreased circulating volume. Hence, the effects of hyperoxia on CO are determined by the balance between volume recruitment (P_{msf}) and change in R_{vr} and baseline heart function, as observed before [32]. Although our results clearly indicate that hyperoxia increases venous resistance by venous vasoconstriction and that left ventricular output resistance (R_{vo}) did not change, we must realize that our description of the circulation is not complete. We cannot describe the part between the site where P_{cc} exists and the site where P_{msf} exists. Therefore, there is a missing part of the circulatory circuit, i.e., the distal arterial compartment, where control of the peripheral circulation is performed by the pre-capillary sphincters.

A recent study with an alternative cardiac output monitor of the arterial pressure wave showed a poor correlation with the thermodilution obtained CO values while changing norepinephrine doses [33]. However, measurements carried out by our group suggest that the Modelflow technique is capable of measuring the effects induced by vasoconstriction in an accurate manner [32], suggesting that vasoactive agents may not importantly affect the precision of your technology. This was also underlined by the CO values measured by the LiDCO-*plus* monitor that showed a similar pattern compared

to the Modelflow technique in our study. Furthermore, the determination of P_{msf} is not dependent on the accuracy of the Modelflow technique. Indeed, extrapolation of the venous return curve to flow zero is independent of absolute cardiac output. The ability to follow changes in cardiac output within a patient has been clearly demonstrated before [18]. We also showed that beat-to-beat changes in Modelflow cardiac output follows cardiac output by beat-to-beat analysis of electromagnetic probe flow signals [19].

Acknowledging that our findings are to be reproduced in a larger cohort and different clinical settings, the following study aspects should be considered. First, the small sample size and the specific subgroup of patients do not warrant a broad generalizability for the observed effects. Hemodynamics in the current patient group may be affected by the effects of the recent bypass and the potential mediators of ischemia reperfusion and inflammation. Other subsets of critically ill patients may respond differently than patients in our cohort who were in a relatively stable condition before starting study procedures. Two patients received small doses of norepinephrine during the experiment to keep the blood pressure in the same order of magnitude as the other included patients but showed stable hemodynamics and the dose was not changed throughout the experiment. Also, excluding these patients from our analyses showed virtually no change in our results.

There may be a time effect in which recovery and stabilization of patients in the ICU after surgery may influence hemodynamics. However, assuming that the effect of hyperoxia was transient and respecting a 15-min time gap between the two exposures, the carryover effect was minimized and each case served as its own control (self-matched) [34]. Adjusted changes in estimates were based on within-subject comparisons of exposure to hyperoxia with exposure to normoxia. Sampling bias was minimized by continuously measuring central circulatory variables, which provide a highly accurate representation of the parameters over the time periods. Cerebral blood flow, microcirculation and parameters assessed from the inspiratory hold procedures were measured intermittently, yet at representative sampling moments during the sequential time points and averaged as appropriate.

Since we could not detect large differences between the outcomes of univariate and multivariate statistical models accounting for repeated measurements, the observed effects may be predominantly attributed to hyperoxic ventilation, rather than to concomitant changes in other parameters. Other covariates that were considered, such as $PaCO_2$, are therefore not a likely explanation for the hemodynamic changes as seen during the experiment. While a short period of supraphysiological arterial oxygenation may disturb the hemodynamic balance, the effects of long-term exposure to hyperoxia are still uncertain but may be essential regarding patient-centered outcomes.

Conclusions

Short-term hyperoxia after cardiac surgery induces significant alterations in systemic circulation mainly by vasoconstriction of both the venous and arterial circulation and an increase of mean systemic filling pressure. The increase in stressed volume and systemic filling pressure by hyperoxia resembles the effects of administering a fluid bolus or norepinephrine. This may have clinically important consequences in critically ill patients when hemodynamic and microcirculatory changes are vital, but the effects were not clearly linked to relevant changes in cardiac output and cerebral blood flow.

Abbreviations
APACHE: Acute Physiology and Chronic Health Evaluation Score; APRV: airway pressure release ventilation; AVA: Automated Vascular Analysis; BFV: blood flow velocity; CABG: coronary artery bypass grafting; CO: cardiac output; CVP: central venous pressure; ICU: intensive care unit; FiO$_2$: fraction of inspired oxygen; Hb: hemoglobin; Ht: hematocrit; HR: heart rate; MAP: mean arterial pressure; MCA: middle cerebral artery; NTR: Netherlands Trial Register; PaCO$_2$: partial pressure of arterial carbon dioxide; PaO$_2$: partial pressure of arterial oxygen; PBR: perfused boundary region; P_{cc}: critical closing pressure; PEEP: positive end-expiratory pressure; P_{insp}: inspiratory pressure; P_{msf}: mean systemic filling pressure; PPV: pulse pressure variation; PV: perfused vessels; PVD: perfused vessel density; RBC: red blood cell; R_{sys}: resistance of the systemic circulation; R_{vo}: resistance for ventricular output; R_{vr}: resistance for venous return; SaO$_2$: arterial oxygen saturation; SAPS: Simplified Acute Physiology Score; SDF: sidestream dark field; Slope$_{voc}$: slope of ventricular output curve; Slope$_{vrc}$: slope of venous return curve; SVV: stroke volume variation; TCD: transcranial Doppler; TVD: total vessel density; V_T: tidal volume; VVD: valid vessel density.

Authors' contributions
HH had full access to the data in the study and takes responsibility for the integrity of the data and the accuracy of the data analysis. RdW assisted in collection of the data and execution of the measurement procedures. DL assisted with the analysis of the microcirculation. JJ assisted in analysis and interpretation of the inspiratory hold maneuvers. HH, RdW, DL, MP, JJ, DvW and EdJ contributed substantially to the study design, interpretation of the data, and writing and critical revision of the manuscript. All authors read and approved the final manuscript.

Author details
[1] Department of Intensive Care Medicine, Leiden University Medical Center, Post Box 9600, Leiden 2300 RC, The Netherlands. [2] Department of Anesthesiology, Leiden University Medical Center, Leiden, The Netherlands. [3] Laboratory of Experimental Intensive Care and Anesthesiology, Academic Medical Center, Amsterdam, The Netherlands. [4] Department of Nephrology, Einthoven Laboratory for Vascular Medicine, Leiden University Medical Center, Leiden, The Netherlands. [5] Department of Cardiothoracic Surgery, Leiden University Medical Center, Leiden, The Netherlands.

Competing interests
The authors declare that they have no competing interests.

Funding
Hendrik J.F. Helmerhorst is supported by the ESICM Young Investigator Award.

References
1. Rachmale S, Li G, Wilson G, Malinchoc M, Gajic O. Practice of excessive F(IO(2)) and effect on pulmonary outcomes in mechanically ventilated patients with acute lung injury. Respir Care. 2012;57(11):1887–93.
2. Helmerhorst HJ, Schultz MJ, van der Voort PH, de Jonge E, van Westerloo DJ. Bench-to-bedside review: the effects of hyperoxia during critical illness. Crit Care. 2015;19(1):284.
3. Sinclair SE, Altemeier WA, Matute-Bello G, Chi E. Augmented lung injury due to interaction between hyperoxia and mechanical ventilation. Crit Care Med. 2004;32(12):2496–501.
4. Li LF, Liao SK, Ko YS, Lee CH, Quinn DA. Hyperoxia increases ventilator-induced lung injury via mitogen-activated protein kinases: a prospective, controlled animal experiment. Crit Care. 2007;11(1):R25.
5. Helmerhorst HJ, Roos-Blom MJ, van Westerloo DJ, de Jonge E. Association between arterial hyperoxia and outcome in subsets of critical illness: a systematic review, meta-analysis, and meta-regression of cohort studies. Crit Care Med. 2015;43(7):1508–19.
6. Farquhar H, Weatherall M, Wijesinghe M, Perrin K, Ranchord A, Simmonds M, Beasley R. Systematic review of studies of the effect of hyperoxia on coronary blood flow. Am Heart J. 2009;158(3):371–7.
7. Rousseau A, Bak Z, Janerot-Sjoberg B, Sjoberg F. Acute hyperoxaemia-induced effects on regional blood flow, oxygen consumption and central circulation in man. Acta Physiol Scand. 2005;183(3):231–40.
8. Kilgannon JH, Jones AE, Shapiro NI, Angelos MG, Milcarek B, Hunter K, Parrillo JE, Trzeciak S, Emergency Medicine Shock Research Network (EMShockNet) Investigators. Association between arterial hyperoxia following resuscitation from cardiac arrest and in-hospital mortality. JAMA. 2010;303(21):2165–71.
9. Wang CH, Chang WT, Huang CH, Tsai MS, Yu PH, Wang AY, Chen NC, Chen WJ. The effect of hyperoxia on survival following adult cardiac arrest: a systematic review and meta-analysis of observational studies. Resuscitation. 2014;85(9):1142–8.
10. Davis DP, Meade W, Sise MJ, Kennedy F, Simon F, Tominaga G, Steele J, Coimbra R. Both hypoxemia and extreme hyperoxemia may be detrimental in patients with severe traumatic brain injury. J Neurotrauma. 2009;26(12):2217–23.
11. Rincon F, Kang J, Maltenfort M, Vibbert M, Urtecho J, Athar MK, Jallo J, Pineda CC, Tzeng D, McBride W, et al. Association between hyperoxia and mortality after stroke: a multicenter cohort study. Crit Care Med. 2014;42(2):387–96.
12. Rincon F, Kang J, Vibbert M, Urtecho J, Athar MK, Jallo J. Significance of arterial hyperoxia and relationship with case fatality in traumatic brain injury: a multicentre cohort study. J Neurol Neurosurg Psychiatry 2014;85(7):799–805.
13. de Jonge E, Peelen L, Keijzers PJ, Joore H, de Lange D, van der Voort PH, Bosman RJ, de Waal RA, Wesselink R, de Keizer NF. Association between administered oxygen, arterial partial oxygen pressure and mortality in mechanically ventilated intensive care unit patients. Crit Care. 2008;12(6):R156.
14. Stub D, Smith K, Bernard S, Nehme Z, Stephenson M, Bray JE, Cameron P, Barger B, Ellims AH, Taylor AJ, et al. Air versus oxygen in ST-segment-elevation myocardial infarction. Circulation. 2015;131(24):2143–50.
15. McGuinness SP, Parke RL, Drummond K, Willcox T, Bailey M, Kruger C, Baker M, Cowdrey KA, Gilder E, McCarthy L, et al. A multicenter, randomized, controlled phase IIb trial of avoidance of hyperoxemia during cardiopulmonary bypass. Anesthesiology. 2016;125(3):465–73.
16. Smit B, Smulders YM, de Waard MC, Boer C, Vonk AB, Veerhoek D, Kamminga S, de Grooth HJ, Garcia-Vallejo JJ, Musters RJ, et al. Moderate hyperoxic versus near-physiological oxygen targets during and after coronary artery bypass surgery: a randomised controlled trial. Crit Care. 2016;20:55.
17. De Backer D, Ortiz JA, Salgado D. Coupling microcirculation to systemic hemodynamics. Curr Opin Crit Care. 2010;16(3):250–4.
18. Jansen JR, Schreuder JJ, Mulier JP, Smith NT, Settels JJ, Wesseling KH. A comparison of cardiac output derived from the arterial pressure wave against thermodilution in cardiac surgery patients. Br J Anaesth. 2001;87(2):212–22.
19. Maas JJ, Geerts BF, Jansen JR. Evaluation of mean systemic filling pressure from pulse contour cardiac output and central venous pressure. J Clin Monit Comput. 2011;25(3):193–201.

20. Maas JJ, Geerts BF, van den Berg PC, Pinsky MR, Jansen JR. Assessment of venous return curve and mean systemic filling pressure in postoperative cardiac surgery patients. Crit Care Med. 2009;37(3):912–8.

21. De Backer D, Hollenberg S, Boerma C, Goedhart P, Buchele G, Ospina-Tascon G, Dobbe I, Ince C. How to evaluate the microcirculation: report of a round table conference. Crit Care. 2007;11(5):R101.

22. Lee DH, Dane MJ, van den Berg BM, Boels MG, van Teeffelen JW, de Mutsert R, den Heijer M, Rosendaal FR, van der Vlag J, van Zonneveld AJ, et al. Deeper penetration of erythrocytes into the endothelial glyco-calyx is associated with impaired microvascular perfusion. PLoS ONE. 2014;9(5):e96477.

23. Vlahu CA, Lemkes BA, Struijk DG, Koopman MG, Krediet RT, Vink H. Dam-age of the endothelial glycocalyx in dialysis patients. J Am Soc Nephrol. 2012;23(11):1900–8.

24. Donati A, Damiani E, Domizi R, Romano R, Adrario E, Pelaia P, Ince C, Singer M. Alteration of the sublingual microvascular glycocalyx in criti-cally ill patients. Microvasc Res. 2013;90:86–9.

25. De Backer D, Donadello K, Sakr Y, Ospina-Tascon G, Salgado D, Scolletta S, Vincent JL. Microcirculatory alterations in patients with severe sepsis: impact of time of assessment and relationship with outcome. Crit Care Med. 2013;41(3):791–9.

26. Maas JJ, de Wilde RB, Aarts LP, Pinsky MR, Jansen JR. Determination of vascular waterfall phenomenon by bedside measurement of mean systemic filling pressure and critical closing pressure in the intensive care unit. Anesth Analg. 2012;114(4):803–10.

27. Bulte DP, Chiarelli PA, Wise RG, Jezzard P. Cerebral perfusion response to hyperoxia. J Cereb Blood Flow Metab. 2007;27(1):69–75.

28. Borzage MT, Bush AM, Choi S, Nederveen AJ, Vaclavu L, Coates TD, Wood JC. Predictors of cerebral blood flow in patients with and without anemia. J Appl Physiol (1985). 2016;120(8):976–81.

29. Bak Z, Sjoberg F, Rousseau A, Steinvall I, Janerot-Sjoberg B. Human car-diovascular dose-response to supplemental oxygen. Acta Physiol (Oxf). 2007;191(1):15–24.

30. Orbegozo Cortes D, Puflea F, Donadello K, Taccone FS, Gottin L, Creteur J, Vincent JL, De Backer D. Normobaric hyperoxia alters the microcirculation in healthy volunteers. Microvasc Res. 2015;98:23–8.

31. de Wit F, van Vliet AL, de Wilde RB, Jansen JR, Vuyk J, Aarts LP, de Jonge E, Veelo DP, Geerts BF. The effect of propofol on haemodynamics: cardiac output, venous return, mean systemic filling pressure, and vascular resist-ances. Br J Anaesth. 2016;116(6):784–9.

32. Maas JJ, Pinsky MR, de Wilde RB, de Jonge E, Jansen JR. Cardiac output response to norepinephrine in postoperative cardiac surgery patients: interpretation with venous return and cardiac function curves. Crit Care Med. 2013;41(1):143–50.

33. Monnet X, Anguel N, Jozwiak M, Richard C, Teboul JL. Third-generation FloTrac/Vigileo does not reliably track changes in cardiac output induced by norepinephrine in critically ill patients. Br J Anaesth. 2012;108(4):615–22.

34. Maclure M. The case-crossover design: a method for studying transient effects on the risk of acute events. Am J Epidemiol. 1991;133(2):144–53.

7

Sepsis risk factors in infants with congenital diaphragmatic hernia

Michaël Levy[1,2], Nolwenn Le Sache[1,2], Mostafa Mokhtari[2], Guy Fagherazzi[3], Gaelle Cuzon[4], Benjamin Bueno[1], Virginie Fouquet[2,5,6], Alexandra Benachi[2,6,7], Sergio Eleni Dit Trolli[1,2,8] and Pierre Tissieres[1,2,6,8*] (iD)

Abstract

Background: Congenital diaphragmatic hernia (CDH) is a rare congenital anomaly and remains among the most challenging ICU-managed disease. Beside severe pulmonary hypertension, lung hypoplasia and major abdominal surgery, infective complications remain major determinants of outcome. However, the specific incidence of sepsis as well as associated risk factors is unknown.

Methods: This prospective, 4-year observational study took place in the pediatric intensive care and neonatal medicine department of the Paris South University Hospitals (Le Kremlin-Bicêtre, France), CDH national referral center and involved 62 neonates with CDH.

Main results: During their ICU stay, 28 patients (45%) developed 38 sepsis episodes. Ventilator-associated pneumonia (VAP: 23/38; 31.9 VAP per 1000 days of mechanical ventilation) and central line-associated blood stream infections (CLABSI: 5/38; 5.5 per 1000 line days) were the most frequently encountered infections. Multivariate analysis showed that gestational age at birth and intra-thoracic position of liver were significantly associated with the occurrence of sepsis. Infected patients had longer duration of mechanical and noninvasive ventilation (16.2 and 5.8 days, respectively), longer delay to first feeding (1.2 days) and a longer length of stay in ICU (23 days), but there was no difference in mortality.

Conclusions: Healthcare-associated infections, and more specifically VAP, are the main infective threat in children with CDH. Sepsis has a significant impact on the duration of ventilator support and ICU length of stay but does not impact mortality. Low gestational age and intra-thoracic localization of the liver are two independent risk factors associated with sepsis.

Keywords: Congenital diaphragmatic hernia, Sepsis, Healthcare-associated infection, Ventilator-associated pneumonia, Central line-associated bloodstream infection

Background

Congenital diaphragmatic hernia (CDH) is a rare congenital anomaly of the diaphragm with an incidence of approximately 1–3.5 per 10,000 births [1–3]. CDH patients suffer from severe respiratory failure caused by a combination of defect in the muscular or tendinous portion of the diaphragm, pulmonary hypoplasia and persistent pulmonary hypertension (PAH) [4]. Once the diaphragm is surgically repaired, lung morbidities are considered to be the main determinant for postnatal outcome, resulting in an overall survival rate up to 84% [5]. With the improvement in neonatal care of children with CDH, other factors than pulmonary hypoplasia and PAH impact on the prognosis like nutrition and infections [6, 7]. It is recognized that following the initial neonatal period, recurrent respiratory infections are frequently reported complications and are responsible for most hospital readmissions [7]. However, there are very few data concerning sepsis and healthcare-associated infection (HCAI) in this population and its impact on prognosis.

*Correspondence: pierre.tissieres@aphp.fr
[1] Pediatric Intensive Care and Neonatal Medicine, Paris South University Hospitals, Assistance Publique Hôpitaux de Paris, 78, Rue du Général Leclerc, 94270 Le Kremlin-Bicêtre, France
Full list of author information is available at the end of the article

The aim of this study is to evaluate the incidence of sepsis and HCAI in children with CDH and to identify the associated risk factors.

Methods

We performed prospective, monocentric study that included all consecutive neonates born with a CDH who were between December 2009 and January 2015 in the neonatal intensive care unit of the Paris South University Hospitals in Kremlin-Bicêtre, France. Our center is a national referral center for CDH management. During the study period, 161 pregnant mothers with prenatally diagnosed CDH were referred from other centers for antenatal evaluation for potential inclusion in fetal tracheal occlusion (FETO) trials (AB; TOTAL Trial 1 NCT007637737; TOTAL Trial 2 NCT01240057). Subsequently, 82 (51%) with the most severe CDH form were selected and oriented to our center for perinatal management. These patients were identified from a prospectively maintained database of all newborn admitted in our unit with congenital diaphragmatic hernia. In addition, patients with sepsis were identified in a prospective HCAI and sepsis surveillance program and matched with the institutional program of medicalization of information systems (PMIS) database using the 10th version of the International Classification of Diseases. All newborns dying within the first 3 days of life were excluded. Additional data missing in the prospective database were retrospectively collected from patient's files. All patients' data were secondarily anonymized. Children representatives were informed. The study was reviewed by the Ethic Committee of the French Society of Intensive Care (Société de Reanimation de Langue Française), which waived the need of parents signed informed consent (CE SRLF-15-38).

The primary endpoint was to describe the incidence of sepsis in children with CDH. Secondary endpoints were the identification of associated risk factors and to evaluate the impact on patients' outcome. The following data were collected for all patients: sex, gestational age at birth, gestational age at diagnosis, birth weight, hernia type (right or left), best observed/expected lung–head ratio (O/E LHR), intra-thoracic position of liver, the period of diagnosis (ante versus postnatal), fetal tracheal occlusion (FETO) during pregnancy, antenatal steroid therapy, delay between delivery and surgery, presence of surgical abdominal plate or chest tube, use of various catheters (umbilical venous and artery catheters, peripheral arterial catheter, centrally inserted central venous catheter (CVC) and peripherally inserted central catheter (PICC). Sepsis was defined as clinical symptoms of infection and/or sudden clinical deterioration together with significant increase in C-reactive protein (CRP) and/

or procalcitonin (PCT). Healthcare-associated infections were defined according to the 2016 update of Center for Disease Control HCAI criteria (Additional file 1: Table S1) [8, 9].

Data on infection were also collected: type of infection, presence of septic shock, identification of bacteria, temperature, CRP, PCT, leukocyte and neutrophil counts, initial antibiotic therapy and duration, time to first negative PCT. The outcome data were durations of mechanical ventilation, duration of high-frequency oscillatory ventilation (HFOV), duration of noninvasive ventilation, time to first day of feeding, weight at day five, presence of PAH, use of pulmonary vasodilators, use of inotrope treatments, length of hospitalization stay and death.

The results of the descriptive analysis were expressed as numbers and percentages for qualitative variables and as mean and standard deviation for quantitative variables. Two-tailed Fisher's exact test for quantitative variables and Chi-square test for qualitative variable were used. Risk of infection was modeled using a multivariate logistical regression analysis. A stepwise selection was used, and the final model was adjusted on all variables associated with a p value below 0.2.

Results

Patients characteristics

Eighty-two children were hospitalized during the study period. Sixteen children died within the first 3 days of life (38% of right CDH, no sepsis), and two additional patients were excluded because the diagnosis was made after the neonatal period (2.4 and 6 months after birth). The 62 remaining newborns (all inborn) were included in the study. Patients' characteristics are described in Table 1. The mean gestational age at birth was 38.4 ± 2.2 weeks and the mean birth weight was 3072 ± 671 g. Ten patients (16%) were preterm. Most patients had left-sided CDH (90%, $n = 56$) and 38.7% of the patients had an intra-thoracic ascension of liver ($n = 24$). 83.9% of the patients ($n = 52$) were diagnosed during pregnancy, the mean age of CDH diagnosis was 27.6 ± 7.4 weeks and the mean of O/E LHR was 42.1%. Seven patients (11.3%) underwent a FETO procedure during pregnancy and nine (14.5%) had antenatal steroids. The mean length of hospitalization was 21.9 ± 27.8 days.

Description of sepsis episodes

Twenty-eight patients (45%) developed 38 sepsis episodes during the hospitalization period. Four patients developed two different sepsis episodes, one patient developed three and one patient developed five episodes during the hospitalization. Clinical and laboratory findings are presented in Table 2. VAP was the main cause of sepsis and accounted for 60.5% of all cases (23/38) with

Table 1 Patients characteristics

	No sepsis (n = 34)	Sepsis (n = 28)	p value*
Gender (male)	26 (76.5%)	19 (67.9%)	0.57
Gestational age at birth (weeks)	38.8 (2.1)	37.8 (2.2)	0.09
Term of birth			
Preterm (<37 weeks)	4 (11.8%)	6 (21.4%)	0.49
Term (≥37 weeks)	30 (88.2%)	22 (78.6%)	0.79
≥37 and <39 weeks	8	11	
≥39 and <42 weeks	22	11	
Birth weight (g)	3092 (633)	3048 (726)	
Gestational age at diagnosis (weeks)	30.0 (7.5)	25.1 (6.3)	<0.01
Type			
Left	31 (91.2%)	25 (89.3%)	0.80
Right	3 (8.8%)	3 (10.7%)	
Best observed/expected LHR (%)	47.2 ± 12.2	37.8 ± 12.5	0.02
Intra-thoracic liver	7 (21.2%)*1	17 (60%)	<0.01
Antenatal diagnosis	26 (76.5%)	26 (92.8%)	0.08
FETO	3 (8.8%)	4 (14.3%)	0.49
Antenatal steroids	1 (2.9%)	8 (28.6%)	<0.01
Time before surgery (days)	2.26 (1.9)	2.14 (1.0)	0.74
Patch repair	4 (12.5%)*2	13 (46.4%)	<0.01
Chest tube	7 (25.9%)*2	4 (12.5%)*1	0.18
Umbilical venous catheter	29 (85.3%)	26 (92.9%)	0.34
Umbilical arterial catheter	4 (11.8%)	3 (10.7%)	0.89
Arterial catheter	2 (5.8%)	5 (17.9%)	0.13
Central venous catheter	17 (50.0%)	26 (92.9%)	<0.01
Peripherally inserted central venous catheter	9 (26.5%)	10 (35.7%)	0.43

Values are expressed as number (%), or mean ± SD

*X X number of missing data; LHR lung-to-head ratio; FETO fetal tracheal occlusion

* Univariate analysis

an incidence density of 31.9 per 1000 days of mechanic ventilation. VAP was followed by CLABSI (5/38, 5.5 per 1000 line days, 13.2% of the infections) and by urinary tract infections and bacteremia with no source identified. Forty-seven centrally inserted CVC were used in 43 patients including 31 left subclavian vein, 15 internal jugular veins and one femoral vein CVC. CLABSI occurred in 3/47 (6.4%) centrally inserted CVC and in 2/19 (10.5%) PICC. Sepsis occurred after a mean of 22.4 ± 33.1 days of hospitalization. The mean time to develop VAP was 25.5 ± 36.1 days, and CLABSI was 35.6 ± 41.9 days. Most patients (65.8%) had fever, while 15.8% had hypothermia at diagnosis. Mean CRP value was 103.2 ± 73.5 mg/L, and mean PCT value was 10.5 ± 21.2 µg/L. The main bacteria identified were *Escherichia coli* (22%), *Staphylococcus epidermidis* (19.5%), *Staphylococcus aureus* (14.6%) and *Enterobacter cloacae* (9.8%). Vancomycin, piperacillin–tazobactam, cefotaxime, gentamicin and amikacin were the main antibiotics used following unit protocoled antibiotic therapy. Antibiotics were adapted to the bacteria and its resistance profile in all cases. Bacteria were

identified in 89% of all sepsis. The mean time to normal PCT was 6.5 ± 3.4 days, and the mean duration of antibiotic therapy was 8.02 ± 2.41 days.

Risk factors for infection

Using univariate comparison (Table 1), infected patients had a significant lower gestational age at diagnosis, lower observed/expected LHR than non-infected patients (O/E LHR range 12.5–65 vs. 27.1–69, respectively) and more use of antenatal steroids. Intra-thoracic liver, use of surgical plate and CVC were also more frequent in infected patients. The difference between the two groups regarding gender, gestational age at birth, proportion of preterm, birth weight, type of hernia, FETO, delay between delivery and surgery, requirement of a chest tube, umbilical venous and arterial catheters, peripheral arterial catheter and PICCs was not significant. After multivariate logistical regression analysis and a stepwise selection of variables (Table 3), the gestational age at birth (in weeks), the birth weight (in grams), an intra-thoracic position of liver and the presence of a centrally inserted CVC were

57

Table 2 Sepsis characterization

Data	N (%) or mean (SD)
Number of sepsis episodes*	38
Type of sepsis	
Meningitis	1 (2.6%)
Ventilator-associated pneumonia	23 (60.5%)
Same side as hernia	6 (26%)
Opposite side as hernia	11 (48%)
Both lungs	6 (26%)
Urinary tract infection	3 (7.9%)
With urinary catheter	1 (2.6%)
Without urinary catheter	2 (5.3%)
Central line-associated bloodstream infection	5 (13.2%)
Central venous catheter	3 (7.9%)
Peripherally inserted central catheter	2 (5.3%)
Bacteremia with no origin found	3 (7.9%)
Early-onset neonatal sepsis	2 (5.3%)
Surgical site infection	1 (2.6%)
Septic shock	7 (18.4%)
Delay between delivery and sepsis (days)	
All infections	22.4 (33.1)
VAP	25.5 (36.1)

N number, SD standard deviation, VAP ventilator-associated pneumonia

* In 28 patients

Table 3 Multivariate analysis of risk factor for sepsis

	Odds ratio	Wald-type 95% CI	p value
Gestational age at birth (weeks)	0.439	0.224–0.862	0.016
Birth weight (grams)	1.003	1.001–1.006	0.012
Right CDH	0.894	0.783–1.022	0.099
Intra-thoracic liver	8.319	1.439–48.104	0.018
Centrally inserted venous catheter	34.582	2.864–417.635	0.005
Peripherally inserted central catheter	3.836	0.627–23,485	0.145

significantly associated with the occurrence of an infection. With every additional week of gestation at birth, the OR of contracting an infection was 0.439 (95% CI 0.224–0.862). Although most children with sepsis had a centrally inserted CVC (26/28), outlining the severity of those patients, very few developed a CLABSI.

Impact of sepsis on patients' outcome
Infected patients had significantly poorer prognosis than non-infected patients (Table 4). Infected patients had longer duration of mechanical ventilation, longer

Table 4 Impact of sepsis on patients' outcomes

	Sepsis (n = 28)	No sepsis (n = 34)	p value or OR (95% CI)
Duration of mechanical ventilation (days)	20.5 (15.6)	4.3 (4.0)	<0.0001
Duration of HFOV (days)	10.2 (9.9)	1.2 (2.4)	<0.0001
Duration of noninvasive ventilation (days)	6.9 (12.3)	1.1 (2.4)	<0.01
Time to first day of feeding (days)	6.0 (2.3)	4.8 (2.0)	0.049
Weight at day 5 (g)	3246 (769)	3076 (644)	0.37
Duration of hospitalization (days)	34.6 (35.9)	11.6 (11.6)	<0.001
Volemic expansion*	21 (75.0%)	14 (41.1%)	4.2 (1.4–12.8)
Inotrope treatment*	24 (85.7%)	17 (50.0%)	5.9 (1.7–21.0)
NO treatment*	20 (71.4%)	9 (26.4%)	6.9 (2.2–21.2)
PAH*	27 (96.4%)	27 (79.4%)	7.0 (0.8–60.0)
Death*	7 (25.0%)	5 (14.7%)	1.9 (0.6–6.9)

Values are expressed as mean (SD) or * number (percent)

OR odd ratio, HFOV high-frequency oscillatory ventilation, NO nitric oxide, PAH pulmonary arterial hypertension defined as tricuspid regurgitation >3 m/s associated with right ventricle and septal signs of PAH

duration of noninvasive ventilation, longer delay to first feeding and longer duration of hospitalization. Infected patients also requested significantly more inotrope treatment, fluid resuscitation and red blood cells transfusion (data not shown). There was no significant difference in death rate in the two groups.

Discussion
The major finding of this study is that lower gestational age at birth is independently associated with sepsis and HCAI in children with CDH, representing a major risk factor for associated morbidities. Similarly, following neonatal congenital heart surgery, HCAI is known to be associated with prolonged length of stay in ICU as well as increased mortality and costs [10–14].

Although HCAI is representing the vast majority of sepsis (30/38), VAP is clearly emerging as the main cause of infection in this subset of neonatal patients. The prevalence of VAP in this population (31.9 per 1000 ventilator days) is higher than in other neonates admitted in our unit during the same period of time (2009–2014) with a mean of 16.5 per 1000 ventilator days (yearly range 9.1–19.3 per 1000). In most studies, rate of VAP varies between 0.2 and 10.9 per 1000 ventilator days, and a recent meta-analysis found a prevalence ranging from 8.1 to 57.1% [9, 15–17]. Beside local prevention bundles application, the mechanism by which neonates with CDH have higher rates of VAP is not clear. A susceptibility to pulmonary infection could be explained by lung hypoplasia including fewer alveoli, reduced vascular bed and a certain degree of reduced ciliary epithelium. The fact that the most severe cases (with liver up) were more prone to infection is in favor of this hypothesis. Hypoplastic lung immunity might not be as efficient as in normal lungs, explaining why children with CDH have an increased sensitivity to the development of VAP. Some indirect observations are supporting this hypothesis. It was shown that adult patients with pulmonary fibrosis have increased bacterial burden due to poorer lung vascularization [18]. Although altered immunity has not been described in neonates with CDH, recently, it was shown that peak inspiratory pressure impacts sphingomyelin degradation in CDH patients outlining the effects of ventilation on lung cell apoptosis and homeostasis [19]. Furthermore, role of mechanical ventilation in potentializing the innate immune response to bacteria and subsequent development of VAP is now well validated [20]. In neonates with CDH and hypoplastic lung, mechanical ventilation is associated with a high risk of barotrauma potentially aggravating secondary bacterial insults on lung parenchyma.

In our CDH cohort, we observed a microbiological shift in VAP pathogen. It is usually considered that in neonatal VAP, the most prevalent monomicrobial pathogens are *P. aeruginosa*, *K. pneumonia* and *S. aureus*, whereas polymicrobial VAP accounted for 6–58% of the cases [9]. In our series, few polymicrobial infections (3/38 episodes) were observed, and we did not found any infection due to *P. aeruginosa* but a high proportion of other Gram-negative bacteria, including *E. coli* and *E. cloacae*. In our patients, CLABSI is the second cause of sepsis. It is difficult to compare CLABSI incidence rate (5.5 par 1000 line days) to the neonatal literature (ranging between 1.43 and 11 per 1000 line days), considering that most studies include neonates from all terms (including very low birth weights) and that most neonatal units are using preferentially PICC and not centrally inserted CVC as routine practice [21–25]. Nevertheless, neonatal CLABSI incidence rates are mainly caused by *S. epidermidis* and *S. aureus* [26]. In our series, although Gram-negative sepsis burden was high (55.2%), there was no CLABSI caused by enterobacteria.

We found that children with older gestational age at delivery have reduced risk of developing an infection in the course of hospitalization. This result leads to the question of the best timing of delivery of neonates with CDH. The CDH Study Group reported increased survival among prenatally diagnosed CDH infants born at early-term ages (37–38 weeks of gestation), compared with infants born at later term ages (39–41 weeks of gestation) hypothesizing an increasing severity of lung hypoplasia with advancing gestational age [27]. However, the results have been challenged, and other studies

found that neonates with CDH seemed to have inferior neonatal and infant mortality with the increase in the gestational age of birth [28–31]. Although most patients are less than 39 and more than 37 weeks of gestational age, our results clearly outline the impact of lower gestational age at delivery as a major perioperative risk factor for infective complications. The intra-thoracic position of liver is also an independent risk factor for infection in our population. Infants with intra-thoracic liver are already known to have poorer neonatal outcome with greater death before discharge and increased risk of extracorporeal membrane oxygenation (ECMO) [32–35]. The importance of liver positioning is crucial for the outcome of patients, and its link to poorer long-term outcome has been well established [32, 36]. Among the 17 infected patients with liver ascension, 12 developed a VAP adding to the probable hypothesis of a specific lung cause to the development of VAP. Controlateral pneumonia, in the so-called healthy lung, reinforces the barotrauma hypothesis and subsequent pathogenesis of VAP and raised the difficult question of optimal pressure/volume target ventilation [20, 37, 38].

Despite its monocentric design, our cohort is characterized by a highly selected case load. Interestingly, mortality (13/62; 21%) in our cohort is corresponding to those of the CDH Euro consortium (25%) as recently shown, outlining the adequacy of our results with larger European CDH centers [38]. Although one can argue that most infections were HCAI, and presumably preventable, our study suggest that neonates managed for CDH have an increased risk of developing sepsis and more specifically VAP compared to the general neonatal ICU patients. During the same period of time, in our unit, VAP incidence in CDH patients (23/62, 37.4%) was much higher than in the rest of patients ventilated for >12 h (68/715, 9.5%). Furthermore, the high incidence of VAP despite local VAP prevention bundles should raise the possibility that children with the most severe form of CDH have an intrinsic susceptibility to VAP. This has to be confirmed in multicenter cohort.

Conclusion

This study shows that neonates hospitalized for CDH have a high incidence of sepsis, mostly related to the development of VAP. We showed that the gestational age independently affects the risk of sepsis development. However, although the impact of sepsis on hospital morbidities is strong, sepsis has no effect on mortality in neonates with CDH. This study urge confirmation and immunologic investigations aimed at studying susceptibility to infections of infants with CDH and particularly the physiopathologic basis of VAP in hypoplastic neonatal lung.

Abbreviations

CDH: congenital diaphragmatic hernia; CLABSI: central line-associated bloodstream infections; CSF: cerebrospinal fluid; CVC: central venous catheter; FETO: fetal tracheal occlusion; HCAI: healthcare-associated infection; HFOV: high-frequency oscillatory ventilation; NO: nitric oxide; O/E LHR: observed/expected lung–head ratio; PICC: peripherally inserted central catheter; PAH: pulmonary arterial hypertension; VAP: ventilator-associated pneumonia.

Authors' contributions

ML, SEDT, PT were involved in study conception and design; ML, NLE, GC, BB, GF, SEDT, MM, VF, AB PT were involved in acquisition, analysis, or interpretation of data. ML and GF were involved in statistical analysis. All authors contributed to drafting and revision of the work. All authors read and approved the final manuscript.

Author details

[1] Pediatric Intensive Care and Neonatal Medicine, Paris South University Hospitals, Assistance Publique Hôpitaux de Paris, 78, Rue du Général Leclerc, 94270 Le Kremlin-Bicêtre, France. [2] Centre de référence Maladie Rare: Hernie de Coupole Diaphragmatique, 94270 Le Kremlin-Bicêtre, France. [3] INSERM U1018, Center for Research in Epidemiology and Population Health (CESP), Paris South University, 94805 Villejuif, France. [4] Bacteriology-Hygiene Unit, Paris South University Hospitals, Assistance Publique Hôpitaux de Paris, Le Kremlin-Bicêtre, France. [5] Pediatric Surgery, Paris South University Hospitals, Assistance Publique Hôpitaux de Paris, Le Kremlin-Bicêtre, France. [6] School of Medicine, Paris South University, UPS11, Le Kremlin-Bicêtre, France. [7] Obstetrics, Gynecology and Reproductive Medicine, Antoine Béclère Hospital, Assistance Publique Hôpitaux de Paris, Clamart, France. [8] Institute of Integrative Biology of the Cell, CNRS, CEA, Univ. Paris Sud, Paris Saclay University, Gif-sur-Yvette, France.

Acknowledgements

None.

Competing interests

The authors declare that they have no competing interests.

Financial disclosure

The authors have no financial relationship relevant to this article to disclose. No honorarium, grant or other form of payment was given to anyone to produce the manuscript.

References

1. Wright JCE, Budd JLS, Field DJ, et al. Epidemiology and outcome of congenital diaphragmatic hernia: a 9-year experience. Paediatr Perinat Epidemiol. 2011;25:144–9.
2. Torfs CP, Curry CJ, Bateson TF, et al. A population-based study of congenital diaphragmatic hernia. Teratology. 1992;46:555–65.
3. McGivern MR, Best KE, Rankin J, et al. Epidemiology of congenital diaphragmatic hernia in Europe: a register-based study. Arch Dis Child Fetal Neonatal Ed. 2015;100:F137–44.
4. Keijzer R, Puri P. Congenital diaphragmatic hernia. Semin Pediatr Surg. 2010;19:180–5.
5. Tsao K, Lally KP. The Congenital Diaphragmatic Hernia Study Group: a voluntary international registry. Semin Pediatr Surg. 2008;17:90–7.
6. Muratore CS, Utter S, Jaksic T, et al. Nutritional morbidity in survivors of congenital diaphragmatic hernia. J Pediatr Surg. 2001;36:1171–6.
7. Tracy S, Chen C. Multidisciplinary long-term follow-up of congenital diaphragmatic hernia: a growing trend. Semin Fetal Neonatal Med. 2014;19:385–91.
8. 2016 CDC's National Healthcare Safety Network Patient Safety Component Manual. http://www.cdc.gov/nhsn/pdfs/pscmanual/pcsmanual_current.pdf.
9. Cernada M, Brugada M, Golombek S, et al. Ventilator-associated pneumonia in neonatal patients: an update. Neonatology. 2014;105:98–107.
10. Murray MT, Krishnamurthy G, Corda R, et al. Surgical site infections and bloodstream infections in infants after cardiac surgery. J Thorac Cardiovasc Surg. 2014;148:259–65.
11. Levy I, Ovadia B, Erez E, et al. Nosocomial infections after cardiac surgery in infants and children: incidence and risk factors. J Hosp Infect. 2003;53:111–6.
12. Pasquali SK, He X, Jacobs ML, et al. Hospital variation in postoperative infection and outcome after congenital heart surgery. Ann Thorac Surg. 2013;96:657–63.
13. Kansy A, Jacobs JP, Pastuszko A, et al. Major infection after pediatric cardiac surgery: external validation of risk estimation model. Ann Thorac Surg. 2012;94:2091–5.
14. Abou Elella R, Najm HK, Balkhy H, et al. Impact of bloodstream infection on the outcome of children undergoing cardiac surgery. Pediatr Cardiol. 2010;31:483–9.
15. Dudeck MA, Horan TC, Peterson KD, et al. National Healthcare Safety Network report, data summary for 2011, device-associated module. Am J Infect Control. 2013;41:286–300.
16. Kawanishi F, Yoshinaga M, Morita M, et al. Risk factors for ventilator-associated pneumonia in neonatal intensive care unit patients. J Infect Chemother. 2014;20:627–30.
17. Tan B, Zhang F, Zhang X, et al. Risk factors for ventilator-associated pneumonia in the neonatal intensive care unit: a meta-analysis of observational studies. Eur J Pediatr. 2014;173:427–34.
18. Molyneaux PL, Cox MJ, Willis-Owen SAG, et al. The role of bacteria in the pathogenesis and progression of idiopathic pulmonary fibrosis. Am J Respir Crit Care Med. 2014;190:906–13.
19. Snoek KG, Reiss IKM, Tibboel J, et al. Sphingolipids in congenital diaphragmatic hernia; results from an international multicenter study. PLoS ONE. 2016;11:e0155136.
20. Ladoire S, Pauchard L-A, Barbar S-D, et al. Impact of the prone position in an animal model of unilateral bacterial pneumonia undergoing mechanical ventilation. Anesthesiology. 2013;118:1150–9.
21. Erdei C, McAvoy LL, Gupta M, et al. Is zero central line-associated bloodstream infection rate sustainable? A 5-year perspective. Pediatrics. 2015;135:e1485–93.
22. Shepherd EG, Kelly TJ, Vinsel JA, et al. Significant reduction of central-line associated bloodstream infections in a network of diverse neonatal nurseries. J Pediatr. 2015;167:41-6.e1–3. doi:10.1016/j.jpeds.2015.03.046.
23. Shalabi M, Adel M, Yoon E, et al. Risk of infection using peripherally inserted central and umbilical catheters in preterm neonates. Pediatrics. 2015;136:1073–924.
24. de Brito CS, de Brito DVD, Abdallah VOS, et al. Occurrence of bloodstream infection with different types of central vascular catheter in critically neonates. J Infect. 2010;60:128–32.
25. Steiner M, Langgartner M, Cardona F, et al. Significant reduction of catheter-associated blood stream infections in preterm neonates after implementation of a care bundle focusing on simulation training of central line insertion. Pediatr Infect Dis J. 2015;34:1193–6.
26. Hooven TA, Polin RA. Healthcare-associated infections in the hospitalized neonate: a review. Early Hum Dev. 2014;90(Suppl 1):S4–6.
27. Stevens TP, van Wijngaarden E, Ackerman KG, et al. Timing of delivery and survival rates for infants with prenatal diagnoses of congenital diaphragmatic hernia. Pediatrics. 2009;123:494–502.
28. Gorincour G, Bouvenot J, Mourot MG, et al. Prenatal prognosis of congenital diaphragmatic hernia using magnetic resonance imaging measurement of fetal lung volume. Ultrasound Obstet Gynecol. 2005;26:738–44.
29. Jani J, Nicolaides KH, Keller RL, et al. Observed to expected lung area to head circumference ratio in the prediction of survival in fetuses with isolated diaphragmatic hernia. Ultrasound Obstet Gynecol. 2007;30:67–71.
30. Hutcheon JA, Butler B, Lisonkova S, et al. Timing of delivery for pregnancies with congenital diaphragmatic hernia. BJOG Int J Obstet Gynaecol. 2010;117:1658–62.
31. Ali K, Grigoratos D, Cornelius V, et al. Outcome of CDH infants following fetoscopic tracheal occlusion—influence of premature delivery. J Pediatr Surg. 2013;48:1831–6.
32. Lusk LA, Wai KC, Moon-Grady AJ, et al. Fetal ultrasound markers of severity predict resolution of pulmonary hypertension in congenital diaphragmatic hernia. Am J Obstet Gynecol. 2015;213(2):216.e1-8.
33. Lazar DA, Ruano R, Cass DL, et al. Defining "liver-up": does the volume of liver herniation predict outcome for fetuses with isolated left-sided congenital diaphragmatic hernia? J Pediatr Surg. 2012;47:1058–62.
34. Mullassery D, Ba'ath ME, Jesudason EC, et al. Value of liver herniation in prediction of outcome in fetal congenital diaphragmatic hernia:

a systematic review and meta-analysis. Ultrasound Obstet Gynecol. 2010;35:609–14.

35. Jani J, Keller RL, Benachi A, et al. Prenatal prediction of survival in isolated left-sided diaphragmatic hernia. Ultrasound Obstet Gynecol. 2006;27:18–22.

36. Takayasu H, Masumoto K, Jimbo T, et al. Analysis of risk factors of long-term complications in congenital diaphragmatic hernia: a single institution's experience. Asian J Surg. 2017;40(1):1–5.

37. Reiss I, Schaible T, van den Hout L, et al. Standardized postnatal management of infants with congenital diaphragmatic hernia in Europe: the CDH EURO Consortium consensus. Neonatology. 2010;98:354–64.

38. Snoek KG, Capolupo I, van Rosmalen J, et al. Conventional mechanical ventilation versus high-frequency oscillatory ventilation for congenital diaphragmatic hernia: a randomized clinical trial (the VICI-trial). Ann Surg. 2016;263:867–74.

8

Noninvasive ventilation with helium–oxygen mixture in hypercapnic COPD exacerbation

Fekri Abroug[1][*], Lamia Ouanes-Besbes[1], Zeineb Hammouda[1], Saoussen Benabidallah[1], Fahmi Dachraoui[1], Islem Ouanes[1] and Philippe Jolliet[2]

Abstract

When used as a driving gas during NIV in hypercapnic COPD exacerbation, a helium–oxygen (He/O_2) mixture reduces the work of breathing and gas trapping. The potential for He/O_2 to reduce the rate of NIV failure leading to intubation and invasive mechanical ventilation has been evaluated in several RCTs. The goal of this meta-analysis is to assess the effect of NIV driven by He/O_2 compared to air/O_2 on patient-centered outcomes in hypercapnic COPD exacerbation. Relevant RCTs were searched using standard procedures. The main endpoint was the rate of NIV failure. The effect size was computed by a fixed-effect model, and estimated as odds ratio (OR) with 95% confidence interval (CI). Additional endpoints were ICU mortality, NIV-related side effects, and the length and costs of ICU stay. Three RCTs fulfilled the selection criteria and enrolled a total of 772 patients (386 patients received He/O_2 and 386 received air/O_2). Pooled analysis showed no difference in the rate of NIV failure when using He/O_2 mixture compared to air/O_2: 17 vs 19.7%, respectively; OR 0.84, 95% CI 0.58–1.22; $p = 0.36$; I^2 for heterogeneity = 0%, and no publication bias. ICU mortality was also not different: OR 0.8, 95% CI 0.45–1.4; $p = 0.43$; $I^2 = 5\%$. However, He/O_2 was associated with less NIV-related adverse events (OR 0.56, 95% CI 0.4–0.8, $p = 0.001$), and a shorter length of ICU stay (difference in means = −1.07 day, 95% CI −2.14 to −0.004, $p = 0.049$). Total hospital costs entailed by hospital stay and NIV gas were not different: difference in means = −279\$, 95% CI −2052–1493, $p = 0.76$. Compared to air/O_2, He/O_2 does not reduce the rate of NIV failure in hypercapnic COPD exacerbation. It is, however, associated with a lower incidence of NIV-related adverse events and a shortening of ICU length of stay with no increase in hospital costs.

Keywords: COPD, Exacerbation, Acute respiratory failure, Noninvasive ventilation, Helium

Background

Noninvasive ventilation (NIV) has become a standard of care in COPD patients with acute exacerbation requiring ventilatory support [1–4]. Avoiding tracheal intubation drastically reduces the rate of ventilator-associated pneumonia (VAP), antibiotic use, the time spent under mechanical ventilation, ICU length of stay, and associated mortality [5–9]. The sustained mastering of the clinical and technological aspects of NIV (defining optimal indications, selection of ventilators and interface, improvements in patient–ventilator synchrony) has been associated with substantial advances in NIV success rates, allowing a wide range of patients to be managed entirely by this technique, thereby minimizing the risk of complications inherent to conventional invasive ventilation [2, 8, 9]. Despite these advances, it is believed that an additional success margin is possible, leading to further reduction in the number of patients still in need of invasive ventilation. One such area of potential progress is the gas used for ventilation [10–12].

*Correspondence: f.abroug@rns.tn
[1] Intensive Care Unit, CHU Fatouma Bourguiba, Research Laboratory LR12SP15, University of Monastir, 5000 Monastir, Tunisia
Full list of author information is available at the end of the article

Compared to air–oxygen (air/O_2), a mixture of helium and oxygen (He/O_2) has been consistently shown to convey numerous beneficial effects in the setting of increased airway resistance owing to its lower density. Indeed, the lower density of helium enhances the transition from a turbulent to a laminar flow, thereby reducing density-dependent components of airway resistance within bronchi with increased resistance, as is the case in COPD exacerbation [10–16]. These effects translate into a reduction in dynamic hyperinflation and a lower work of breathing [10, 15, 17]. These studies provide sound scientific grounds to anticipate a reduction in NIV failure rate when using He/O_2 instead of air/O_2 in COPD exacerbation requiring ventilatory support [10]. This hypothesis has been tested in randomized controlled trials (RCTs).

The aim of the present systematic review and meta-analysis is to compare the effect of He/O_2 and air/O_2 NIV on patient-centered clinical outcomes.

Methods
Search strategy and study selection
Relevant studies were searched in MEDLINE, EMBASE, and Science Citation Index with the restriction of randomized clinical trial for article type published up to September 20, 2016, with the following MeSH terms: ["non-invasive ventilation" or "Bilevel"] AND [("pulmonary disease, chronic obstructive"[MeSH Terms] OR ("pulmonary"[All Fields] AND "disease"[All Fields] AND "chronic"[All Fields] AND "obstructive"[All Fields]) OR "chronic obstructive pulmonary disease"[All Fields] OR "copd"[All Fields]) AND "exacerbation"[All Fields] AND ["heliox" or "helium–oxygen" or "helium"]. We have also conducted a manual search in journals and contacted authors of trials.

Study selection
We included all randomized controlled clinical trials designed to evaluate the efficacy and safety of NIV using a mixture of helium and oxygen to ventilate COPD patients with acute hypercapnic respiratory failure. Standard treatment (e.g., bronchodilators and antibiotics) had to be comparable in control and intervention arms. Patients included in these studies were adults aged 18 and older with COPD diagnosed on clinical criteria and respiratory function tests.

Data extraction and study characteristics
Two independent evaluators (FA and LOB) selected studies according to the inclusion criteria and extracted the following: type and baseline characteristics of included patients, the criteria for NIV, type and composition of He/O_2 mixture (78/22 or 65/35%), time to the first NIV session and its duration, total duration of He/O_2

administration, minimum NIV duration with a given gas mixture during the first 24 h, composition of the gas administered between NIV sessions (whether helium/O_2 or air/O_2), type of associated medications, and criteria for primary and secondary endpoints. Disagreements were resolved by consensus.

Data were extracted to allow quality assessment of the included studies. The risk of bias tool from the Cochrane Handbook was used [18].

Data synthesis
In this meta-analysis, the primary endpoint was the rate of NIV failure during the index ICU stay. The secondary endpoints included the intubation rate per se as the definition of NIV failure was not uniform; in one study, the failure rate was a composite of necessity of intubation and/or death without intubation during the ICU stay [19]. Additional endpoints were ICU mortality, the length of ICU stay, and the costs of ICU stay. Safety was assessed through the number of serious adverse events related to He/O_2 mixture, and the number of episodes of complication related to NIV. The latter consisted of facial skin necrosis, gastric distension, pneumothorax, and nosocomial pneumonia. NIV failure was not considered an NIV adverse effect since it was counted separately as the primary outcome.

Statistical analysis
For binary outcomes (NIV failure rate, intubation rate, mortality, NIV complications, and adverse effects of He/O_2 mixture), we reported the effect sizes estimates as odds ratios (ORs) with 95% confidence intervals (CIs). For the length of ICU stay, and the difference in costs of the total hospitalization per patient, results were expressed as difference of means and 95% CIs. Only two out of three included studies reported the total costs per patient, which consisted of both the costs of hospital stay and those of the gas used for noninvasive ventilation. The first study was a Swiss one [20], and expressed the expenses in US$, while the second was a multicenter study and reported detailed costs in French patients relying on diagnosis-related group (DRG) tools [19]. In the latter, costs were expressed in euros, and converted to US$ (1€ = 1.1386US$).

Statistical significance was set at $p < 0.05$ for hypothesis testing and $p < 0.1$ for heterogeneity testing. We measured heterogeneity and expressed it as I^2, with suggested thresholds for low ($I^2 = 25–49\%$), moderate ($I^2 = 50–74\%$), and high ($I^2 \geq 75\%$) values. We used a fixed-effect model which assumes that studies included in the meta-analysis should share a common effect size, since patients' characteristics and the evaluated intervention are similar in all studies. To assess publication bias, we visually examined the funnel plot for NIV failure and performed the Egger test of the intercept which uses precision to predict the standardized effect. All statistical tests were two-sided.

The meta-analysis was conducted using the Comprehensive Meta-Analysis (CMA) program version 2 software (Biostat, Englewood, NJ, USA). This meta-analysis was conducted in accordance with the PRISMA guidelines.

Results

Search results and trials characteristics

The literature search initially identified 164 citations. Among these studies, only 15 dealt with the use of He/O_2 for NIV in COPD exacerbation. Of these, three randomized controlled studies evaluating the efficacy of NIV using He/O_2 in acute COPD exacerbation were included in the final analysis [19–21]. The selection process is illustrated by the flowchart in Fig. 1. The included studies enrolled a total of 772 patients. The main clinical characteristics of included studies are depicted in Table 1.

Quality assessment

The three studies were randomized, controlled, non-blinded studies. The risk of bias regarding random sequence generation and allocation concealment was low in the study by Maggiore et al. [21] and unclear in the remaining two. Blinding of patients was possible in the three studies. All studies were open-label regarding physicians' assessment of outcomes, which were either hard outcomes such as ICU mortality, or relied on pre-defined objective criteria such as the main efficacy criteria (tracheal intubation). In the most recent study by Jolliet et al. [19], an adjudication and safety committee determined in a blinded manner whether intubation criteria were met in every case. All included studies had low bias for incomplete data. There was no selective outcome reporting bias in the three studies (Table 2).

The studies included a majority of males (65%) with a mean age of 69 $\pm$ 14 years (Table 1). All studies included COPD patients (mean baseline FEV1 = 808 $\pm$ 110 ml), experiencing severe exacerbation requiring ventilatory support. COPD diagnosis

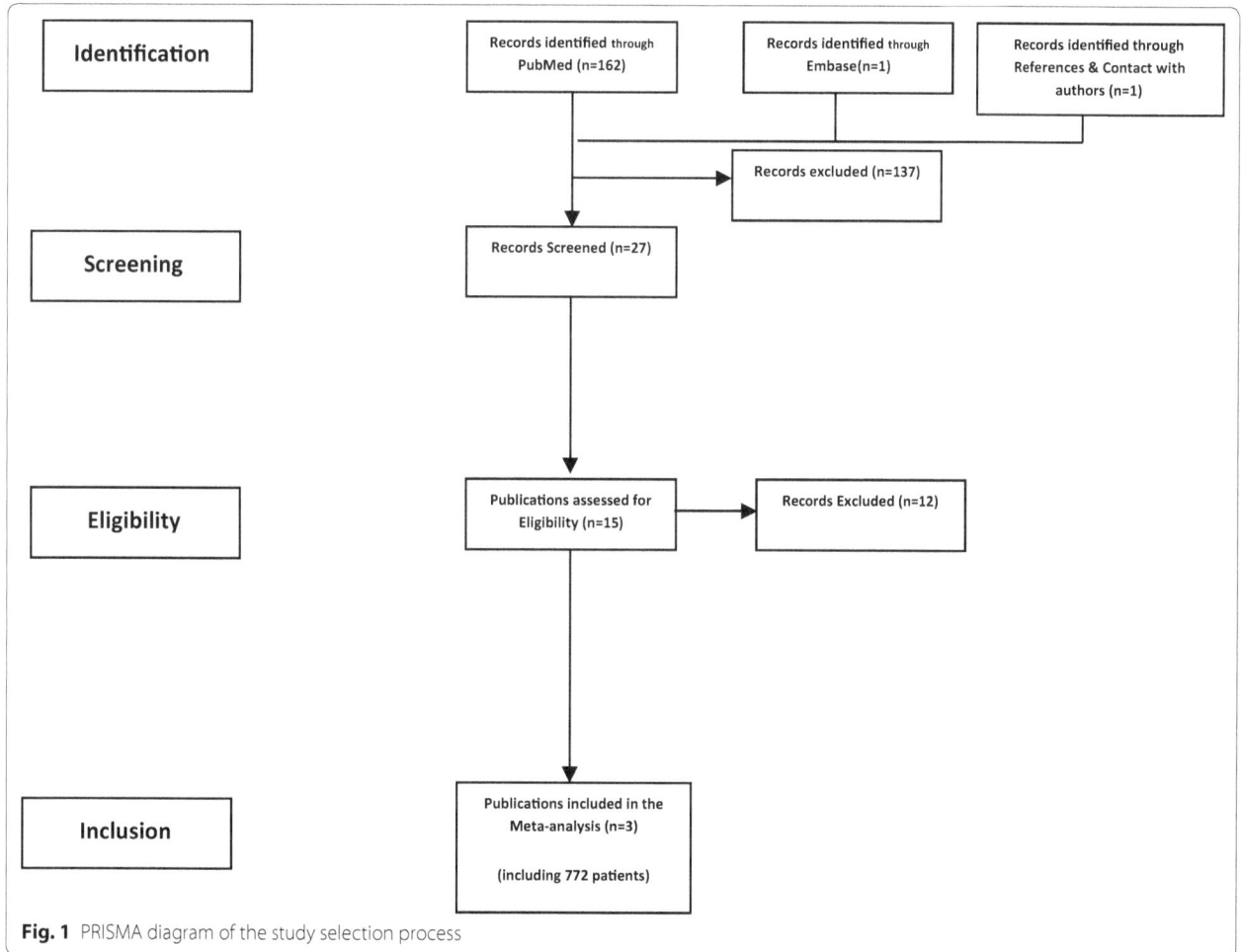

Fig. 1 PRISMA diagram of the study selection process

Table 1 Characteristics of included studies

RCT	Sample size		Baseline FEV1 (ml/s)	He/O$_2$ mixture	Ventilator type/ helium canister connection	Ventilation mode/ daily duration/ study duration	Interface	Between NIV sessions gas	NIV failure criteria	Baseline pH		Baseline PaCO$_2$ (mmHg)		Predicted mortality rate (%)	SMR	Predicted NIV failure rate (%)	Observed NIV failure rate (%)	
	He/O$_2$	Air/O$_2$								He/O$_2$	Air/O$_2$	He/O$_2$	Air/O$_2$				He/O$_2$	Air/O$_2$
Jolliet_2003	59	64	740 ± 362	78/22	ICU ventilator with connection to the air inlet	NIPSV/≥ 6H/until recovery	Oronasal mask	Air/O$_2$	Intubation	7.32 ± 0.06	7.30 ± 0.07	65 ± 13	63 ± 15	24	0.33	45	13.5	20.3
Maggiore_2010	102	102	900 ± 400	65/35	ICU ventilator with connection to the O$_2$ inlet	NIPSV/≥ 6H/until recovery	Facial full mask	Air/O$_2$	Intubation	7.28 ± 0.07	7.28 ± 0.06	73 ± 18	72 ± 15	15	0.67	40	24.5	30.4
Jolliet_2016	225	220	785 ± 360	78/22	ICU ventilator with dedicated connection	NIPSV/≥ 6H/≤ 72H	Oronasal mask	He/O$_2$	Intubation or death in the ICU	7.29 ± 0.05	7.30 ± 0.06	71 ± 16	68 ± 17	15	0.37	25	14.7	14.5

FEV1 forced expiratory volume in 1 s, *NIPSV* noninvasive pressure support ventilation, *SMR* standardized mortality ratio

Table 2 Quality assessment of RCTs

Study	Random sequence generation	Allocation concealment	Blinding of patients	Blinding of outcome assessment	Incomplete outcome data		Selective outcome reporting
					He/O$_2$ group	Air/O$_2$ group	
Jolliet_2003	UNCLEAR Stated only that patients were randomized	UNCLEAR	LOW Patients blind to the type of driving gas	UNCLEAR Hard outcomes such as mortality and pre-defined criteria of intubation	LOW All results are based on all patients (ITT)	LOW All results are based on all patients (ITT)	LOW No apparent selective reporting
Maggiore_2010	LOW Computer-generated randomization	LOW Randomization under-taken at central site with a computer-generated allocation sequence	LOW Patients blind to the type of driving gas	UNCLEAR Hard outcomes such as mortality and pre-defined criteria of intubation	LOW All results are based on all patients (ITT)	LOW All results are based on all patients (ITT)	LOW No apparent selective reporting
Jolliet_2016	UNCLEAR Stated only that eligible patients were rand-omized	UNCLEAR	LOW Patients blind to the type of driving gas	UNCLEAR Hard outcomes such as mortality and pre-defined criteria of intubation	LOW All results are based on all patients (ITT)	LOW All results are based on all patients (ITT)	LOW No apparent selective reporting

was either known or suspected on smoking status, clinical and radiologic signs, and respiratory function tests. The need for ventilatory support and ICU admission relied on the association of respiratory acidosis (pH ≤ 7.35 and $PaCO_2$ ≥ 45 mmHg), and a respiratory rate ≥25 b/min. In the group of patients receiving He/O_2, the gas mixture composition varied among studies with similar formulations: He/O_2 78/22% in both studies conducted by Jolliet et al. [19, 20], and a 65/35% formulation in the study by Maggiore et al. [21]. In the most recent study by Jolliet et al., the group of patients allocated to He/O_2 also received this mixture continuously during the first 72 h after inclusion, both during NIV sessions and during spontaneous breathing between NIV sessions [19]. In the previous studies, patients belonging to both study arms inhaled an air/O_2 mixture between NIV sessions.

Overall, the severity of the index exacerbation was high as inferred from the baseline arterial pH (7.3 as a mean in two studies and 7.28 in one study) and from the predicted mortality derived from mortality prediction systems (SAPS and APACHE scores): between 15 and 24% in the three studies. NIV failure was defined as the need for tracheal intubation in the studies by Jolliet and Maggiore [20, 21], and by the need for intubation or death in the ICU without intubation, in the ECHO [ICU] trial [19].

Data analysis
Comparison of NIV gas mixtures involved 386 patients who received He/O_2 and 386 ventilated with air/O_2.

Primary endpoint
Pooled analysis shows no statistically significant difference in the rate of NIV failure when using He/O_2 mixture

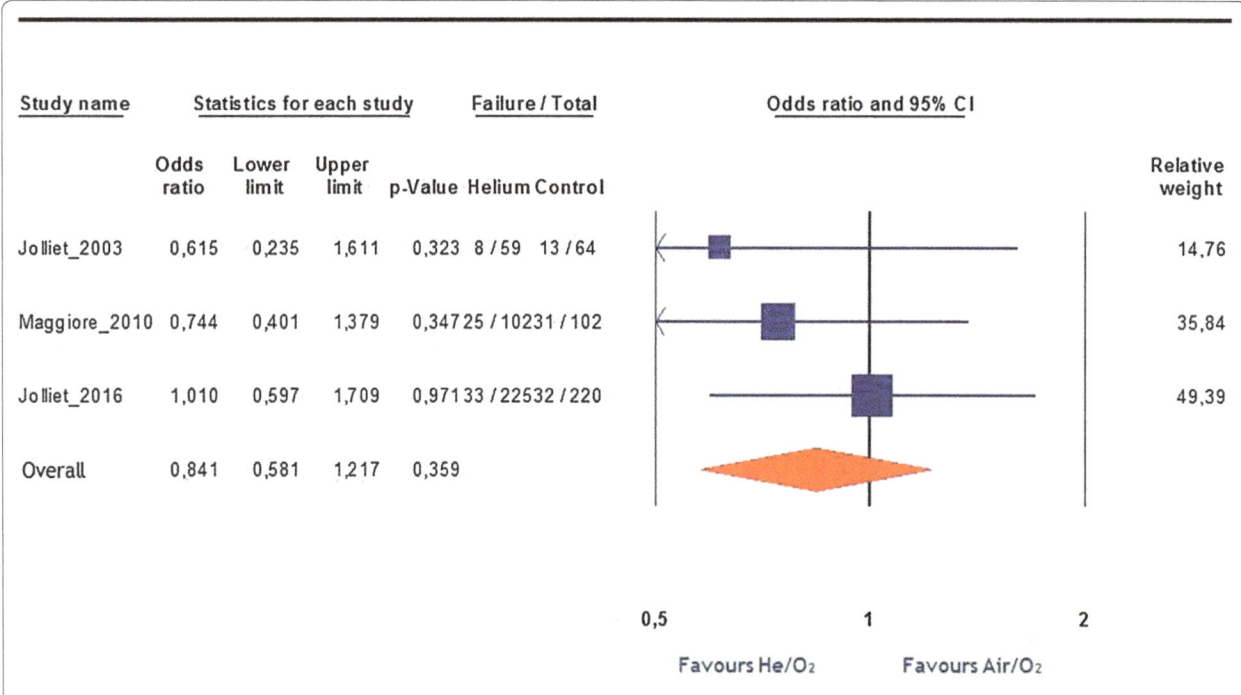

Fig. 2 Effects of He/O_2 mixture on NIV failure rate. Blue squares represent odds ratios (ORs) in individual trials with the size proportional to the weight of the study. The 95% confidence intervals (CIs) for individual trials are denoted by *lines*. The contribution of each included study to the pooled estimate (weight) is plotted as a percentage in the *right column*. The combined overall effect is represented by the *red diamond*

compared to air/O_2: 17 vs. 19.7%, respectively; OR 0.84, 95% CI 0.58 to 1.22; p = 0.36 (Fig. 2). Overall, there was no heterogeneity (I^2 = 0%). There was no obvious publication bias detected by visual inspection of the "funnel plot." The Egger test was also non-significant (regression intercept = −2.18, p = 0.3). We also computed the aggregate effect on the need for tracheal intubation *per se*, as it was a common definition of NIV failure in the included studies. The pooled analysis of the intubation rate reported in the three studies yielded no statistically significant difference between patients ventilated with He/O_2 or air/O_2: OR 0.81, 95% CI 0.56–1.17; p = 0.27; I^2 = 0%.

Secondary endpoints

Overall, the ICU mortality rate was not statistically different between the He/O_2 and air/O_2 groups: OR 0.8, 95% CI 0.45–1.4; p = 0.43; I^2 = 5% (Fig. 3).

No adverse event attributable to He/O_2 was reported. Regarding NIV complications (facial skin necrosis,

gastric distension, pneumothorax, and nosocomial pneumonia), there was a statistically significant difference, with less events in the He/O_2 patients: OR 0.56, 95% CI 0.4–0.8, p = 0.001, I^2: 0.02 (Fig. 4).

The length of ICU stay was also significantly lower in the He/O_2 group compared to the standard treatment group: difference in means = −1.07 day 95% CI −2.14 to −0.004, p = 0.049, I^2: 0% (Fig. 5). Regarding total hospital costs incurred by hospital stay and NIV gas (air or helium), there was no statistical difference between both study groups: difference in mean = −279$ by fixed-effect model, 95% CI −2052 to 1493, p = 0.76, I^2: 85% (Fig. 6).

Discussion

The current meta-analysis of controlled studies evaluating the use of He/O_2 as a driving gas for NIV in hypercapnic COPD exacerbation found no significant reduction in either the failure rate of NIV or ICU mortality. However,

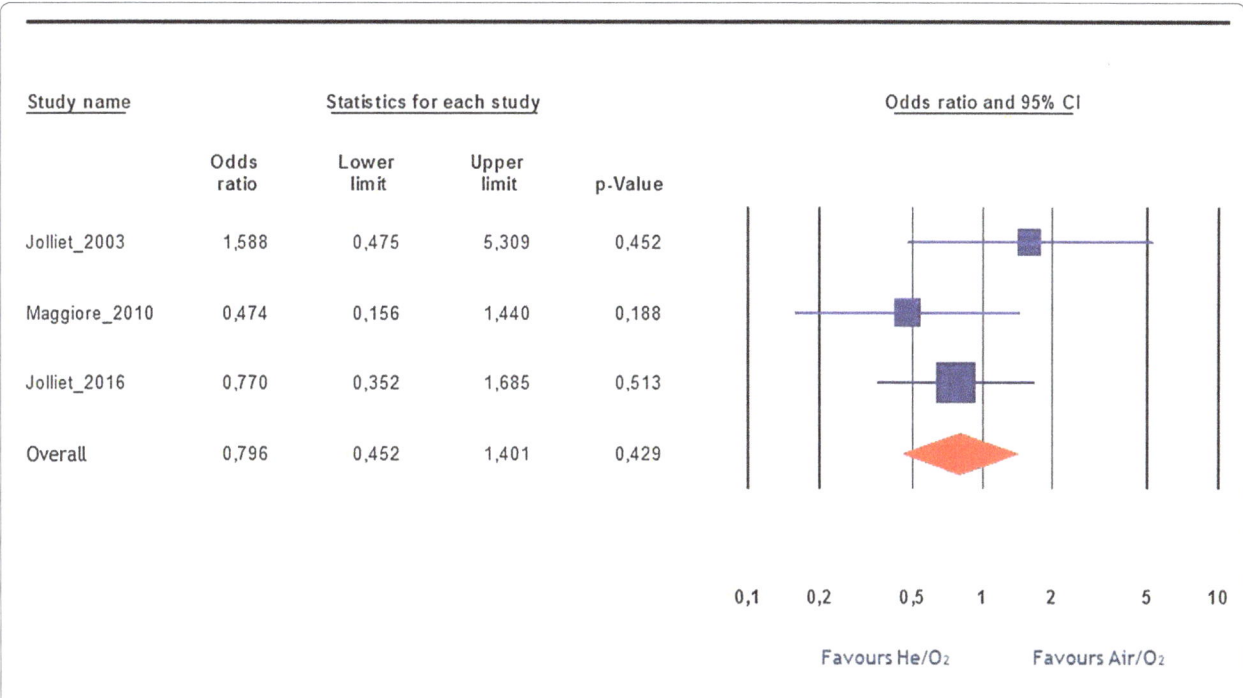

Fig. 3 Effects on ICU mortality rate. *Blue squares* represent odds ratios (ORs) in individual trials, while the *red diamond* represents the combined overall effects. I^2 test for heterogeneity: 5%

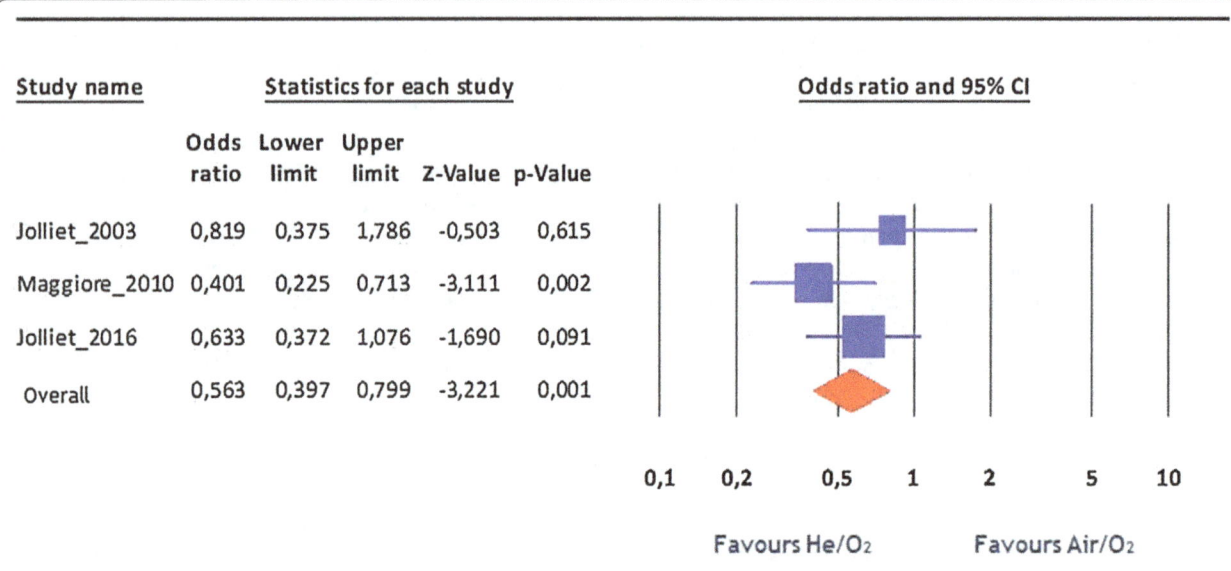

Fig. 4 Rate of NIV complications. *Blue squares* represent odds ratios (ORs) in individual trials, while the *red diamond* represents the combined overall effects. I^2 test for heterogeneity: 0.02%

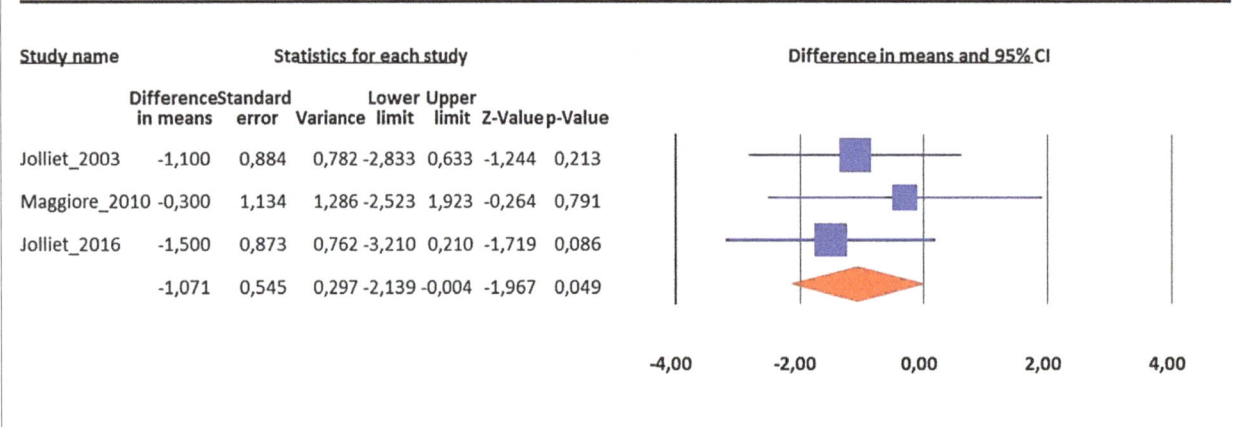

Fig. 5 Length of ICU stay. Estimates are expressed as difference in means and 95% confidence. The length of stay was significantly lower in the He/O_2 with no heterogeneity between included studies (I^2: 0%)

He/O_2 significantly reduced the length of ICU stay and the rate of NIV-associated complications.

Beyond the lack of statistical heterogeneity in the main or secondary outcomes analysis, one of the strengths of the current meta-analysis is the lack of clinical heterogeneity incurred by the three included studies. Indeed, the included patients were fairly similar between the first and last study with similar levels of baseline FEV1, pH

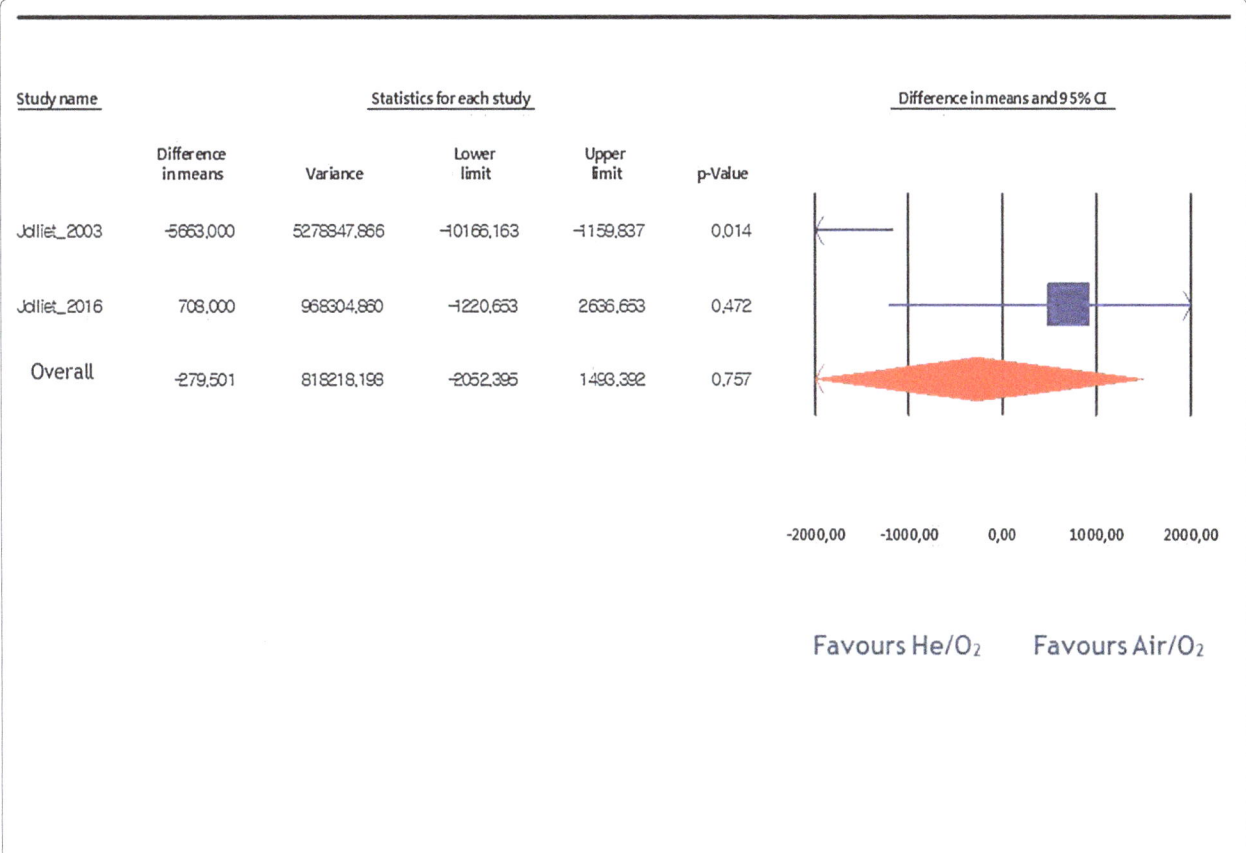

Study name	Statistics for each study					Difference in means and 95% CI
	Difference in means	Variance	Lower limit	Upper limit	p-Value	
Jolliet_2003	-5663,000	5278347,866	-10166,163	-1159,837	0,014	
Jolliet_2016	708,000	968304,860	-1220,653	2636,653	0,472	
Overall	-279,501	818218,198	-2052,395	1493,392	0,757	

Favours He/O₂   Favours Air/O₂

Fig. 6 Difference in total costs (per patient) of the initial admission. There was no statistical difference between study groups with a high heterogeneity level between studies (I²: 85%)

at inclusion, predicted mortality, etc. In addition, given the relevance of the ventilatory strategy to NIV success/failure, the investigators applied a so-called bundle ventilatory strategy that sought to conform both to evolving technological advances (quality of the interface, compatibility of accessories and ventilators with helium gas) and to clinical standards (mode and ventilatory settings, NIV sessions duration, interaction with patients). Moreover, in each new study, researchers tried to tackle shortcomings of the preceding one as reflected by the extension of the duration of administration of the gas to NIV-free periods in the most recent study [19]. The participating research teams also had comparable levels of performance and mastering of NIV techniques, and have clearly benefited from the learning curve of NIV implementation. This observation is reflected by a steady reduction in the failure rate recorded in the three studies, a fact that negatively impacted subsequent study design. Indeed, in the three RCTs that evaluated He/O$_2$ in hypercapnic

COPD exacerbation, there was a recurrent overestimation of the NIV failure rate in the control group, leading to an underestimation of the sample size, thereby yielding substantially underpowered trials. Yet, the first two RCTs conducted by Jolliet et al. [20] and Maggiore et al. [21] exhibited a reduction in the intubation rate with He/O$_2$ which went well beyond what could be considered as a minimal clinically relevant effect. In fact, these studies were conducted at times when the "learning curve" of NIV in real life was still in its ascending limb [22]. For example, Jolliet et al. [20] assumed an intubation rate of 45%, the rate assumed by Maggiore et al. [21] was 40%, while these assumptions were reduced to 25% in the recent and largest study conducted by Jolliet et al. [19]. However, the observed intubation rate recorded in the control group of each study was actually much lower, amounting to 20, 30.4, and 14.5%, respectively [19–21]. Of note, the ECHO^{ICU} study, which was the largest study on the evaluation of He/O$_2$ mixture in hypercapnic COPD exacerbation, recorded the lowest rate of primary outcome event, i.e., NIV failure and tracheal intubation [19].

Should a new study be conducted in order to provide a definitive answer on the benefit of He/O$_2$ in hypercapnic COPD exacerbation? Besides the cumbersome logistics (ventilators with helium option, gas cylinders blended with the needed He/O$_2$ mixture, specific high-concentration facial masks using He/O$_2$), the sample size needed to detect a clinically relevant reduction in the NIV failure rate (considering that recorded with standard air/O$_2$, 14.5%) would amount to no less than 1000 patients in each arm, with a type 1 and type 2 errors of 5 and 10%, respectively [19].

We cannot readily account for the observed reduction in the rate of NIV complications by the use of He/O$_2$ mixture. Explanation cannot be based solely on differences in the properties of the two inhaled mixtures with the change in the flow pattern from turbulent to laminar. Explanation must remain a matter of speculation at the present time.

The initial assumption of systematically substituting air/O$_2$ by He/O$_2$ in patients with hypercapnic COPD exacerbation seems actually unreasonable in the light of the downward trend in the failure rates reported in the most recent studies, particularly those issued from well-trained teams [2, 5]. He/O$_2$ mixture becomes in this context a much less attractive option given its constraining logistics and high costs. However, real-life surveys have recently reported significantly higher failure rates than those observed by Jolliet et al. in the most recent RCT, where the experienced participating teams and a potential study effect probably had a positive impact. The cost–benefit trade-off could under these conditions still lean toward the use of He/O$_2$ [1, 9, 23, 24]. Nonetheless, it seems unrealistic to propose He/O$_2$ invariably to all patients with hypercapnic COPD exacerbation [25]. Because the response to He/O$_2$ mixture breathing has a large variability between subjects according to diseases phenotypes, every effort should be made to identify a subgroup of patients who might derive a real clinical benefit from the physiological effects of He/O$_2$, which may make the small difference that would reduce the intubation rate further [15, 26–29]. Indeed, the use of He/O$_2$ instead of air/O$_2$ in such patients may reduce the work of breathing and dynamic hyperinflation to a sufficient level to avert intubation. Clinical indicators that are well correlated with the work of breathing, and capable of detecting impending respiratory muscle fatigue, are therefore warranted and need to be validated in the clinical setting [30–32]. Identifying such a subgroup of potential responders to He/O$_2$ mixture can also be addressed in a specifically designed RCT, or through an individual patient data meta-analysis.

Conclusion

in the light of the results uncovered by the current meta-analysis, there is insufficient evidence to recommend the systematic use of He/O$_2$ in all patients with hypercapnic COPD exacerbation requiring NIV despite the reduction in the ICU length of stay and NIV side effects, given the constraining logistics. One may argue that with standard air/O$_2$ we have probably reached an acceptable level of NIV failure. However, a subset of patients (which remains to be clearly delineated) at high risk of NIV failure might benefit from the use of He/O$_2$, and efforts should now be directed at identifying such a subgroup.

Abbreviations

CI: Confidence interval; COPD: Chronic obstructive pulmonary disease; DRG: Diagnosis-related group; ICU: Intensive care unit; NIV: Noninvasive ventilation; OR: Odds ratio; PRISMA: Preferred Reporting Items for Systematic Reviews and Meta-Analysis; RCT: Randomized controlled trial; VAP: Ventilator-associated pneumonia.

Authors' contributions

FA, LOB, and PJ conducted the literature searches, selected the studies, and extracted the data. ZH, SB, FD, and IO screened the abstracts, selected the studies meeting the inclusion criteria, and extracted the data. All authors assessed the study quality. FA prepared the initial and subsequent drafts of the manuscript. FA and LOB carried out the statistical analyses. All authors read and approved the final manuscript..

Author details

[1] Intensive Care Unit, CHU Fatouma Bourguiba, Research Laboratory LR12SP15, University of Monastir, 5000 Monastir, Tunisia. [2] Département des Centres Interdisciplinaires et de Logistique Médicale, Lausanne, Switzerland.

Competing interests

FA, LOB, and PJ were investigators in the ECHO^{ICU} trial which was sponsored by Air Liquide Santé International. There is no potential competing interests relevant to this article for the other authors.

References

1. Lindenauer PK, Stefan MS, Shieh MS, Pekow PS, Rothberg MB, Hill NS. Hospital patterns of mechanical ventilation for patients with exacerbations of COPD. Ann Am Thorac Soc. 2015;12(3):402–9.
2. Stefan MS, Nathanson BH, Higgins TL, Steingrub JS, Lagu T, Rothberg MB, et al. Comparative Effectiveness of Noninvasive and Invasive Ventilation in Critically Ill Patients With Acute Exacerbation of Chronic Obstructive Pulmonary Disease. Crit Care Med. 2015;43(7):1386–94.
3. Stefan MS, Shieh MS, Pekow PS, Hill N, Rothberg MB, Lindenauer PK. Trends in mechanical ventilation among patients hospitalized with acute exacerbations of COPD in the United States, 2001 to 2011. Chest. 2015;147(4):959–68.
4. Lindenauer PK, Stefan MS, Shieh MS, Pekow PS, Rothberg MB, Hill NS. Outcomes associated with invasive and noninvasive ventilation among patients hospitalized with exacerbations of chronic obstructive pulmonary disease. JAMA Intern Med. 2014;174(12):1982–93.
5. Ouanes I, Ouanes-Besbes L, Ben Abdallah S, Dachraoui F, Abroug F. Trends in use and impact on outcome of empiric antibiotic therapy and non-invasive ventilation in COPD patients with acute exacerbation. Ann Intensive Care. 2015;5(1):30.
6. Girou E, Brun-Buisson C, Taille S, Lemaire F, Brochard L. Secular trends in nosocomial infections and mortality associated with noninvasive ventilation in patients with exacerbation of COPD and pulmonary edema. JAMA. 2003;290(22):2985–91.
7. Girou E, Schortgen F, Delclaux C, Brun-Buisson C, Blot F, Lefort Y, et al. Association of noninvasive ventilation with nosocomial infections and survival in critically ill patients. JAMA. 2000;284(18):2361–7.

8. Brochard L, Mancebo J, Wysocki M, Lofaso F, Conti G, Rauss A, et al. Noninvasive ventilation for acute exacerbations of chronic obstructive pulmonary disease. N Engl J Med. 1995;333(13):817–22.

9. Chandra D, Stamm JA, Taylor B, Ramos RM, Satterwhite L, Krishnan JA, et al. Outcomes of noninvasive ventilation for acute exacerbations of chronic obstructive pulmonary disease in the United States, 1998-2008. Am J Respir Crit Care Med. 2012;185(2):152–9.

10. Jolliet P, Tassaux D, Thouret JM, Chevrolet JC. Beneficial effects of helium:oxygen versus air:oxygen noninvasive pressure support in patients with decompensated chronic obstructive pulmonary disease. Crit Care Med. 1999;27(11):2422–9.

11. Morice AH. Helium/oxygen and severe COPD. Lancet. 2000;356(9244):1785–6.

12. Laden G. Helium/oxygen and severe COPD. Lancet. 2001;357(9255):559–60.

13. Allan PF, Thomas KV, Ward MR, Harris AD, Naworol GA, Ward JA. Feasibility study of noninvasive ventilation with helium-oxygen gas flow for chronic obstructive pulmonary disease during exercise. Respir Care. 2009;54(9):1175–82.

14. Hussain O, Collins EG, Adiguzel N, Langbein WE, Tobin MJ, Laghi F. Contrasting pressure-support ventilation and helium-oxygen during exercise in severe COPD. Respir Med. 2011;105(3):494–505.

15. Jaber S, Fodil R, Carlucci A, Boussarsar M, Pigeot J, Lemaire F, et al. Noninvasive ventilation with helium-oxygen in acute exacerbations of chronic obstructive pulmonary disease. Am J Respir Crit Care Med. 2000;161(4 Pt 1):1191–200.

16. Pecchiari M, Pelucchi A, D'Angelo E, Foresi A, Milic-Emili J, D'Angelo E. Effect of heliox breathing on dynamic hyperinflation in COPD patients. Chest. 2004;125(6):2075–82.

17. Tassaux D, Gainnier M, Battisti A, Jolliet P. Helium-oxygen decreases inspiratory effort and work of breathing during pressure support in intubated patients with chronic obstructive pulmonary disease. Intensive Care Med. 2005;31(11):1501–7.

18. Higgins JPT AD, Sterne JAC, editors. Chapter 8: Assessing risk of bias in included studies. Cochrane Handbook for Systematic Reviews of Interventions Version 510: Cochrane 2011; 2011.

19. Jolliet P, Ouanes-Besbes L, Abroug F, Ben Khelil J, Besbes M, Garnero A, et al. A Multicenter Randomized Trial Assessing the Efficacy of Helium/Oxygen in Severe Exacerbations of Chronic Obstructive Pulmonary Disease. American journal of respiratory and critical care medicine. 2016.

20. Jolliet P, Tassaux D, Roeseler J, Burdet L, Broccard A, D'Hoore W, et al. Helium-oxygen versus air-oxygen noninvasive pressure support in decompensated chronic obstructive disease: a prospective, multicenter study. Crit Care Med. 2003;31(3):878–84.

21. Maggiore SM, Richard JC, Abroug F, Diehl JL, Antonelli M, Sauder P, et al. A multicenter, randomized trial of noninvasive ventilation with helium-oxygen mixture in exacerbations of chronic obstructive lung disease. Crit Care Med. 2010;38(1):145–51.

22. Schnell D, Timsit JF, Darmon M, Vesin A, Goldgran-Toledano D, Dumenil AS, et al. Noninvasive mechanical ventilation in acute respiratory failure: trends in use and outcomes. Intensive Care Med. 2014;40(4):582–91.

23. Gacouin A, Jouneau S, Letheulle J, Kerjouan M, Bouju P, Fillatre P, et al. Trends in Prevalence and Prognosis in Subjects With Acute Chronic Respiratory Failure Treated With Noninvasive and/or Invasive Ventilation. Respiratory care. 2015;60(2):210–8.

24. Toft-Petersen AP, Torp-Pedersen C, Weinreich UM, Rasmussen BS. Trends in assisted ventilation and outcome for obstructive pulmonary disease exacerbations. A nationwide study. PLoS one. 2017;12(2):e0171713.

25. Carr J, Jung B, Chanques G. Jaber S. Helium as a therapeutic gas: An old idea needing some new thought. European Respiratory Monograph; 2012. p. 124–32.

26. Mutlu GM, Budinger GRS. Not much turbulence: addition of heliox to noninvasive ventilation fails to improve outcomes in patients with exacerbations of chronic obstructive pulmonary disease. Crit Care Med. 2010;38(1):319–20.

27. Burgel PR, Paillasseur JL, Peene B, Dusser D, Roche N, Coolen J, et al. Two distinct chronic obstructive pulmonary disease (COPD) phenotypes are associated with high risk of mortality. PLoS ONE. 2012;7(12):e51048.

28. Adler D, Pepin JL, Dupuis-Lozeron E, Espa-Cervena K, Merlet-Violet R, Muller H, et al. Comorbidities and Subgroups of Patients Surviving Severe Acute Hypercapnic Respiratory Failure in the ICU. American journal of respiratory and critical care medicine. 2016.

29. Turner AM, Tamasi L, Schleich F, Hoxha M, Horvath I, Louis R, et al. Clinically relevant subgroups in COPD and asthma. European respiratory review: an official journal of the European Respiratory Society. 2015;24(136):283–98.

30. Roche N, Chavaillon JM, Maurer C, Zureik M, Piquet J. A clinical in-hospital prognostic score for acute exacerbations of COPD. Respir Res. 2014;15:99.

31. Quintana JM, Esteban C, Unzurrunzaga A, Garcia-Gutierrez S, Gonzalez N, Barrio I, et al. Predictive score for mortality in patients with COPD exacerbations attending hospital emergency departments. BMC Med. 2014;12:66.

32. Contou D, Fragnoli C, Córdoba-Izquierdo A, Boissier F, Brun-Buisson C, Thille AW. Noninvasive ventilation for acute hypercapnic respiratory failure: intubation rate in an experienced unit. Respiratory care. 2013;58(12):2045–52.

9

Nebulized antibiotics in mechanically ventilated patients: a challenge for translational research from technology to clinical care

Stephan Ehrmann[1,2]* ⓘ, Jean Chastre[3], Patrice Diot[2,4] and Qin Lu[5]

Abstract

Nebulized antibiotic therapy directly targets airways and lung parenchyma resulting in high local concentrations and potentially lower systemic toxicities. Experimental and clinical studies have provided evidence for elevated lung concentrations and rapid bacterial killing following the administration of nebulized antibiotics during mechanical ventilation. Delivery of high concentrations of antibiotics to infected lung regions is the key to achieving efficient nebulized antibiotic therapy. However, current non-standardized clinical practice, the difficulties with implementing optimal nebulization techniques and the lack of robust clinical data have limited its widespread adoption. The present review summarizes the techniques and clinical constraints for optimal delivery of nebulized antibiotics to lung parenchyma during invasive mechanical ventilation. Pulmonary pharmacokinetics and pharmacodynamics of nebulized antibiotic therapy to treat ventilator-associated pneumonia are discussed and put into perspective. Experimental and clinical pharmacokinetics and pharmacodynamics support the use of nebulized antibiotics. However, its clinical benefits compared to intravenous therapy remain to be proved. Future investigations should focus on continuous improvement of nebulization practices and techniques. Before expanding its clinical use, careful design of large phase III randomized trials implementing adequate therapeutic strategies in targeted populations is required to demonstrate the clinical effectiveness of nebulized antibiotics in terms of patient outcomes and reduction in the emergence of antibiotic resistance.

Keywords: Nebulizers and vaporizers (MeSH), Pneumonia, ventilator-associated (MeSH), Colistin (MeSH), Amikacin (MeSH)

Background

Effective antimicrobial therapy requires adequate drug concentrations at the site of the infection. This is often not possible when using intravenous therapy among intensive care unit (ICU) patients who require mechanical ventilation due to altered pharmacokinetics and poor lung tissue penetration of many antimicrobial agents [1, 2]. Outcome is often suboptimal, with clinical response rates of lower than 60%, even for antibiotic-susceptible bacterial pneumonia [3]. The situation is particularly challenging when bacteria with a minimum inhibitory concentration (MIC) close to the resistance breakpoint are involved [4]. Raising the systemic antibiotic dose leads to increased toxicity. Nebulized antibiotic therapy directly targets airways and lung parenchyma, thereby resulting in increased local concentrations and hence potentially improving efficacy and minimizing toxicities [5, 6]. For patients suffering from cystic fibrosis, for whom maintaining intravenous access can be challenging and who frequently develop lung infections with bacteria exhibiting reduced antibiotic sensitivity, these theoretical advantages have led to large-scale clinical implementation of nebulized antibiotic therapy and improved patient-centered outcomes [7, 8]. In the setting of critically ill patients undergoing mechanical ventilation, despite similar theoretical advantages to treat ventilator-associated pneumonia (VAP), practical issues regarding

*Correspondence: stephanehrmann@gmail.com
[1] Médecine Intensive Réanimation, Réseau CRICS-TRIGGERSEP, Centre Hospitalier Régional et Universitaire de Tours, Tours, France
Full list of author information is available at the end of the article

the use of nebulized drugs and an overall lack of robust clinical data have limited their widespread adoption.

The present review summarizes current practical constraints for optimal delivery of nebulized antibiotics to the lung parenchyma during invasive mechanical ventilation, and the resulting pharmacokinetics and pharmacodynamics. Current clinical practice is put into perspective with evidence that has become available from recent clinical studies so as to provide a better understanding of the relevance of future phase III trials.

Practical constraints to optimizing nebulized antibiotic delivery during mechanical ventilation

Delivery of high concentrations of antibiotics to infected lung regions is the key to achieving efficient nebulized antibiotic therapy. The antibiotic dose placed in the nebulizer should take into account the significant extrapulmonary drug deposition (i.e., the residual antibiotic volume remaining in the nebulizer chamber, ventilator circuit and endotracheal tube deposition, and exhaled particles). Poor implementation may result in extrapulmonary deposition as high as 97% [9]. Key practical factors need to be taken into account to optimize delivery.

Particle size

The optimal mass median aerodynamic diameter that allows for distal lung deposition ranges from 0.5 to 3 µm [10]. Particles larger than 5 µm are subject to pronounced deposition in the ventilator circuit and the large airways.

Nebulizer

Table 1 displays advantages and drawbacks of available nebulizers. Jet nebulizers appear to be less efficient than ultrasonic and vibrating mesh nebulizers for antibiotic delivery [11, 12]. The large residual volume of medication

remaining in the chamber at the end of nebulization, as well as high-speed turbulent flow due to the gas driving the nebulizer, underlies these results. Vibrating mesh nebulizers appear to be advantageous compared to ultrasonic devices due to a smaller residual volume and because the temperature of the medication does not increase significantly during nebulization [13].

Drug concentration

Medication dilution and the nebulizer fill volume influence particle size and drug delivery. For a given dose, a larger fill volume with a diluted solution can overcome the residual volume issues mentioned above [14]. Nevertheless, dilution increases the duration of the nebulization, and as a result, issues with antibiotic stability may arise. For example, solubilized colistimethate sodium (CMS) is not stable and its antimicrobial efficacy decreases over time [15]. Conversely, a highly concentrated or viscous solution increases the particle size, potentially decreasing lung deposition [16]; it may also induce obstruction or damage when used with a vibrating mesh nebulizer.

Nebulizer position

A nebulizer operating continuously during both insufflation and expiration should be placed in the inspiratory limb, 15–40 cm upstream of the Y-piece [11, 17]. The optimal distance from the Y-piece depends on bias flow and the circuit section. Indeed, the bias flow flushes aerosol into the expiratory limb during expiration, inducing aerosol loss (Fig. 1) [11, 18]. Breath-actuated nebulization, which occurs only during insufflation, offers theoretical advantages in light of the reduced expiratory loss. A nebulizer placement closer to the Y-piece may hence be an option [18]. Moreover, breath-actuated jet nebulizers

Table 1 Advantages and disadvantages of three types of nebulizers

	Jet nebulizer	Ultrasonic nebulizer	Vibrating mesh nebulizer
Mechanism of aerosol generation	Compressed gas and Venturi effect	High-frequency drug solution agitation by a piezoelectric crystal	High-frequency mesh vibrations pumping the drug solution trough tapered holes
Residual volume	Large	Medium	Small
Medication restriction	None	Degradation of heat-sensitive drugs	Highly concentrated or viscous solutions may cause damage to the nebulizer
Ergonomics	Not portable, need of compressed gas Loud Disposable Potential interference with the ventilator	Bulky Silent Need for decontamination No interference with the ventilator	Portable, small size Silent Disposable No interference with the ventilator

The particle sizes generated depend on each individual nebulizer model rather than the nebulizer type, and they are substantially impacted by the measurement conditions (e.g., temperature and humidity). For example, some specific jet nebulizers may deliver large particles (>5 µm for proximal targeting), whereas others deliver nanoparticles. All nebulizers available for clinical use produce sufficient droplets in the 1–5 µm size range of for pulmonary delivery during mechanical ventilation

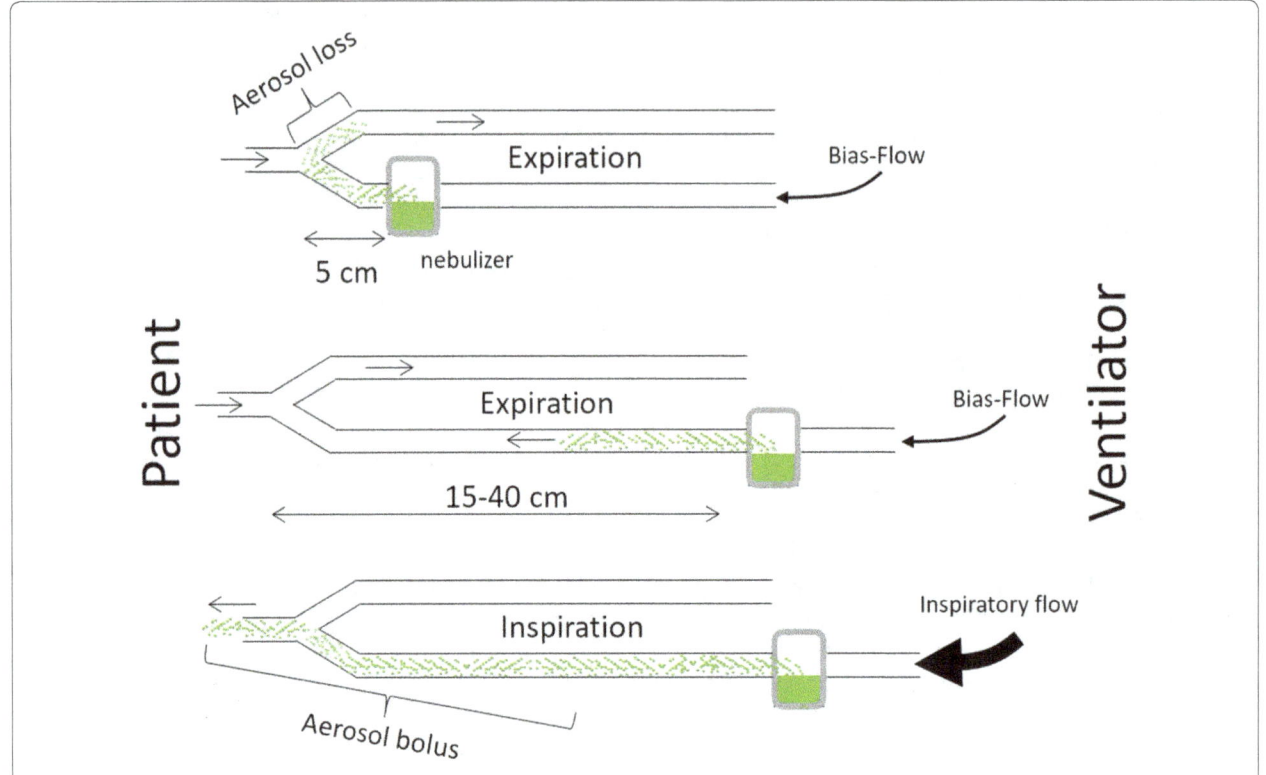

Fig. 1 Influence of the nebulizer position on aerosol losses during expiration. Nebulizer positioning upstream in the inspiratory limb enables the latter to act as a spacer/reservoir, thereby storing aerosol during expiration for an aerosol bolus delivery at the next insufflation

enable tidal volume control, as opposed to using driving gas external to the ventilator, which is a practice that should be avoided [19]. Breath-synchronized vibrating mesh nebulizers are currently undergoing investigation, and they may overcome the poor synchronization observed with current jet systems [19]. However, breath synchronization comes at the cost of increased treatment durations [20], and direct comparison with continuous nebulization performed under optimal conditions requires further studies.

Circuit humidification and filter

Humidified gas increases the size of the aerosol particles through hygroscopic water absorption. Decreased efficiency has been demonstrated to occur in heated and humidified as compared to dry ventilator circuits [21, 22]. As heat and moisture exchangers present a complete barrier to aerosol delivery, they should be removed during nebulization, thus interrupting passive humidification. When using an active heated humidifier, switching it off during nebulization may be an option. However, the decrease in humidity and temperature may be slow and the benefit on nebulization is questionable [23]. An effective way to reduce humidity during nebulization is to use a dedicated dry ventilator circuit during nebulization.

Although nebulization by itself exerts some form of humidification, caution should be taken when nebulization lasts more than 1 h to avoid damage to the ciliated epithelium and endotracheal tube occlusion [24].

Ventilator settings

Theoretically, a laminar low inspiratory flow is required to promote distal lung aerosol deposition [25]. Ventilator settings that enhance nebulization efficacy include a low respiratory frequency, low inspiratory flow and increased inspiratory time [14, 26]. Volume-controlled ventilation with constant low inspiratory flow increases efficacy compared to pressure-controlled ventilation (high peak flow followed by deceleration) [17, 27]. An end inspiratory pause may facilitate the settling of aerosol particles in the lung [26]. Complete ventilator synchrony may reduce turbulence and improve efficacy. Tolerance of such specific ventilator settings in patients who are awake may be poor and the benefit-to-risk ratio of temporary sedation during nebulization should be evaluated on a case-by-case basis.

These practical constraints present a substantial hurdle in regard to performing clinical trials and ultimately for the feasibility of large-scale nebulized antibiotic therapy in daily clinical routine.

Pharmacokinetics and pharmacodynamics

The efficacy of antibiotic therapy depends on pharmacokinetic and pharmacodynamic criteria. Antibiotics with poor diffusion through biological membranes are appropriate candidates for nebulization, as intravenous infusion results in low lung concentrations. Indeed, low concentrations of tobramycin were detected in lung epithelial lining fluids (ELF) following intravenous infusion of 7–10 mg/kg of this drug [28]. Even when the intravenous amikacin dose is increased to 25–30 mg/kg, the target level is rarely reached [2, 29]. Similarly, in regard to polymyxins, several studies have shown a lack of lung tissue penetration of colistin when CMS was administered intravenously [30, 31]. This issue remains controversial, however. Markou et al. [32] were able to detect colistin in lung ELF in two patients after 4 and 12 days, respectively, of intravenous CMS. The pharmacological complexity of CMS and colistin should be pointed out. CMS under in vivo physiological conditions is hydrolyzed into 32 different compounds, among which colistin A and colistin B represent 85% of the mixture and exert most of the antibacterial activity. CMS itself has no antibacterial activity. It is hence difficult to characterize the kinetics of the formation and absorption of colistin after CMS infusion or nebulization.

From a pharmacodynamic point of view, aminoglycosides and colistin are concentration-dependent antibiotics with a post-antibiotic effect. They are particularly suitable for nebulization as high lung concentrations can be expected and only 1 to 3 daily administrations are required. Time-dependent antibiotics, such as β-lactams or glycopeptides, require drug concentrations to be maintained above the MIC throughout the dosing interval. Continuous or closely repeated administration is hence required [33, 34], which could limit the clinical feasibility of nebulized delivery of such drugs.

Nephrotoxicity associated with CMS and aminoglycosides after intravenous infusion represents an additional rationale for their nebulized delivery. Given the lack of a proven benefit and increased nephrotoxicity, a recent Cochrane systematic review discouraged the use of intravenous aminoglycoside in combination with β-lactam antibiotics for treating sepsis [35]. Conversely, systemic uptake, albeit not negligible [36, 37], is limited after nebulization. Therefore, nebulization of hydrophilic drugs such as aminoglycosides, polymyxins and glycopeptides presents a favorable pharmacokinetic profile, thus potentially limiting nephrotoxicity [1].

These theoretical favorable pharmacokinetic and pharmacodynamic profiles, summarized in Fig. 2, have been documented in experimental and clinical studies involving optimized nebulization techniques for amikacin and colistin.

Experimental evidence of favorable pulmonary pharmacokinetics

The efficacy of 45 mg/kg/24 h nebulized amikacin has been studied in ventilated piglets with pneumonia due to *Escherichia coli*. The amikacin concentrations measured in the infected lung parenchyma were significantly higher than the MIC and 3–30 times higher than after intravenous infusion [5]. No pulmonary or systemic accumulation was observed over three days in piglets with normal kidneys [5, 38]. The efficacy of 8 mg/kg/12 h nebulized CMS has been studied in ventilated piglets with pneumonia due to *Pseudomonas aeruginosa*. Peak concentrations in the infected lung parenchyma were significantly higher than the MIC [30]. In an experimental sheep model, no colistin was quantifiable in the ELF after intravenous infusion of CMS, whereas high ELF colistin concentrations were measured after nebulization [39]. Improved bacterial killing after nebulization was also observed in these animal studies compared to intravenous administration of the drug [5, 30, 39].

These experimental studies, documenting high lung parenchymal antibiotic concentrations after nebulization of high doses and implementing optimized techniques, laid the foundations for clinical pharmacokinetic studies.

Clinical evidence of favorable pulmonary pharmacokinetics

It was recently shown that in patients with healthy lungs, 10–15% of the nebulizer charge is deposited in the lungs [17]. Such a level of delivery is compatible with high drug concentrations in the lung, although a substantial level of heterogeneity within the lung and a predominantly proximal deposition pattern were observed.

In patients with VAP, nebulized amikacin (400 mg/12 h) achieved median lung ELF concentrations 100 times higher than the maximum serum concentration [40]. Similarly, Niederman et al. [41] measured very high amikacin concentrations in the tracheal aspirate of patients suffering from VAP after nebulized amikacin (400 mg/12 h). In both studies [40, 41], a vibrating mesh nebulizer synchronized with inspiration was used [42]; patients were ventilated in pressure-controlled or volume-controlled mode, and heated humidification was performed during the nebulization. Despite the use of an only partially optimized nebulization technique and a relatively low amikacin dose compared to experimental data, it is likely that high amounts of amikacin were delivered to the lungs given the specific synchronized device that was used [42]. Systemic absorption remained low. Another group tested a combination nebulization of low-dose amikacin (100–500 mg) and fosfomycin (40–200 mg) in patients with VAP [43]. Although the continuously operating vibrating mesh nebulizer was optimally placed in the ventilator

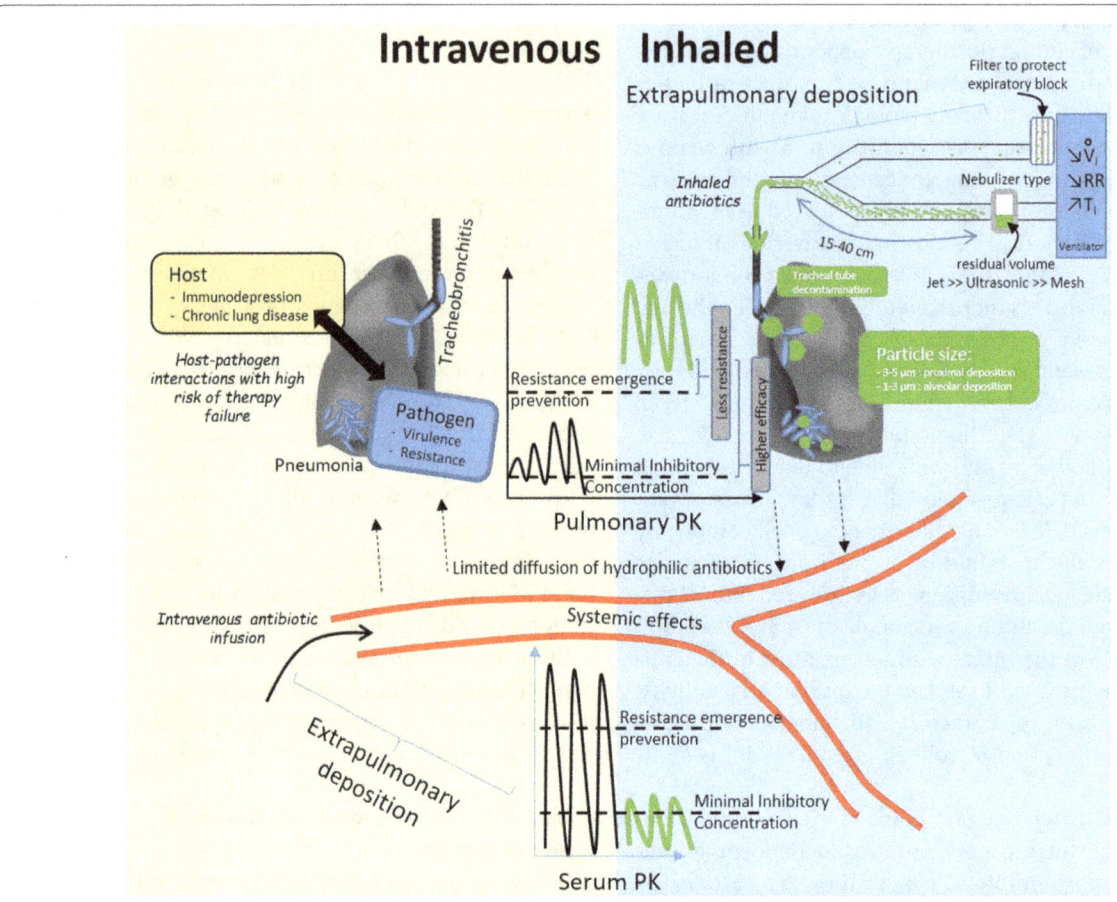

Fig. 2 Differences between intravenous and nebulized antibiotic therapy. Intravenous infusion (*yellow panel, left bottom corner*) leads to high extrapulmonary concentrations and potential toxicities. Diffusion to the lung is limited and resulting concentrations that may not exceed minimal inhibitory concentration can lead to treatment failure in challenging host–pathogen combinations. Nebulized delivery (*blue panel, right top corner*), implementing an optimized technique (detailed in Table 3) results in higher pulmonary concentrations that are above the resistance emergence prevention threshold, thus reducing the likelihood of resistant strain selection. These concentrations are well above the minimal inhibitory concentration, thus resulting in improved efficacy of concentration-dependent antibiotics, even with difficult-to-treat pathogens; systemic side effects may be reduced. Nebulization requires carful implementation so as to avoid potential respiratory side effects. *PK* pharmacokinetics, V_i inspiratory flow, *RR* respiratory rate, T_i inspiratory time

circuit, the ventilator settings were not controlled. Again, very high antibiotic concentrations were measured in bronchial secretions, even in patients receiving the lowest amikacin doses (concentrations above 5000 μg/mL, amounting to 40 times the serum peak concentration). Using higher amikacin doses with a different nebulizer in patients with VAP, Peticollin et al. [37] showed that nebulized doses of up to 60 mg/kg may be safe as they were associated with serum concentrations that were lower than those observed after intravenous infusion of a standard dose. Inter- and intra-patient pharmacokinetic variabilities of serum concentrations were very high in this study. Similarly, high inter-patient variations of amikacin concentrations were observed at the lung level with a factor of 100 in ELF and bronchial secretions [40].

In patients with VAP or ventilator-associated tracheobronchitis (VAT) who were administered 1 million international units (MIU, i.e., 80 mg) of CMS via a vibrating mesh nebulizer under optimal conditions every 8 h, peak ELF concentrations were high but then dropped below the sensitivity breakpoint at 4 h, thus indicating that this dose may not be optimal for treating pneumonia [44] (Table 2). Nebulization of CMS at a single dose of 2 MIU, implementing the same optimal nebulization technique, has been reported to yield significantly higher ELF colistin concentrations than after intravenous administration [45]. Steady-state plasma concentrations of colistin, indirectly reflecting alveolar deposition, were significantly higher in studies evaluating high doses of nebulized CMS (4–5 MIU/8 h) [46, 47] compared to 2 MIU/8 h [45].

Table 2 Colistin ELF and plasma concentrations after nebulization with different doses

Study	Athanassa [44] ($n = 20$)[a]	Boisson [45] ($n = 12$)[a]	Bihan [46] ($n = 1$)[b]	Lu [6] ($n = 16$)[b]
Nebulized dose	1 MIU	2 MIU	4 MIU	5 MIU
Nebulizer	Vibrating mesh nebulizer, continuous delivery, optimized conditions			
Colistin assay	HPLC	LC–MS/MS	LC–MS/MS	HPLC
VAP/VAT	VAT	VAP	VAP	VAP
Lung ELFmax (mg/L)	6.73 (4.8–10.1)	1137	NA	NA
Lung ELFmin (mg/L)	2.0 (1.0–3.8)	9.53	NA	NA
Plasma Cmax (mg/L)	1.6 (1.5–1.9)	0.73	2.9	2.2 ± 1.3
Plasma Cmin (mg/L)	0.3 (0.3–0.5)	0.15	2.4	1.4 ± 0.9

Data are presented as mean $\pm$ SD, medians (25–75% interquartile) or maximum and minimum values

HPLC High-performance liquid chromatography, VAP ventilator-associated pneumonia; VAT ventilator-associated tracheobronchitis, ELF epithelial lining fluid, LC–MS/MS liquid chromatography–tandem mass spectrometry, Cmax maximum plasma concentration, Cmin minimum plasma concentration

[a] Blood sampled after the first dose; [b] blood sample performed at steady-state

Systemic exposure of CMS and colistin was significantly lower after nebulization compared to intravenous infusion [6, 45], indicating a reduced risk of nephrotoxicity [47]. The various methods used to measure deposition and the concentration of nebulized antibiotics at the site of infection have several technical limitations. The measurement of ELF concentrations of antibiotics could be skewed by contamination as a result of lysis of ELF cells and technical constraints of bronchoalveolar lavage [48], as well as reliable assessment of the unbound drug concentration in the lung. Further development and research, including use of micro-dialysis, are required to better characterize local antibiotic concentrations [49]. Lastly, the inter-subject variability of pharmacokinetics may not have been fully captured given the limited sample size of currently available studies.

Clinical efficacy

One randomized controlled trial studied the efficacy of nebulized antibiotic therapy only to treat VAP caused by *P. aeruginosa* as compared to intravenous therapy [34]. Forty patients were allocated to receive either nebulized ceftazidime (15 mg/kg every 3 h) and amikacin (25 mg/kg once per day) or intravenous ceftazidime (90 mg/kg daily continuous infusion) and amikacin (15 mg/kg once per day). Antibiotics were delivered implementing strict optimized nebulization practice via a vibrating mesh nebulizer (a continuous delivery system), ventilator settings were optimized and the humidifier was switched off during the nebulization. In this phase II study, patients who only received nebulized antibiotics had a 70% cure rate compared to 55% for those receiving only intravenous antibiotics. The difference was not statistically significant, however. Interestingly, effective therapy was also observed in patients infected by bacteria with intermediate susceptibility to the nebulized antibiotics.

Furthermore, in patients for whom the treatment failed, new or persistent bacterial growth was caused exclusively by susceptible strains in the nebulized group, whereas 50% of the recurrent strains had become intermediately or fully resistant in the intravenous group. High antibiotic lung concentrations well above the MIC and higher than the concentration preventing the emergence of resistance may explain these results (Fig. 2). The median peak plasma concentration after amikacin nebulization was 8.9 mg/L, thus reflecting significant systemic diffusion, with 25% of patients presenting a trough amikacin concentration above 5.9 µg/mL. It is difficult, however, to translate this exclusively nebulized antibiotic therapy into routine practice, as ceftazidime nebulization every 3 h may be considered cumbersome and outweigh potential benefits.

Testing another clinical strategy, Palmer et al. [50] assessed the effects of nebulized antibiotics as an adjunctive therapy to intravenous antibiotics in patients with VAT and/or VAP [51]. Patients with Gram-positive bacteria were treated with vancomycin at 120 mg/8 h and those with Gram-negative organisms were treated with gentamicin at 80 mg/8 h or amikacin at 400 mg/8 h. Antibiotics were delivered via a breath-actuated jet nebulizer with active humidification turned off. Adjunction of nebulized antibiotics to systemic therapy rapidly sterilized bronchial secretions and decreased the VAT/VAP incidence, thus revealing a favorable prophylactic effect on the transition from VAT to VAP and a curative effect for patients with VAP. Nebulization was associated with a faster resolution of signs of infection and weaning, as well as reduced use of systemic antibiotics. Similar to the work by Lu et al. [34], the emergence of drug-resistant bacteria was reduced for patients receiving nebulized antibiotics [51]. Kollef et al. [52] tested a strategy of low-dose nebulized amikacin (300 mg/12 h) combined with fosfomycin (120 mg/12 h) as adjuncts to intravenous antibiotics in patients with VAP. Whereas no significant effect on clinical outcomes was observed, nebulized antibiotics were associated with a faster sterilization of bronchial secretions and again a significantly reduced emergence of drug-resistant bacteria.

The systemic antibiotic sparing effect of nebulized antibiotics was also observed in the earlier mentioned work by Niederman et al. [41]. For 69 patients with VAP, nebulized amikacin (400 mg/12 h or/24 h) reduced the number of systemic antibiotics per patient per day at the end of the 14-day therapy. However, no benefit in terms of clinical responses was observed, and this may have been due to a very high cure rate in the control group.

In these studies, various doses of nebulized amikacin were used (twice as many high-dose versus low-dose studies) and aerosols were delivered with different nebulizers although close attention was often paid to optimize the nebulization technique. Nebulized amikacin allowed for effective treatment of bronchial and parenchymal infections, even when involving bacteria with high MIC, and it consistently reduced the emergence of resistant bacteria. Clinical cure, evaluated as a secondary endpoint in these trials, depends in part on the therapeutic efficacy in the control group. Further clinical phase III studies are required to prove the clinical benefit of nebulized amikacin.

As colistin is the most frequently nebulized antibiotic in ICUs, there is some information in regard to clinical bedside safety and efficacy as well as large retrospective databases. However, only a small number of prospective controlled studies have evaluated nebulized colistin in mechanically ventilated patients implementing optimized technique. High-dose nebulized CMS (5 MIU/8 h with strict optimized technique) has been evaluated in patients with VAP caused by multidrug-resistant (MDR) *P. aeruginosa* and *Acinetobacter baumannii* [6]. Patients with VAP caused by sensitive strains and treated with standard intravenous antibiotics served as controls. The clinical cure rate was 66% in the sensitive strain group and 67% in MDR strain group. By testing a nearly exclusively nebulized therapy strategy (a minority of patients received an intravenous aminoglycoside complement), this study very much indicates that nebulization of high-dose CMS may be effective to treat MDR bacterial VAP. Conversely, in patients suffering from VAP primarily due to sensitive bacteria, a randomized trial testing nebulized colistin as an adjunctive therapy to intravenous antibiotics appeared to yield negative results [53]. A recent randomized trial evaluated high doses of nebulized colistin using an optimized technique either as adjunct to intravenous antibiotics for VAP due to sensitive bacteria or as an exclusively nebulized therapy in case of MDR bacteria. Patients in the nebulized group had a significantly lower

incidence of acute renal failure, a higher level of oxygenation and a shortened time to bacterial eradication than those in the control group receiving intravenous colistin [54], although the overall clinical cure rate was not significantly different. The fact that patients infected with MDR bacteria and treated exclusively with nebulized colistin had similar outcomes as patients infected with sensitive bacteria who were treated with intravenous antibiotics in addition to nebulized colistin can be considered to be an encouraging result [54].

Three groups of investigators used databases with information regarding patients suffering from colistin-only susceptible bacterial VAP to evaluate whether nebulized CMS as adjunct to intravenous CMS is beneficial. One study observed no additional benefit of combined nebulized and intravenous CMS therapy [55], whereas the two others observed a higher cure rate compared to intravenous therapy alone [56, 57]. Furthermore, clinical use of intravenous colistin is still a matter of debate [58, 59].

Meta-analyses of the clinical studies have yielded conflicting results and further clinical evidence from randomized trials is required, while more extensive evaluation of renal toxicity related to the administration of high dose of CMS or amikacin intravenously or by nebulization is also needed [60–65]. The currently available evidence cannot be considered to be sufficient for implementation of nebulized antibiotics as a straightforward therapeutic option.

Aside from investigating curative nebulized antibiotics to treat patients suffering from VAT and/or VAP, some authors have also tested nebulized colistin, ceftazidime or aminoglycosides for prophylaxis in intubated patients. Two small-sized studies obtained positive results with such a preemptive nebulized therapy in terms of the VAP frequency, and they also observed no significant change in the bacterial antibiotic sensitivity pattern [66, 67]. Further studies are required to assess this benefit as well as the risk of antibiotic resistance selection pressure.

Current practice

The spread of MDR associated with the favorable data outlined above led to implementation of nebulized antibiotic therapy in the clinical setting despite the lack of large-scale patient-centered evidence. Among 816 international intensivists surveyed electronically, one-third reported that they usually or frequently nebulize colistin [68]. In an observational study in 80 ICUs, every fifth intubated patient received an aerosol, and 5% involved nebulized antibiotics [69]. Nebulized antibiotics (80% colistin) were delivered to 1% of the ICU patients in 17% of the study centers. A subsequent international survey that specifically investigated the use of nebulized antibiotics in ICUs highlighted very heterogeneous indications ranging from prophylactic or empirical therapy to documented lung infections in immunocompetent and immunocompromised patients, for VAT and VAP [70]. The use of jet nebulizers appears to be predominant, and practical implementations were far from the optimized efficacy conditions described above. Overall practice was considered to be adequate in only one-third of the ICUs, with no effect of longer experience in using nebulized antibiotics on the rate of adequate practice [71].

This practice pattern challenges the conclusions drawn from some prospective and retrospective studies without standardized nebulization procedures. In many patients, the amount of drug delivered beyond the tip of the endotracheal tube may be negligible, and low drug pulmonary concentrations may enhance the selection of drug-resistant bacteria. The observed practices illustrate the difficulties of implementing optimal nebulization techniques in patients outside of controlled clinical research settings, and this may have implications for future trial designs and the dissemination of knowledge.

Safety and good practices

In order to guarantee adequate safety and aerosol therapy efficiency during mechanical ventilation, standard operating procedures should be implemented including a checklist for physicians and nurses [34, 72]. Adequate staff training is essential. Key points for good practice with nebulization during mechanical ventilation are summarized in Table 3. Antibiotic nebulization in mechanically ventilated patients is generally well tolerated [6, 34, 69]. Aside from potential toxicities related to systemic absorption, specific nebulization-related side effects need to be considered, however.

Ventilator dysfunction and circuit obstructions

A filter needs to be positioned between the expiratory limb and the ventilator to protect the latter from expired particles and to prevent dysfunction (Fig. 2). A new filter should be used before each nebulization to prevent progressive obstruction. Mechanical filters appear to be the most effective [73–75]. Obstruction of the expiratory filter is the most serious complication that can arise as it can lead to cardiac arrest [34]. In case of interruption of humidification during the nebulization, its resumption is an important safety condition in order to avoid tracheal tube obstruction.

Direct mucosal toxicity

Long-term bronchial toxicity and alveolar damage that can result from high local antibiotic concentrations have received scant attention. Whereas a transient benign cough is common, bronchospasm is a more severe, albeit infrequent, side effect that has been reported to occur during antibiotic nebulization [6, 34, 40]. Preventive bronchodilation appears to be unnecessary, although the occurrence of bronchospasm imposes aerosol interruption and bronchodilator nebulization. Tobramycin, colistin and aztreonam are commercially available as solutions for inhalation, whereas amikacin solutions for inhalation, including liposomal forms, are still undergoing investigation [76]. Medications for inhalation should be pyrogen-free, isotonic and sterile, and their pH should be adjusted to that of the airway epithelium (pH 6). Importantly, preservatives and sulfites should be avoided, as they have been specifically associated with adverse effects when inhaled.

Circuit manipulation and oxygenation

Circuit manipulation for nebulization must follow the usual hygiene standards; the availability of single-patient-use nebulizers contributes to hygiene control. Desaturation and hypoxemia have been reported in patients receiving frequent repeated nebulization [34] due to alveolar derecruitment induced by disconnection of the patient from the ventilator.

Monitoring

Bronchospasm and obstruction of expiratory filters are first detected as an increase in the peak airway pressure.

Table 3 Key good practices for optimal antibiotic nebulization during mechanical ventilation

Organization	Use standard operating procedures and a checklist. Ensure adequate staff training
Nebulizer	Use nebulizers with a small residual volume Do not operate jet nebulizers with gas external to the ventilator
Medication solution	Use solutions for inhalation
Nebulizer position	Position the nebulizer (continuous delivery) upstream in the inspiratory limb at 15–40 cm of the Y-piece
Humidification	Remove the heat and moisture exchanger during nebulization; if using a heated humidifier, consider switching it off or use of a dry circuit
Ventilator settings	Volume-controlled constant flow ventilation. Use low respiratory rate, low inspiratory flow and a long inspiratory time
Safety	Place a new filter between the expiratory limb and the ventilator for each nebulization Monitor patients closely during the nebulization, particularly in regard to airway pressure, arterial pressure and oxygen saturation Check for resumption of humidification at the end of the nebulization

These complications emphasize the need for close monitoring of the peak airway pressure and oxygenation during nebulization [77]. Systemic absorption of antibiotics may be substantial in patients with renal failure, and drug monitoring is recommended when aminoglycosides are used [36, 37].

Perspectives

Since 2007, six meta-analyses have been published in regard to nebulized antibiotics as a treatment for lung infections among ventilated patients [60–65], and two meta-analyses evaluated prophylactic nebulized antibiotics [78, 79]. None of them have allowed a definitive conclusion to be reached in regard to possible benefits. As a result, a recent review recommended that use of nebulized antibiotics should be avoided in clinical practice, due to a low level of evidence for their efficacy and the risks of adverse events [80]. Despite this low-quality evidence, recent VAP management guidelines recommend adjunctive nebulized antibiotic therapy for bacteria that are only susceptible to antibiotics when there is evidence for limited efficacy of the intravenous route, i.e., aminoglycosides and colistin. Adjunctive nebulized antibiotic therapy as a treatment of last resort is also recommended [4]. Careful design of future large randomized trials to turn the favorable pharmacokinetic/pharmacodynamic profile of nebulized antibiotics into improved clinical outcomes and reduced toxicity in patients with VAP is needed (Fig. 2). The following considerations should be taken into account in order to comprehensively integrate both technical issues and clinical complexity in a translational research effort.

Target population

Patients with a high rate of intravenous treatment failure are most susceptible to benefit from this approach. Thus, patients and/or ICUs at high risk of the emergence of MDR bacteria represent target populations for nebulized antibiotics. Defining populations at high risk of toxicity (mainly patients with acute kidney injury) may also be a worthwhile challenge.

Therapeutic strategy

Intravenous therapy is effective and well tolerated in most patients with VAP caused by β-lactam-susceptible bacteria. The benefit of withholding this therapy is elusive. In patients with late-onset VAP caused by difficult-to-treat bacteria with frequent recurrence, in the light of the questionable benefit of intravenous aminoglycosides, nebulized aminoglycosides as adjunct to systemic therapy may be considered [4, 81]. For the most severely affected patients, who are at very high risk of death, and who are afflicted with pneumonia due to MDR bacteria

for which intravenous antibiotics are likely to fail [4, 81], adjunctive high-dose nebulized antibiotics may be beneficial. In patients with VAP due to MDR bacteria that are only susceptible to aminoglycosides or colistin, an exclusive nebulized strategy may be considered. At the other end of the severity spectrum, in patients at risk of developing pneumonia, but who do not yet exhibit parenchymal infection, the benefits of intravenous preemptive antibiotic therapy remain debatable [82–85]. An exclusively nebulized therapeutic strategy may thus warrant evaluation.

Continuous improvement of nebulization technique

This is urgently needed to implement easy, safe and reproducible techniques as well as to standardize nebulization practices for clinical trials and to thereafter translate the results into clinical practice. A paradigm change may occur in the future with the development of inhaled anti-infective nanoparticle antibody or phage therapies.

Conclusions

Experimental and clinical pharmacokinetics and pharmacodynamics support the feasibility and possible benefits of nebulized antibiotic therapy to treat VAP in mechanically ventilated patients. Before expanding its clinical use, optimization of nebulization techniques and standardization of nebulization procedures are urgently needed. Large phase III randomized trials are required to demonstrate the clinical effectiveness and benefits in terms of improvements in patient outcomes and reduction in the emergence of antibiotic resistance.

Abbreviations

CMS: colistimethate sodium; ELF: epithelial lining fluid; ICU: intensive care unit; MDR: multidrug-resistant; MIC: minimum inhibitory concentration; MIU: million international units; VAP: ventilator-associated pneumonia; VAT: ventilator-associated tracheobronchitis.

Authors' contributions

All of the authors contributed to the manuscript design, drafting and review for important intellectual content. All authors read and approved the final manuscript.

Author details

[1] Médecine Intensive Réanimation, Réseau CRICS-TRIGGERSEP, Centre Hospitalier Régional et Universitaire de Tours, Tours, France. [2] Centre d'études des Pathologies Respiratoires, INSERM U1100, Faculté de Médecine de Tours, Université François Rabelais de Tours, Tours, France. [3] Service de Réanimation Médicale, Institut de Cardiologie, Assistance Publique-Hôpitaux de Paris, Pitié-Salpêtrière Hospital, UPMC (University Pierre and Marie Curie) Paris-6, Paris, France. [4] Pneumologie, Centre Hospitalier Régional et Universitaire de Tours, Tours, France. [5] Multidisciplinary Critical Care Unit, Department of Anesthesiology and Critical Care Medicine, Assistance Publique-Hôpitaux de Paris, Pitié-Salpêtrière Hospital, UPMC (University Pierre and Marie Curie) Paris-6, Paris, France.

Acknowledgements

None.

Competing interests

SE has received research grants from Fisher & Paykel, Aerogen, Hamilton, Firalis and Consulting/Lecture fees from La diffusion technique française, Aerogen, Baxter and Bayer. JC has received honoraria for lectures or for being on the advisory board from Bayer/Nektar, Medimmune/Astrazeneca, Pfizer, Arsanis, Cubist/Merck, Aridis and Astellas. PD and QL have no competing interests to declare.

References

1. Rodvold KA, George JM, Yoo L. Penetration of anti-infective agents into pulmonary epithelial lining fluid: focus on antibacterial agents. Clin Pharmacokinet. 2011;50:637–64.
2. de Montmollin E, Bouadma L, Gault N, Mourvillier B, Mariotte E, Chemam S, et al. Predictors of insufficient amikacin peak concentration in critically ill patients receiving a 25 mg/kg total body weight regimen. Intensive Care Med. 2014;40:998–1005.
3. Kollef MH, Chastre J, Clavel M, Restrepo MI, Michiels B, Kaniga K, et al. A randomized trial of 7-day doripenem versus 10-day imipenem-cilastatin for ventilator-associated pneumonia. Crit Care. 2012;16:R218.
4. Kalil AC, Metersky ML, Klompas M, Muscedere J, Sweeney DA, Palmer LB, et al. Management of adults with hospital-acquired and ventilator-associated pneumonia: 2016 Clinical practice guidelines by the Infectious Diseases Society of America and the American Thoracic Society. Clin Infect Dis. 2016;63:e61–111.
5. Goldstein I, Wallet F, Nicolas-Robin A, Ferrari F, Marquette CH, Rouby JJ. Lung deposition and efficiency of nebulized amikacin during *Escherichia coli* pneumonia in ventilated piglets. Am J Respir Crit Care Med. 2002;166:1375–81.
6. Lu Q, Luo R, Bodin L, Yang J, Zahr N, Aubry A, et al. Efficacy of high-dose nebulized colistin in ventilator-associated pneumonia caused by multidrug-resistant *Pseudomonas aeruginosa* and *Acinetobacter baumannii*. Anesthesiology. 2012;117:1335–47.
7. Dalhoff A. Pharmacokinetics and pharmacodynamics of aerosolized antibacterial agents in chronically infected cystic fibrosis patients. Clin Microbiol Rev. 2014;27:753–82.
8. Mogayzel PJ Jr, Naureckas ET, Robinson KA, Mueller G, Hadjiliadis D, Hoag JB, Lubsch L, Hazle L, Sabadosa K, Marshall B. Cystic fibrosis pulmonary guidelines. Chronic medications for maintenance of lung health. Am J Respir Crit Care Med. 2013;187:680–9.
9. MacIntyre NR, Silver RM, Miller CW, Schuler F, Coleman RE. Aerosol delivery in intubated, mechanically ventilated patients. Crit Care Med. 1985;13:81–4.
10. Brain JD, Valberg PA. Deposition of aerosol in the respiratory tract. Am Rev Respir Dis. 1979;120:1325–73.
11. Ari A, Atalay OT, Harwood R, Sheard MM, Aljamhan EA, Fink JB. Influence of nebulizer type, position, and bias flow on aerosol drug delivery in simulated pediatric and adult lung models during mechanical ventilation. Respir Care. 2010;55:845–51.
12. Harvey CJ, O'Doherty MJ, Page CJ, Thomas SH, Nunan TO, Treacher DF. Comparison of jet and ultrasonic nebulizer pulmonary aerosol deposition during mechanical ventilation. Eur Respir J. 1997;10:905–9.
13. Ferrari F, Liu ZH, Lu Q, Becquemin MH, Louchahi K, Aymard G, et al. Comparison of lung tissue concentrations of nebulized ceftazidime in ventilated piglets: ultrasonic versus vibrating plate nebulizers. Intensive Care Med. 2008;34:1718–23.
14. O'Doherty MJ, Thomas SH, Page CJ, Treacher DF, Nunan TO. Delivery of a nebulized aerosol to a lung model during mechanical ventilation. Effect of ventilator settings and nebulizer type, position, and volume of fill. Am Rev Respir Dis. 1992;146:383–8.
15. Wallace SJ, Li J, Rayner CR, Coulthard K, Nation RL. Stability of colistin methanesulfonate in pharmaceutical products and solutions for administration to patients. Antimicrob Agents Chemother. 2008;52:3047–51.
16. Boe J, Dennis JH, O'Driscoll BR, Bauer TT, Carone M, Dautzenberg B, et al. Adaptations of the European Respiratory Society guidelines by the Aerosol Therapy Group of the French Lung Society on the use of aerosol therapy through nebulization. Rev Mal Respir. 2004;21:1033–8.
17. Dugernier J, Reychler G, Wittebole X, Roeseler J, Depoortere V, Sottiaux T, et al. Aerosol delivery with two ventilation modes during mechanical ventilation: a randomized study. Ann Intensive Care. 2016;6:73.
18. Miller DD, Amin MM, Palmer LB, Shah AR, Smaldone GC. Aerosol delivery and modern mechanical ventilation: in vitro/in vivo evaluation. Am J Respir Crit Care Med. 2003;168:1205–9.
19. Ehrmann S, Lyazidi A, Louis B, Isabey D, Le Pennec D, Brochard L, et al. Ventilator-integrated jet nebulization systems: tidal volume control and efficiency of synchronization. Respir Care. 2014;59:1508–16.
20. Rau JL, Ari A, Restrepo RD. Performance comparison of nebulizer designs: constant-output, breath-enhanced, and dosimetric. Respir Care. 2004;49:174–9.
21. Ari A, Areabi H, Fink JB. Evaluation of aerosol generator devices at 3 locations in humidified and non-humidified circuits during adult mechanical ventilation. Respir Care. 2010;55:837–44.
22. Boukhettala N, Poree T, Diot P, Vecellio L. In vitro performance of spacers for aerosol delivery during adult mechanical ventilation. J Aerosol Med Pulm Drug Deliv. 2015;28:130–6.
23. Lin HL, Fink JB, Zhou Y, Cheng YS. Influence of moisture accumulation in inline spacer on delivery of aerosol using metered-dose inhaler during mechanical ventilation. Respir Care. 2009;54:1336–41.
24. Villafane MC, Cinnella G, Lofaso F, Isabey D, Harf A, Lemaire F, et al. Gradual reduction of endotracheal tube diameter during mechanical ventilation via different humidification devices. Anesthesiology. 1996;85:1341–9.
25. Dhand R. Maximizing aerosol delivery during mechanical ventilation: go with the flow and go slow. Intensive Care Med. 2003;29:1041–2.
26. Dhand R. Special problems in aerosol delivery: artificial airways. Respir Care. 2000;45:636–45.
27. Dugernier J, Wittebole X, Roeseler J, Michotte JB, Sottiaux T, Dugernier T, et al. Influence of inspiratory flow pattern and nebulizer position on aerosol delivery with a vibrating-mesh nebulizer during invasive mechanical ventilation: an in vitro analysis. J Aerosol Med Pulm Drug Deliv. 2015;28:229–36.
28. Carcas AJ, Garcia-Satue JL, Zapater P, Frias-Iniesta J. Tobramycin penetration into epithelial lining fluid of patients with pneumonia. Clin Pharmacol Ther. 1999;65:245–50.
29. Taccone FS, Laterre PF, Spapen H, Dugernier T, Delattre I, Layeux B, et al. Revisiting the loading dose of amikacin for patients with severe sepsis and septic shock. Crit Care. 2010;14:R53.
30. Lu Q, Girardi C, Zhang M, Bouhemad B, Louchahi K, Petitjean O, et al. Nebulized and intravenous colistin in experimental pneumonia caused by *Pseudomonas aeruginosa*. Intensive Care Med. 2010;36:11471155.
31. Imberti R, Cusato M, Villani P, Carnevale L, Iotti GA, Langer M, et al. Steady-state pharmacokinetics and BAL concentration of colistin in critically ill patients after IV colistin methanesulfonate administration. Chest. 2010;138:1333–9.
32. Markou N, Fousteri M, Markantonis SL, Boutzouka E, Tsigou E, Baltopoulo G. Colistin penetration in the alveolar lining fluid of critically ill patients treated with IV colistimethate sodium. Chest. 2011;139:232–4.
33. Ferrari F, Lu Q, Girardi C, Petitjean O, Marquette CH, Wallet F, et al. Nebulized ceftazidime in experimental pneumonia caused by partially resistant *Pseudomonas aeruginosa*. Intensive Care Med. 2009;35:1792–800.
34. Lu Q, Yang J, Liu Z, Gutierrez C, Aymard G, Rouby JJ. Nebulized ceftazidime and amikacin in ventilator-associated pneumonia caused by *Pseudomonas aeruginosa*. Am J Respir Crit Care Med. 2011;184:106–15.
35. Paul M, Lador A, Grozinsky-Glasberg S, Leibovici L. Beta lactam antibiotic monotherapy versus beta lactam-aminoglycoside antibiotic combination therapy for sepsis. Cochrane Database Syst Rev. 2014;1:CD003344.
36. Badia JR, Soy D, Adrover M, Ferrer M, Sarasa M, Alarcon A, et al. Disposition of instilled versus nebulized tobramycin and imipenem in ventilated intensive care unit (ICU) patients. J Antimicrob Chemother. 2004;54:508–14.
37. Petitcollin A, Dequin PF, Darrouzain F, Vecellio L, Boulain T, Garot D, et al. Pharmacokinetics of high-dose nebulized amikacin in ventilated critically ill patients. J Antimicrob Chemother. 2016;71:3482–6.
38. Ferrari F, Goldstein I, Nieszkowszka A, Elman M, Marquette CH, Rouby JJ. Lack of lung tissue and systemic accumulation after consecutive daily aerosols of amikacin in ventilated piglets with healthy lungs. Anesthesiology. 2003;98:1016–9.

39. Landersdorfer CB, Nguyen TH, Lieu LT, Nguyen G, Bischof RJ, Meeusen EN, et al. Substantial targeting advantage achieved by pulmonary administration of colistin methanesulfonate in a large-animal model. Antimicrob Agents Chemother. 2017;61:e01934-16.

40. Luyt CE, Clavel M, Guntupalli K, Johannigman J, Kennedy JI, Wood C, et al. Pharmacokinetics and lung delivery of PDDS-aerosolized amikacin (NKTR-061) in intubated and mechanically ventilated patients with nosocomial pneumonia. Crit Care. 2009;13:R200.

41. Niederman MS, Chastre J, Corkery K, Fink JB, Luyt CE, Garcia MS. BAY41-6551 achieves bactericidal tracheal aspirate amikacin concentrations in mechanically ventilated patients with Gram-negative pneumonia. Intensive Care Med. 2012;38:263–71.

42. Dhand R, Sohal H. Pulmonary drug delivery system for inhalation therapy in mechanically ventilated patients. Expert Rev Med Devices. 2008;5:9–18.

43. Montgomery AB, Vallance S, Abuan T, Tservistas M, Davies A. A randomized double-blind placebo-controlled dose-escalation phase 1 study of aerosolized amikacin and fosfomycin delivered via the PARI investigational eFlow(R) inline nebulizer system in mechanically ventilated patients. J Aerosol Med Pulm Drug Deliv. 2014;27:441–8.

44. Athanassa ZE, Markantonis SL, Fousteri MZ, Myrianthefs PM, Boutzouka EG, Tsakris A, et al. Pharmacokinetics of inhaled colistimethate sodium (CMS) in mechanically ventilated critically ill patients. Intensive Care Med. 2012;38:1779–86.

45. Boisson M, Jacobs M, Gregoire N, Gobin P, Marchand S, Couet W, et al. Comparison of intrapulmonary and systemic pharmacokinetics of colistin methanesulfonate (CMS) and colistin after aerosol delivery and intravenous administration of CMS in critically ill patients. Antimicrob Agents Chemother. 2014;58:7331–9.

46. Bihan K, Lu Q, Enjalbert M, Apparuit M, Langeron O, Rouby JJ, et al. Determination of colistin and colistimethate levels in human plasma and urine by high-performance liquid chromatography-tandem mass spectrometry. Ther Drug Monit. 2016;38:796–803.

47. Sorli L, Luque S, Grau S, Berenguer N, Segura C, Montero MM, et al. Trough colistin plasma level is an independent risk factor for nephrotoxicity: a prospective observational cohort study. BMC Infect Dis. 2013;13:380.

48. Kiem S, Schentag JJ. Interpretation of epithelial lining fluid concentrations of antibiotics against methicillin resistant staphylococcus aureus. Infect Chemother. 2014;46:219–25.

49. Mukker JK, Singh RS, Derendorf H. Pharmacokinetic and pharmacodynamic implications in inhalable antimicrobial therapy. Adv Drug Deliv Rev. 2015;85:57–64.

50. Palmer LB, Smaldone GC, Chen JJ, Baram D, Duan T, Monteforte M, et al. Aerosolized antibiotics and ventilator-associated tracheobronchitis in the intensive care unit. Crit Care Med. 2008;36:2008–13.

51. Palmer LB, Smaldone GC. Reduction of bacterial resistance with inhaled antibiotics in the intensive care unit. Am J Respir Crit Care Med. 2014;189:1225–33.

52. Kollef MH, Ricard JD, Roux D, Francois B, Ischaki E, Rozgonyi Z, et al. A randomized trial of the amikacin fosfomycin inhalation system for the adjunctive therapy of Gram-negative ventilator-associated pneumonia: IASIS Trial. Chest. 2016. doi:10.1016/j.chest.2016.11.026.

53. Rattanaumpawan P, Lorsutthitham J, Ungprasert P, Angkasekwinai N, Thamlikitkul V. Randomized controlled trial of nebulized colistimethate sodium as adjunctive therapy of ventilator-associated pneumonia caused by Gram-negative bacteria. J Antimicrob Chemother. 2010;65:2645–9.

54. Abdellatif S, Trifi A, Daly F, Mahjoub K, Nasri R, Ben Lakhal S. Efficacy and toxicity of aerosolised colistin in ventilator-associated pneumonia: a prospective, randomised trial. Ann Intensive Care. 2016;6:26.

55. Kofteridis DP, Alexopoulou C, Valachis A, Maraki S, Dimopoulou D, Georgopoulos D, et al. Aerosolized plus intravenous colistin versus intravenous colistin alone for the treatment of ventilator-associated pneumonia: a matched case-control study. Clin Infect Dis. 2010;51:1238–44.

56. Korbila IP, Michalopoulos A, Rafailidis PI, Nikita D, Samonis G, Falagas ME. Inhaled colistin as adjunctive therapy to intravenous colistin for the treatment of microbiologically documented ventilator-associated pneumonia: a comparative cohort study. Clin Microbiol Infect. 2010;16:1230–6.

57. Tumbarello M, De Pascale G, Trecarichi EM, De Martino S, Bello G, Maviglia R, et al. Effect of aerosolized colistin as adjunctive treatment on the outcomes of microbiologically documented ventilator-associated pneumonia caused by colistin-only susceptible gram-negative bacteria. Chest. 2013;144:1768–75.

58. Dalfino L, Puntillo F, Mosca A, Monno R, Spada ML, Coppolecchia S, et al. High-dose, extended-interval colistin administration in critically ill patients: is this the right dosing strategy? A preliminary study. Clin Infect Dis. 2012;54:1720–6.

59. Poudyal A, Howden BP, Bell JM, Gao W, Owen RJ, Turnidge JD, et al. In vitro pharmacodynamics of colistin against multidrug-resistant Klebsiella pneumoniae. J Antimicrob Chemother. 2008;62:1311–8.

60. Florescu DF, Qiu F, McCartan MA, Mindru C, Fey PD, Kalil AC. What is the efficacy and safety of colistin for the treatment of ventilator-associated pneumonia? A systematic review and meta-regression. Clin Infect Dis. 2012;54:670–80.

61. Ioannidou E, Siempos II, Falagas ME. Administration of antimicrobials via the respiratory tract for the treatment of patients with nosocomial pneumonia: a meta-analysis. J Antimicrob Chemother. 2007;60:1216–26.

62. Valachis A, Samonis G, Kofteridis DP. The role of aerosolized colistin in the treatment of ventilator-associated pneumonia: a systematic review and metaanalysis. Crit Care Med. 2015;43:527–33.

63. Zampieri FG, Nassar AP Jr, Gusmao-Flores D, Taniguchi LU, Torres A, Ranzani OT. Nebulized antibiotics for ventilator-associated pneumonia: a systematic review and meta-analysis. Crit Care. 2015;19:150.

64. Russell CJ, Shiroishi MS, Siantz E, Wu BW, Patino CM. The use of inhaled antibiotic therapy in the treatment of ventilator-associated pneumonia and tracheobronchitis: a systematic review. BMC Pulm Med. 2016;16:40.

65. Sole-Lleonart C, Rouby JJ, Blot S, Poulakou G, Chastre J, Palmer LB, et al. Nebulization of antiinfective agents in invasively mechanically ventilated adults: a systematic review and meta-analysis. Anesthesiology. 2017;126:890–908.

66. Karvouniaris M, Makris D, Zygoulis P, Triantaris A, Xitsas S, Mantzarlis K, et al. Nebulised colistin for ventilator-associated pneumonia prevention. Eur Respir J. 2015;46:1732–9.

67. Wood GC, Boucher BA, Croce MA, Hanes SD, Herring VL, Fabian TC. Aerosolized ceftazidime for prevention of ventilator-associated pneumonia and drug effects on the proinflammatory response in critically ill trauma patients. Pharmacotherapy. 2002;22:972–82.

68. Ehrmann S, Roche-Campo F, Sferrazza Papa GF, Isabey D, Brochard L, Apiou-Sbirlea G. Aerosol therapy during mechanical ventilation: an international survey. Intensive Care Med. 2013;39:1048–56.

69. Ehrmann S, Roche-Campo F, Bodet-Contentin L, Razazi K, Dugernier J, Trenado-Alvarez J, et al. Aerosol therapy in intensive and intermediate care units: prospective observation of 2808 critically ill patients. Intensive Care Med. 2016;42:192–201.

70. Sole-Lleonart C, Roberts JA, Chastre J, Poulakou G, Palmer LB, Blot S, et al. Global survey on nebulization of antimicrobial agents in mechanically ventilated patients: a call for international guidelines. Clin Microbiol Infect. 2016;22:359–64.

71. Sole-Lleonart C, Rouby JJ, Chastre J, Poulakou G, Palmer LB, Blot S, et al. Intratracheal administration of antimicrobial agents in mechanically ventilated adults: an international survey on delivery practices and safety. Respir Care. 2016;61:1008–14.

72. Rello J, Rouby JJ, Sole-Lleonart C, Chastre J, Blot S, Luyt CE, et al. Key conceptional considerations on nebulization of antimicrobial agents to mechanically ventilated patients. Clin Microbiol Infect. 2017. doi:10.1016/j.cmi.2017.03.018.

73. Mostofi R, Wang B, Haghighat F, Bahloul A, Jaime L. Performance of mechanical filters and respirators for capturing nanoparticles—limitations and future direction. Ind Health. 2010;48:296–304.

74. Rengasamy S, BerryAnn R, Szalajda J. Nanoparticle filtration performance of filtering facepiece respirators and canister/cartridge filters. J Occup Environ Hyg. 2013;10:519–25.

75. Tonnelier A, Lellouche F, Bouchard PA, L'Her E. Impact of humidification and nebulization during expiratory limb protection: an experimental bench study. Respir Care. 2013;58:1315–22.

76. Antoniu S, Azoicai D. Novel amikacin inhaled formulation for the treatment of lower respiratory tract infections. Drugs Today (Barc). 2013;49:683–92.

77. Rouby JJ, Bouhemad B, Monsel A, Brisson H, Arbelot C, Lu Q. Aerosolized antibiotics for ventilator-associated pneumonia: lessons from experimental studies. Anesthesiology. 2012;117:1364–80.

78. Falagas ME, Siempos II, Bliziotis IA, Michalopoulos A. Administration of antibiotics via the respiratory tract for the prevention of ICU-acquired pneumonia: a meta-analysis of comparative trials. Crit Care. 2006;10:R123.
79. Roquilly A, Marret E, Abraham E, Asehnoune K. Pneumonia prevention to decrease mortality in intensive care unit: a systematic review and meta-analysis. Clin Infect Dis. 2015;60:64–75.
80. Rello J, Solé-Lleonart C, Rouby JJ, Chastre J, Blot S, Poulakou G, et al. Use of nebulized antimicrobials for the treatment of respiratory infections in invasively mechanically ventilated adults: a position paper from the european society of clinical microbiology and infectious diseases. Clin Microbiol Infect. 2017. doi:10.1016/j.cmi.2017.04.011.
81. American Thoracic Society. Guidelines for the management of adults with hospital-acquired, ventilator-associated, and healthcare-associated pneumonia. Am J Respir Crit Care Med. 2005;171:388–416.
82. Hurley JC. Topical antibiotics as a major contextual hazard toward bacteremia within selective digestive decontamination studies: a meta-analysis. BMC Infect Dis. 2014;14:714.
83. Nseir S, Di Pompeo C, Pronnier P, Beague S, Onimus T, Saulnier F, et al. Nosocomial tracheobronchitis in mechanically ventilated patients: incidence, aetiology and outcome. Eur Respir J. 2002;20:1483–9.
84. Nseir S, Martin-Loeches I, Makris D, Jaillette E, Karvouniaris M, Valles J, et al. Impact of appropriate antimicrobial treatment on transition from ventilator-associated tracheobronchitis to ventilator-associated pneumonia. Crit Care. 2014;18:R129.
85. Vincent JL, Jacobs F. Effect of selective decontamination on antibiotic resistance. Lancet Infect Dis. 2011;11:337–8.

10

Opioid-associated iatrogenic withdrawal in critically ill adult patients

Pan Pan Wang[1], Elaine Huang[2], Xue Feng[3], Charles-André Bray[2], Marc M. Perreault[4,5], Philippe Rico[6,7], Patrick Bellemare[6,7], Paul Murgoi[5], Céline Gélinas[8,9], Annie Lecavalier[10], Dev Jayaraman[11], Anne Julie Frenette[3,4] and David Williamson[3,4]*

Abstract

Background: Opioids and benzodiazepines are frequently used in the intensive care unit (ICU). Regular use and prolonged exposure to opioids in ICU patients followed by abrupt tapering or cessation may lead to iatrogenic withdrawal syndrome (IWS). IWS is well described in pediatrics, but no prospective study has evaluated this syndrome in adult ICU patients. The objective of this study was to determine the incidence of IWS caused by opioids in a critically ill adult population. This multicenter prospective cohort study was conducted at two level-1 trauma ICUs between February 2015 and September 2015 and included 54 critically ill patients. Participants were eligible if they were 18 years and older, mechanically ventilated and had received more than 72 h of regular intermittent or continuous intravenous infusion of opioids. For each enrolled patient and per each opioid weaning episode, presence of IWS was assessed by a qualified ICU physician or senior resident according to the 5th edition of Diagnostic and Statistical Manual of Mental Disorders criteria for opioid withdrawal.

Results: The population consisted mostly of males (74.1%) with a median age of 50 years (25th–75th percentile 38.2–64.5). The median ICU admission APACHE II score was 22 (25th–75th percentile 12.0–28.2). The overall incidence of IWS was 16.7% (95% CI 6–27). The median cumulative opioid dose prior to weaning was higher in patients with IWS (245.7 vs. 169.4 mcg/kg, fentanyl equivalent). Patients with IWS were also exposed to opioids for a longer period of time as compared to patients without IWS (median 151 vs. 125 h). However, these results were not statistically significant.

Conclusions: IWS was occasionally observed in this very specific population of mechanically ventilated, critically ill ICU patients. Further studies are needed to confirm these preliminary results and identify risk factors.

Keywords: Iatrogenic withdrawal syndrome, Opioids, DSM-V, Mechanical ventilation, Critically ill, Intensive care unit, Adult

Background

Opioids and benzodiazepines are frequently used in the intensive care unit (ICU) to treat pain, agitation and facilitate mechanical ventilation [1, 2]. Prolonged stimulation of μ, κ and δ receptors by opioids in the central nervous system and in the peripheral tissues leads to down-regulation of intracellular second-messenger signaling, thus inducing tolerance. If the inhibitory stimulus is abruptly removed, a set of symptoms including central nervous stimulation (e.g., agitation, irritability, tremors, increased wakefulness), sympathetic nervous system hyper-activation (e.g., fever, hypertension, tachycardia, tachypnea, sweating) and gastrointestinal disturbance (e.g., vomiting, nausea, diarrhea) can occur. This phenomenon is

*Correspondence: david.williamson@umontreal.ca
[3] Pharmacy Department, Hôpital du Sacré-Coeur de Montréal, 5400 Gouin West, Montreal, QC H4J 1C5, Canada
Full list of author information is available at the end of the article

known as acute iatrogenic withdrawal syndrome (IWS) [3].

IWS is well described in the pediatric ICU (PICU) population [4–8]. An incidence ranging from 10 to 57% has been reported in children receiving mechanical ventilation and continuous infusion of opioids for more than 24 h [7, 8]. Withdrawal symptoms in the pediatric population, as described by the Finnegan Neonatal Abstinence Scale, include irritability, tremors, clonus, yawning, sneezing, delirium, hypertonicity, seizures and hallucinations [9]. In more severe cases, sympathetic activation may result in tachycardia, hypertension, tachypnea, sweating, fever, as well as gastrointestinal symptoms such as feeding intolerance with vomiting and diarrhea [9, 10]. As a result, IWS can complicate patient recovery [11, 12].

In adult ICU patients, a retrospective study reported an incidence of 32% (9 of 28 patients) for analgesic and sedative medications IWS [13]. In that study, IWS evaluation was based on a modified version of the Himmelsbach scale [13]. To our knowledge, there are no published prospective studies evaluating the incidence and risk factors for opioid-associated IWS in the adult ICU population.

The primary objective of this study was to prospectively evaluate the incidence of IWS in mechanically ventilated adult ICU patients receiving opioids. Possible risk factors for opioid-associated IWS in this patient population were also assessed.

Methods

Study design

The study was a prospective observational cohort conducted in two level-1 trauma centers in Montreal, Canada (clinicalTrials.gov. NCT02318290). Enrollment occurred between February 2015 and September 2015. The study was reviewed and approved by the institutional research ethics committees of each participating site.

Participants

Participants were eligible if they were 18 years and older, mechanically ventilated and had received regular intermittent or continuous intravenous infusion of opioids for more than 72 h. Patients were considered as receiving regular intermittent opioids if more than half of the scheduled "as-needed" doses within the previous 24 h were administered. Initially, participants were included after 96 h of mechanical ventilation and opioids administration. This inclusion criterion was later amended to 72 h due to the limited number of eligible patients. Initial consent was obtained from next of kin, and whenever possible, participation was later confirmed by the patient.

Patients were excluded if they were unable to speak English or French, had physical communication barriers, suffered from severe brain injury defined as Glasgow Coma Scale (GCS) ≤ 8 or moderate brain injury (GCS 9–12) with elevated intracranial pressure (ICP > 20 mmHg requiring osmotherapy). Other exclusion criteria included imminent and predictable death, active neurological condition such as status epilepticus, encephalopathy, chronic substance abuse (chronic alcohol use defined as ≥ 2 drinks per day and/or ≥ 14 drinks per week for men and ≥ 9 drinks per week for women, regular use of heroin, γ-hydroxybutyric acid, cocaine or amphetamines), chronic use of opioids prior to ICU admission (defined as regular use for a chronic medical reason reported by next of kin or per home medication list), spinal cord injury, and extubation during the first 72 h.

Procedures and data collection

Patient demographics collected at enrollment included age, gender, past medical history, reason of ICU admission (according to ICD-10 classification) and Acute Physiology and Chronic Health Evaluation II score (APACHE II). Opioids, concomitant sedatives (benzodiazepines, propofol and dexmedetomidine), other co-analgesics, length of ICU stay, and duration of mechanical ventilation were prospectively collected using standardized case report forms. All opioids and benzodiazepines doses were converted into fentanyl and midazolam equivalents, respectively.

There were no standardized opioid weaning protocols at either site. Patient management including all decisions related to analgesia, sedation, weaning and agitation was left to the discretion of the treating team. An opioid weaning episode was defined as a sustained over 4-h $\geq 10\%$ decrease from the previous stable infusion rate (defined as stable for at least 4 h). Upon weaning, the patient was assessed once daily by an ICU physician to detect the potential development of IWS using the Diagnostic and Statistical Manual 5th edition (DSM-V) criteria for opioid withdrawal [14]. The DSM-V criteria include the presence of either cessation or reduction in opioid use that has been heavy and prolonged (adapted to >72 h in our study) and ≥ 3 of the following criteria developing within minutes to several days following cessation or reduction: dysphoric mood, nausea or vomiting, muscle aches, lacrimation or rhinorrhea, pupillary dilatation, piloerection, sweating, yawning, fever, insomnia [15]. IWS was diagnosed if ≥ 3 of the criteria were observed after weaning, and the symptoms could not be explained by another medical condition such as delirium or infection. For each enrolled patient-weaning episode, a second ICU physician or fellow participated in a blinded assessment. A patient was classified as IWS-positive if at least one of the DSM-V evaluations was positive. Patients were followed until death or transfer to another unit. In addition, patients that remained in the ICU were followed for 48 h after the first of the following events: (1) a DSM-V-positive result; (2) an extubation; (3) 14 days after a successful weaning process. Delirium was assessed using daily Confusion Assessment Method for the intensive care unit (CAM-ICU) evaluations.

Statistical analysis

Descriptive data are expressed as proportions and continuous variables as medians with 25th–75th percentiles. The incidence of IWS is defined as the proportion of patients with a positive IWS diagnosis and is presented with 95% confidence intervals. The Mann–Whitney U test was used to compare demographics, cumulative dose of opioids, and duration of exposure to opioids between the IWS-positive and the IWS-negative groups. Chi-square or Fisher's exact tests, as appropriate, were used to compare exposure to concomitant medications. A two-sided p value <0.05 was considered statistically

significant. The last observation carried forward (LOCF) was used to analyze missing observations. Listwise deletion was used for missing demographic data. An independent accredited statistician validated the statistical analyses. Data analysis was performed with IBM SPSS Statistics v. 21.0.

Results

Patient characteristics

All patients admitted to ICU within the study period were screened. Of the 1520 patients screened, 54 were included in the study (Fig. 1). Ten and forty-four patients had received opioids for at least 72 and 96 h, respectively. Main reasons for exclusion were short duration of mechanical ventilation, opioid administration less than 72 h (1300 patients) and imminent death (41 patients).

The study population was mainly comprised of men (74.1%) and Caucasians (81.5%) with a median age of 50 years (25th–75th percentile 38.2–64.5) (Table 1). The

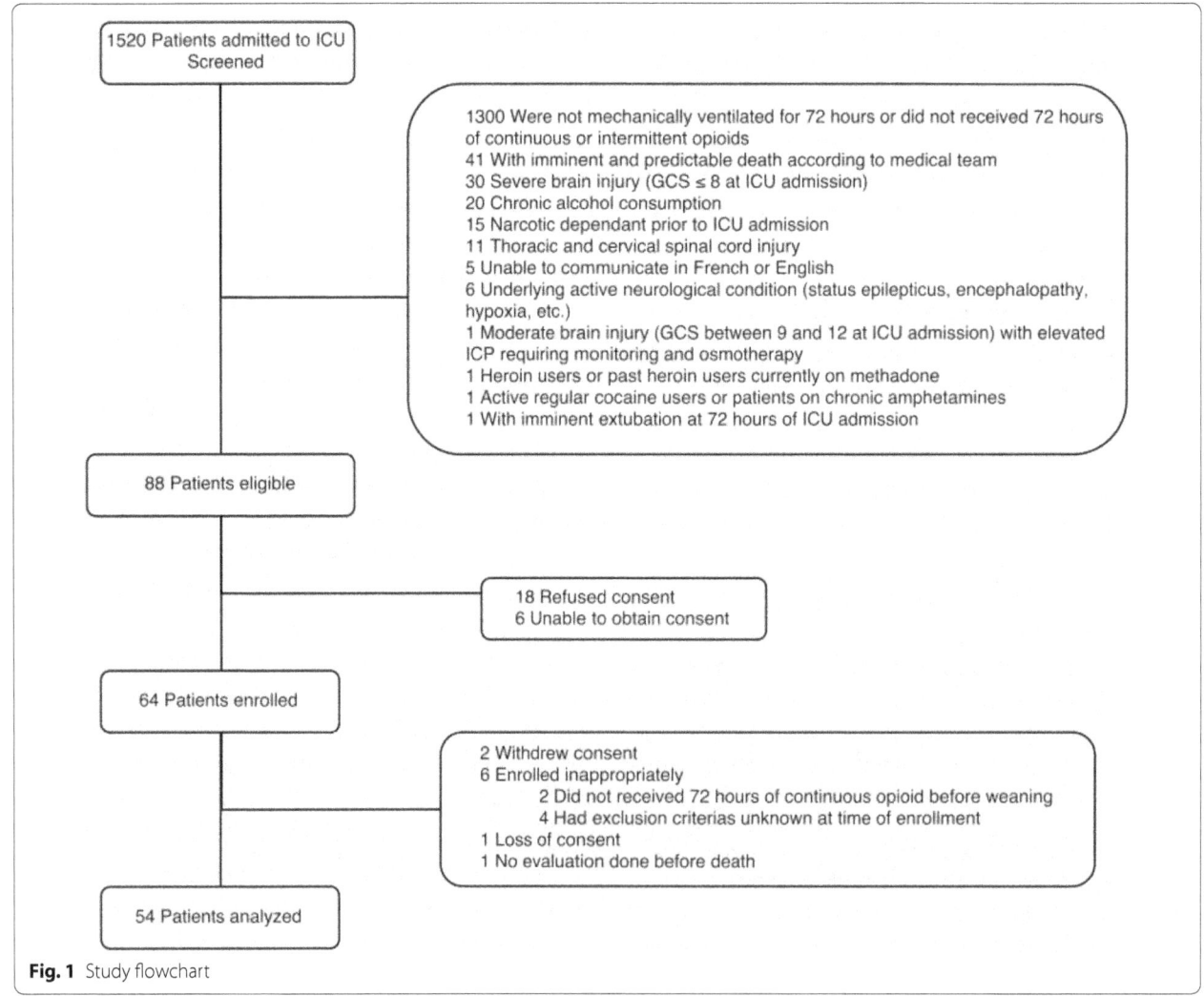

Fig. 1 Study flowchart

Table 1 Patient demographics

Characteristics	IWS-negative (n = 45)	IWS-positive (n = 9)	All patients (n = 54)
Median age (year) (25th–75th percentile)	53 (40.5–66)	46 (26–59)	50 (38.2–64.5)
Male, no (%)	34 (75.6)	6 (66.3)	40 (74.1)
Median APACHE II (25th–75th percentile)	22 (15.5–28.5)	25 (13–31)	22 (12–28.2)
Median weight (kg) (25th–75th percentile)	85 (79–100)	75 (67.2–95.7)	83.5 (75.8–98.4)
Creatinine ICU adm (μmol/L) (25th–75th percentile)	122 (87–179.5)	106 (72–315)	116 (87–209)
Length of mechanical ventilation (h)	188 (120–358)	286 (197–789.5)	226.5 (124.3–380.3)
Median length of ICU stay, days (IQR)	17 (9.5–22.5)	21 (11–42.5)	17.5 (10–23)
Reason of admission (ICD-10) n (%)			
External causes of morbidity (e.g., trauma)	17 (37.8)	4 (44.4)	21 (38.9)
Diseases of the respiratory system	8 (17.8)	0	8 (14.8)
Symptoms and signs not elsewhere classified	4 (8.9)	3 (33.3)	7 (13.0)
Circulatory system	7 (15.6)	0	7 (13.0)
Digestive system	3 (6.7)	0	3 (5.6)
Musculoskeletal/connective tissues	2 (4.4)	1 (11.1)	3 (5.6)
Nervous system	1 (2.2)	1 (11.1)	2 (3.7)
Other categories	3 (6.6)	0 (0)	3 (5.6)

median APACHE II score was 22.0 (25th–75th percentile 12.0–28.2). The most frequent reasons of admission according to ICD-10 classification were external causes of morbidity (e.g., trauma and injuries) (38.9%) and diseases of the respiratory system (14.8%). Prior to admission, 13 (24.1%) patients reported non-chronic alcohol consumption (<14 drinks per week in men and <9 drinks in women). Thirteen patients (24.1%) were tobacco smokers, and 1 patient (1.9%) was a sporadic recreational amphetamine user. Two patients (3.7%) had received sporadic opioid doses due to acute medical conditions prior to hospital admission.

When compared to IWS-negative patients, IWS-positive patients were slightly younger (median age of 46 vs. 53 years; $p = 0.34$), had nonsignificantly higher APACHE II scores (median 25 vs. 22 points; $p = 0.96$), had longer durations of mechanical ventilation (median 286 vs. 188 h; $p = 0.08$) and had longer ICU stays (median 21 vs. 17 days; $p = 0.21$) (Tables 1, 2).

Incidence of IWS

Incidence of IWS was 16.7% (9 out of 54 patients) (95% CI, 6–27%). Onset of IWS ranged from 1 to 11 days following opioid cessation or dose reduction (median = 2 days; 25th–75th percentile 1–4). The agreement between two raters for the 38 evaluations of IWS-based DSM-V criteria was concordant in 90.1% of cases.

Table 2 Opioid exposure and mechanical ventilation

Study group	IWS-negative (n = 45) Median (25th–75th percentile) [min, max]	IWS-positive (n = 9) Median (25th–75th percentile) [min, max]	p value
Cumulative opioid dose prior to weaning (mcg/kg)	169.4 (117,7–234,2) [11.7, 865.6]	245.7 (135,7–437,6) [72.4, 722.4]	$p = 0.32$
Duration of opioid infusion until the first wean (h)[a]	125 (88–243) [57, 564]	151 (81–397) [76, 428]	$p = 0.47$
Duration of mechanical ventilation (h)[b]	188 (122–340) [59, 1201]	286 (207–566) [111, 1245]	$p = 0.08$
Weaning rate (%)	75 (50–100) [12.50, 100]	100 (40–100) [20, 100]	$p = 0.98$

Weaning rate is defined as the difference between the previous stable infusion rate and the new stable infusion rate

[a] The last observation carried forward method was used for 1 patient in each group; opioid begin date = ICU admission date

[b] The last observation carried forward was used for 3 patients in IWS-negative group and 1 in IWS-positive group

Risk factors for IWS

Although not statistically significant ($p = 0.32$), the cumulative opioid dose (fentanyl equivalent) prior to weaning was greater in IWS-positive (median 245.7 mcg/kg; 25th–75th percentile 135.7–437.6) than in IWS-negative patients (median 169.4 mcg/kg; 25th–75th percentile 117.6–234.2) (Table 2). Likewise, duration of continuous opioid prior to weaning was longer in the IWS-positive group (median 151 h; 25th–75th percentile 81–397) compared to the IWS-negative group (median 125 h; 25th–75th percentile 88–243) ($p = 0.47$). Peak daily opioid dose prior to weaning was also higher in IWS-positive patients (median 4175 mcg; 3130–4997.5 25th–75th percentile) than in IWS-negative patients (3550 mcg; 2737.5–4650 25th–75th percentile). However, this difference was not statistically significant ($p = 0.24$). The percentage in opioid dose reduction at the time of IWS evaluation compared to baseline was similar ($p = 0.98$) between IWS-positive (median 100%; IQR 40–100) and IWS-negative patients (median 75%; IQR 50–100).

Benzodiazepines (100 vs. 71.1%; $p = 0.254$) and clonidine (22.2 vs. 15.6%; $p = 0.469$) were used more frequently in the IWS-positive group than in the IWS-negative group, but it did not reach statistical significance. Antipsychotics (100 vs. 57.8%; $p = 0.013$) were significantly used more frequently in the IWS-positive group than in the IWS-negative group (Table 3). When only considering exposed patients, the benzodiazepine cumulative daily dose was more important in patients diagnosed with IWS (median 12.91 vs. 5.84 mg/kg; $p = 0.235$). In comparison, propofol (97.8 vs. 88.9%; $p = 0.308$) and dexmedetomidine (31.1 vs. 22.2%; $p = 0.463$) were used more frequently in the IWS-negative group.

Delirium

The overall incidence of delirium during the study was 35.2% (19/54 patients). Delirium was concomitantly identified in 4 of the 9 patients who were identified with IWS (44%).

Discussion

To our knowledge, this is the first prospective study to evaluate the incidence of IWS in an adult ICU population and to explore its potential risk factors. We reported an IWS incidence of 16.7% (95% CI 6–27%) in our study population. IWS is probably uncommon in the general ICU population. However, it may be more frequent in patients with prolonged mechanical ventilation requiring long-term opioids. Other authors have reported a higher incidence of IWS (32%) [13]. A much shorter duration of mechanical ventilation (12 vs. 39 days in patients with IWS) and a shorter study inclusion opioid exposure (72 vs. 96 h) in our patients could explain this discrepancy [13]. Also, some IWS cases may have been missed because of short-term follow-up. On the other hand, the prospective observational design of this study may have sensitized the physicians to the possible presence of IWS in patients and to its potential prevention. This could potentially have influenced the observed incidence.

In our study, only about 1% of the screened patients were opioid dependent prior to admission. It would be fair to expect opioid withdrawal to be more common in a population with higher rates of opioid use and abuse. Another possible explanation for a lower IWS incidence is our relatively short follow-up for some of the included patients. In the PICU population, withdrawal symptoms have been reported up to 6 days following ≥10% weaning of opioids and/or benzodiazepines [6]. Similarly, in the retrospective study by Cammarano et al., 9 out of 28 patients experienced withdrawal, of which 2 developed IWS in the ICU and 7 on the ward [13]. In our study, the median onset of IWS was 2 days after opioid weaning. However, 25 of the 45 IWS-negative patients (55.6%) were not followed for more than 48 h after extubation as per protocol, and many were rapidly discharged from the

Table 3 Concomitant medications received until end of follow-up

Characteristics	IWS-negative ($n = 45$)	IWS-positive ($n = 9$)
Median cumulative dose of benzodiazepine (mg/kg) (25th–75th percentiles)	5.84 (1.29–13.64) ($n = 29$)	12.91 (3.92–14.10) ($n = 8$)
Propofol	44 (97.8)	8 (88.9)
Dexmedetomidine	14 (31,1)	2 (22.2)
Benzodiazepine	32 (71.1)	9 (100)
Acetaminophen	45 (100)	9 (100)
Pregabalin	5 (11.1)	1 (11.1)
Clonidine	7 (15.6)	2 (22.2)
Antipsychotics	26 (57.8)	9 (100)*

*$p = <0.05$

ICU to other care units. The later occurrence of IWS in these patients is therefore unknown. As the collaborating physicians were no longer the patients-treating physicians once patients left the ICU, we were unable to prospectively evaluate IWS after ICU discharge.

As previously reported in the PICU population, the most probable risk factors for IWS are the cumulative opioid dose and the duration of continuous exposure to opioids [15]. Although the differences did not reach statistical significance, the median cumulative opioid dose adjusted for weight, the median daily peak dose of opioid and the median duration of opioid exposure were higher in the IWS-positive group than in the IWS-negative group. A pediatric study also identified a rapid opioid dose decrease as a risk factor for IWS [7]. This observation was not confirmed by our study. It was also impossible to distinguish the possible association of IWS with specific opioid agents, since all but 3 patients (6% receiving morphine) were on fentanyl infusions.

In PICU studies, IWS has been associated with increased morbidity, hospital costs and psychological distress [7]. Our data suggest similar associations as patients in the IWS-positive group were more heavily sedated (cumulative benzodiazepine dose 12.91 vs. 5.84 mg/kg), were mechanically ventilated for a longer period and had longer ICU stays.

This study has several strengths including its prospective design. As there is currently no validated tool to identify opioid withdrawal syndrome in the adult ICU population, the diagnosis was performed using the DSM-V criteria for opioid withdrawal. IWS diagnosis was also corroborated by clinical judgment, taking into account other differential diagnosis for the featured symptoms. Systematically using the CAM-ICU, delirium was concomitantly diagnosed in 44% of our patients presenting IWS. However, the overlapping of delirium with IWS remains unstudied.

This study also has several limitations including its small sample size. The agreement between raters analysis for the diagnosis of IWS using the DSM-V was also limited to concordance because of the low prevalence of IWS. The reliability and accuracy of the DSM-V for the diagnosis of IWS in an adult ICU population remain to be studied. While others have studied both opioid- and benzodiazepine-related IWS, we focused on opioid-associated IWS [13, 15]. The administration of benzodiazepines was treated as a potential confounding factor. The specific contribution of benzodiazepine exposure to IWS could not be isolated, as benzodiazepines and opioids are often co-administered. Frequency of benzodiazepine use was not statistically different in patients with and without IWS. However, we cannot exclude the contribution of benzodiazepine to IWS in the exposed patients.

The results of this study can only be extrapolated to a subset of patients admitted to the ICU. Of note, 86% of the initially screened patients were excluded due to the absence of mechanical ventilation or because of insufficient opioid exposure. Finally, 38% of the eligible patients refused or withdrew consent to participate, which also weakens the external validity of the study. In summary, more studies are needed for greater recognition of the syndrome and appropriate prevention of IWS in the adult population.

Conclusion

IWS is occasionally observed in critically ill adult patients mechanically ventilated and receiving opioids for more than 72 h. Higher cumulative dose and longer exposure of opioid may have contributed to the increased risk of IWS. Future studies with a larger sample size and a longer follow-up period are needed to confirm these preliminary results.

Abbreviations

APACHE II: Acute Physiology and Chronic Health Evaluation II score; CAM-ICU: Confusion Assessment Method for the intensive care unit; DSM-V: 5th edition of Diagnostic and Statistical Manual of Mental Disorders; ICU: intensive care unit; IWS: iatrogenic withdrawal syndrome; LOCF: last observation carried forward; PICU: pediatric intensive care unit; WAAICUP-1: Withdrawal Assessment in Adult ICU Population-1.

Authors' contributions

PPW, EH, XF and CB were involved in the study design, study realization, data collection, data analysis and manuscript drafting. MMP, AJF, PM and DW were involved in the study design, study realization, data analysis and manuscript drafting. PR, PB, AL and DJ participated in the study realization and reviewed the manuscript for important intellectual content. CG was involved in the study design and reviewed the manuscript for important intellectual content. All authors read and approved the final manuscript.

Author details

[1] Pharmacy Department, Lakeshore General Hospital, Montreal, Canada. [2] Pharmacy Department, Hôpital de Verdun, Montreal, Canada. [3] Pharmacy Department, Hôpital du Sacré-Coeur de Montréal, 5400 Gouin West, Montreal, QC H4J 1C5, Canada. [4] Faculté de Pharmacie, Université de Montréal, Montreal, Canada. [5] Pharmacy Department, McGill University Health Center, Montreal, Canada. [6] Critical Care Department, Hôpital du Sacré-Coeur de Montréal, Montreal, Canada. [7] Faculté de Médecine, Université de Montréal, Montreal, Canada. [8] Ingram School of Nursing, McGill University, Montreal, QC, Canada. [9] Centre for Nursing Research and Lady Davis Institute, Jewish General Hospital, Montreal, Canada. [10] Department of Adult Critical Care, Jewish General Hospital, McGill University, Montreal, QC, Canada. [11] Department of Critical Care, Montreal General Hospital, McGill University Health Center, Montreal, Canada.

Acknowledgements

The authors would like to thank our colleagues from The Montreal General Hospital: Anissa Capilnean, Vlad Rosu, Patricia Sandu and Amanda Martone for their partnership. We would like to express our gratefulness to ICU nursing and physician staff for their collaboration at both sites. We would also thank Simon Lessard for participating in the conception and writing of the protocol.

Competing interests

The authors declare that they have no competing interests.

Funding
This project is supported by an investigator-initiated grant from Hospira/Pfizer Canada.

References
1. Barr J, Fraser GL, Puntillo K, Ely EW, Gelinas C, et al. Clinical practice guidelines for the management of pain, agitation, and delirium in adult patients in the intensive care unit. Crit Care Med. 2013;41:263–306.
2. Jacobi J, Fraser GL, Coursin DB, Riker RR, Fontaine D, et al. Clinical practice guidelines for the sustained use of sedatives and analgesics in the critically ill adult. Crit Care Med. 2002;30:119–41.
3. Devlin JW, Mallow-Corbett S, Riker RR. Adverse drug events associated with the use of analgesics, sedatives, and antipsychotics in the intensive care unit. Crit Care Med. 2010;38:S231–43.
4. Fernandez-Carrion F, Gaboli M, Gonzalez-Celador R, Gomez de Quero-Masia P, Fernandez-de Miguel S, et al. Withdrawal syndrome in the pediatric intensive care unit. Incidence and risk factors. Med Intensiva/Sociedad Espanola de Medicina Intensiva y Unidades Coronarias. 2013;37:67–74.
5. Franck LS, Naughton I, Winter I. Opioid and benzodiazepine withdrawal symptoms in paediatric intensive care patients. Intensive Crit Care Nurs. 2004;20:344–51.
6. Hughes J, Gill A, Leach HJ, Nunn AJ, Billingham I, et al. A prospective study of the adverse effects of midazolam on withdrawal in critically ill children. Acta Paediatr. 1994;83:1194–9.
7. Birchley G. Opioid and benzodiazepine withdrawal syndromes in the paediatric intensive care unit: a review of recent literature. Nurs Crit Care. 2009;14:26–37.
8. Katz R, Kelly HW, Hsi A. Prospective study on the occurrence of withdrawal in critically ill children who receive fentanyl by continuous infusion. Crit Care Med. 1994;22:763–7.
9. Finnegan LP, Connaughton JF Jr, Kron RE, Emich JP. Neonatal abstinence syndrome: assessment and management. Addict Dis. 1975;2:141–58.
10. Tobias JD. Tolerance, withdrawal, and physical dependency after long-term sedation and analgesia of children in the pediatric intensive care unit. Crit Care Med. 2000;28:2122–32.
11. Biswas AK, Feldman BL, Davis DH, Zintz EA. Myocardial ischemia as a result of severe benzodiazepine and opioid withdrawal. Clin Toxicol. 2005;43:207–9.
12. Franck LS, Vilardi J, Durand D, Powers R. Opioid withdrawal in neonates after continuous infusions of morphine or fentanyl during extracorporeal membrane oxygenation. Am J Criti Care. 1998;7:364–9.
13. Cammarano WB, Pittet JF, Weitz S, Schlobohm RM, Marks JD. Acute withdrawal syndrome related to the administration of analgesic and sedative medications in adult intensive care unit patients. Crit Care Med. 1998;26:676–84.
14. American Psychiatric Association. 2013. *Diagnostic and statistical manual of mental disorders: DSM-5*. Washington, DC: American Psychiatric Publishing. xliv, 947 pages pp.
15. Ista E, van Dijk M, Gamel C, Tibboel D, de Hoog M. Withdrawal symptoms in critically ill children after long-term administration of sedatives and/or analgesics: a first evaluation. Crit Care Med. 2008;36:2427–32.

11

Prognostic impact of isolated right ventricular dysfunction in sepsis and septic shock

Saraschandra Vallabhajosyula[1,2,3,4], Mukesh Kumar[3,5], Govind Pandompatam[2], Ankit Sakhuja[2], Rahul Kashyap[3,5], Kianoush Kashani[2,3,6], Ognjen Gajic[2,3], Jeffrey B. Geske[1] and Jacob C. Jentzer[1,2]*

Abstract

Background: Echocardiographic myocardial dysfunction is reported commonly in sepsis and septic shock, but there are limited data on sepsis-related right ventricular dysfunction. This study sought to evaluate the association of right ventricular dysfunction with clinical outcomes in patients with severe sepsis and septic shock.

Methods: Historical cohort study of adult patients admitted to all intensive care units at the Mayo Clinic from January 1, 2007 through December 31, 2014 for severe sepsis and septic shock, who had an echocardiogram performed within 72 h of admission. Patients with prior heart failure, cor-pulmonale, pulmonary hypertension and valvular disease were excluded. Right ventricular dysfunction was defined by the American Society of Echocardiography criteria. Outcomes included 1-year survival, in-hospital mortality and length of stay.

Results: Right ventricular dysfunction was present in 214 (55%) of 388 patients who met the inclusion criteria—isolated right ventricular dysfunction was seen in 100 (47%) and combined right and left ventricular dysfunction in 114 (53%). The baseline characteristics were similar between cohorts except for the higher mechanical ventilation use in patients with isolated right ventricular dysfunction. Echocardiographic findings demonstrated lower right ventricular and tricuspid valve velocities in patients with right ventricular dysfunction and lower left ventricular ejection fraction and increased mitral E/e' ratios in patients with combined right and left ventricular dysfunction. After adjustment for age, comorbidity, illness severity, septic shock and use of mechanical ventilation, isolated right ventricular dysfunction was independently associated with worse 1-year survival—hazard ratio 1.6 [95% confidence interval 1.2–2.1; $p = 0.002$) in patients with sepsis and septic shock.

Conclusions: Isolated right ventricular dysfunction is seen commonly in sepsis and septic shock and is associated with worse long-term survival.

Keywords: Sepsis, Septic shock, Right ventricle, Sepsis-related myocardial dysfunction, Mortality

Background

Sepsis-related myocardial dysfunction is frequently seen in patients with severe sepsis and septic shock [1–3]. Left ventricular (LV) systolic and diastolic dysfunction have been extensively studied in these patients and have demonstrated a variable correlation with clinical outcomes [1, 2]. In contrast, the evaluation and clinical consequences of right ventricular (RV) dysfunction in septic patients has received lesser attention [4]. RV dysfunction in sepsis is multifactorial and can be due to direct myocardial depression, hemodynamic derangements or increase in RV afterload due to hypoxemia, hypercapnia and mechanical ventilation for acute respiratory failure [5]. RV dysfunction is reported in 30–60% of all septic patients and is frequently associated with concomitant LV dysfunction [6, 7]. With the increasing use and evolution of echocardiographic methods for assessment of RV function, such

*Correspondence: Jentzer.Jacob@mayo.edu
[1] Department of Cardiovascular Medicine, Mayo Clinic, 200 First Street SW, Rochester, MN 55905, USA
Full list of author information is available at the end of the article

as semiquantitative RV size and performance, tissue Doppler imaging (TDI) and strain imaging, there is greater evidence of RV dysfunction occurring in sepsis [3, 7].

In this study, the clinical profile and outcomes of patients with RV dysfunction in severe sepsis and septic shock were evaluated. We hypothesized that patients with RV dysfunction would have worse long-term survival and higher hospital mortality. Among patients with RV dysfunction, patients with combined RV and LV dysfunction were hypothesized to have a worse prognosis compared to those with isolated RV dysfunction.

Methods

This historical cohort study screened all adult patients who were admitted to the intensive care units (ICU) at Mayo Clinic Rochester with severe sepsis and septic shock from January 1, 2007 through December 31, 2014. Patients with a formal, clinically indicated transthoracic echocardiogram within 72 h of ICU admission were included in this study. The characteristics of these ICU populations have been described previously [8, 9]. This study was approved by the Mayo Clinic Institutional Review Board as minimal risk to subjects and all activities were carried out in accordance with the modified Declaration of Helsinki. Patients with denial of Minnesota research authorization, known pregnancy, documented history of complex congenital heart disease, patent foramen ovale, moderate or greater valvular stenosis or regurgitation, prior heart failure, asymptomatic LV dysfunction, prior cor-pulmonale, pulmonary hypertension or recent acute coronary syndrome (<1 week) were excluded from the study.

Data: sources, definitions and management

The 2001 American College of Chest Physicians/Society of Critical Care Medicine consensus criteria were used to define sepsis [10]. Sepsis was defined as suspicion of infection and 2/4 positive systematic inflammatory response syndrome criteria. Severe sepsis was defined as sepsis with consequent organ hypoperfusion and dysfunction as defined by lactate ≥ 4.0 mmol/L and/or systolic blood pressure ≤ 90 mmHg. Septic shock was defined as fluid-resistant hypotension (systolic blood pressure ≤ 90 mmHg despite ≥ 30 mL/kg crystalloid resuscitation) and/or use of vasopressors (norepinephrine, epinephrine, dopamine, vasopressin or phenylephrine) [11].

Patients with severe sepsis and septic shock were detected using previously validated automated search algorithms [11–13]. This algorithm has 80% sensitivity and 96% specificity for detection of severe sepsis. Demographic and clinical information was automatically abstracted from the electronic health records saved in the integrated Multidisciplinary Epidemiology and Translational Research in Intensive Care Laboratory DataMart [9, 14]. Prior acute or chronic heart failure, prior cor-pulmonale and pulmonary hypertension were evaluated using a combination of International Classification of Diseases, Clinical Modification version 9.0 diagnostic codes, pre-hospitalization echocardiogram and hemodynamic catheterization data. Laboratory, imaging and physiological parameters closest to ICU admission were abstracted. Hemodynamics, vital sign data, ventilator parameters and fluid data are collected in real time every 15 min into the DataMart and were used to coordinate data abstraction closest to the timing of echocardiography. Pre-admission echocardiography within the last 1 year was used to exclude prior ventricular dysfunction, and a combination of pre-admission echocardiogram and first hospital echocardiogram was used to exclude congenital and valvular heart disease. The severity of illness was measured using Acute Physiology and Chronic Health Evaluation III (APACHE-III) and SOFA scores. All patients with sepsis and septic shock have blood cultures and lactate levels checked, and receive 30 ml/kg intravenous fluid and antimicrobial therapy within 3 h of sepsis onset as detected by electronic search algorithm. This is a part of an ongoing quality improvement initiative in the ICUs at Mayo Clinic [11, 15].

American Society of Echocardiography (ASE) criteria were utilized for echocardiographic assessment [16]. New onset RV dysfunction was assessed using multimodality parameters as defined by the ASE criteria, i.e., specifically semiquantitative size and function, tricuspid annular plane systolic excursion (TAPSE) <16 mm by M-mode, tricuspid lateral annulus tissue Doppler systolic velocity <0.15 cm/s and RV fractional area change <35% [17]. LV dysfunction was defined as either LV systolic or diastolic dysfunction, or both. LV systolic dysfunction was defined as LV ejection fraction $\leq 50\%$ [16]. LV diastolic function was classified according to standard ASE criteria, and grades II–IV were considered as diastolic dysfunction [18]. Three independent investigators (SV, MK and GP) reviewed the relevant variables and, when needed, performed manual chart reviews to ensure accuracy and fidelity of data.

The primary outcome was 1-year survival, and secondary outcomes included in-hospital mortality, ICU length of stay, ICU-free days and hospital length of stay. Mortality data were abstracted from the Mayo Clinic databases, state of Minnesota electronic death certificates and the Rochester Epidemiology Project death data system [19].

Statistical analysis

Continuous data are presented as median (interquartile range [IQR]), and categorical data are presented as counts (percentages). Unpaired t test and Chi-square test were used to evaluate continuous and categorical outcomes. Odds ratio (OR) with corresponding 95% confidence intervals (CI) was used to report categorical variables in the univariate and multivariate analyses. Logistic regression and cox-proportional hazards models were used for the multivariate analysis of in-hospital mortality and 1-year survival, respectively. For the multivariate analyses, outcomes of in-hospital and 1-year mortality were analyzed using models designed from predictors with $p < 0.10$ in the univariate analysis and judgment of clinically relevant variables. Variables were assessed for collinearity prior to inclusion in the model, and only independent variables were included. The outcomes of in-hospital mortality and 1-year survival were reported using OR (95% CI) and hazard ratio (HR) (95% CI). Sensitivity analyses were performed for cohorts of patients with and without RV and/or LV dysfunction. Two-tailed $p < 0.05$ was considered statistically significant, and Bonferroni correction was used for multiple comparisons (p*k). All statistical analyses were performed with JMP version 10.0.1 (SAS Institute, Cary, NC).

Results

Of 1757 patients with severe sepsis and septic shock admitted to the ICUs at Mayo Clinic from 2007 to 2014, 388 (22.1%) met the eligibility criteria (Fig. 1). Using multimodality parameters, RV dysfunction was noted in 214 (55.2%) patients (Fig. 2). The patients were divided into three cohorts—isolated RV dysfunction (100; 25.8%), combined RV and LV dysfunction (114; 29.4%) and no RV dysfunction (174; 44.8%). Detailed baseline and echocardiographic parameters of the cohorts are described in Tables 1 and 2. The three cohorts differed in their severity of hypercapnia, use of mechanical ventilation and mean airway pressures during mechanical ventilation, but were comparable in all other characteristics. Patients with isolated RV dysfunction had higher associated use of invasive mechanical ventilation. RV size and function criteria were similar between isolated RV and combined RV/LV dysfunction. In keeping with the study definitions, patients with isolated RV and combined RV dysfunction had significantly lower TAPSE, and tricuspid annulus peak systolic TDI velocities than patients without RV

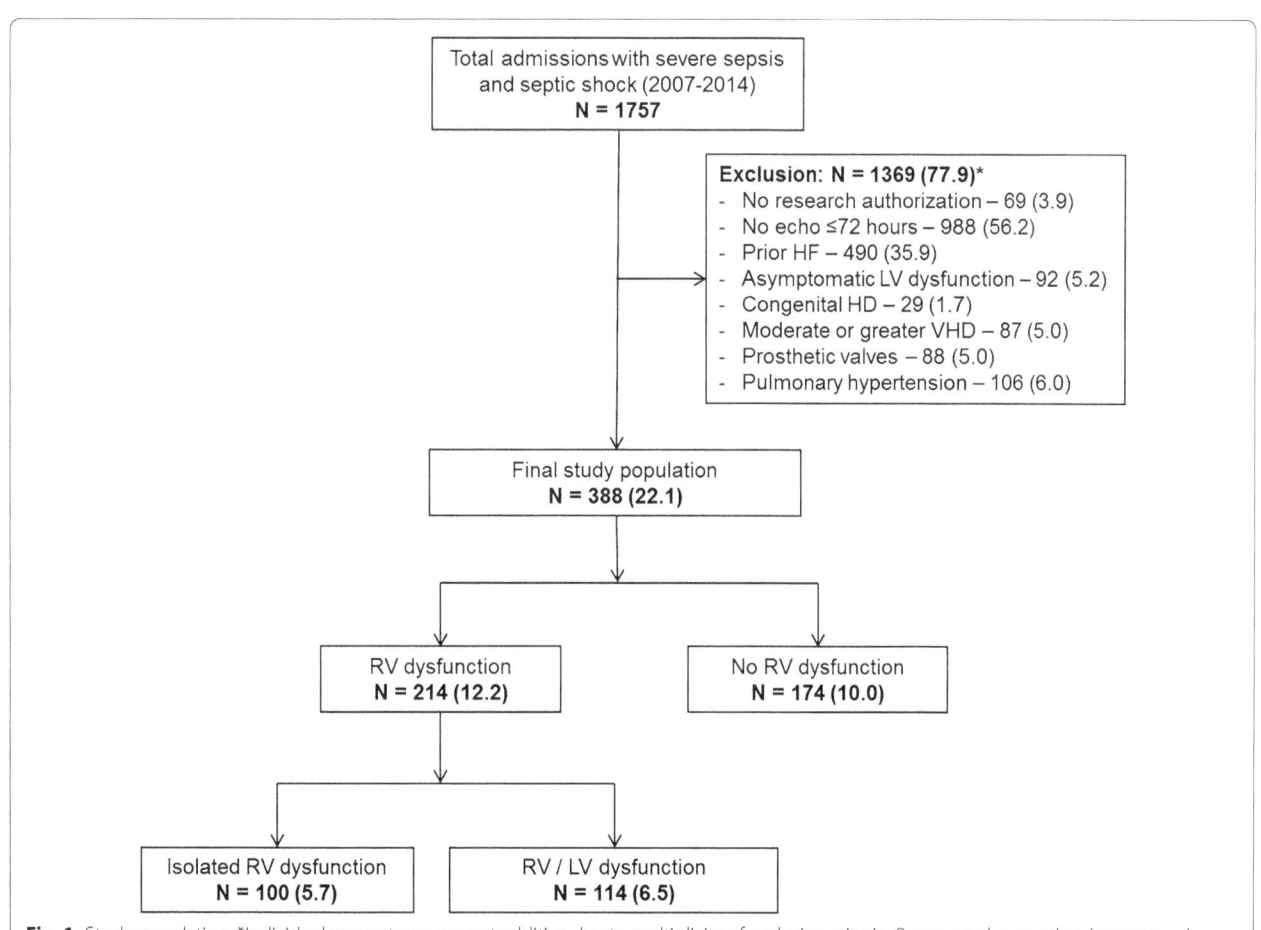

Fig. 1 Study population. *Individual percentages are not additive due to multiplicity of exclusion criteria. *Represented as*: number (percentage). *Abbreviations*: *HD* heart disease, *HF* heart failure, *LV* left ventricular, *RV*, right ventricular, *VHD* valvular heart disease

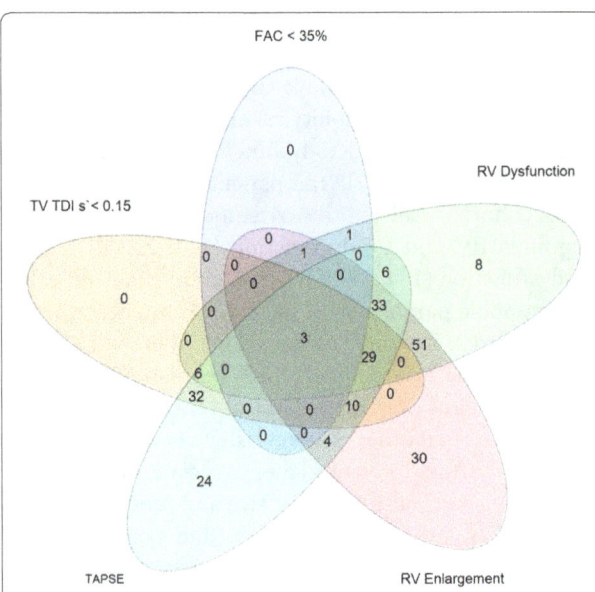

Fig. 2 Right ventricular dysfunction using multimodality parameters. *Abbreviations*: *FAC* fractional area change, *RV* right ventricular, *s′* systolic velocity, *TAPSE* tricuspid annular plane systolic excursion, *TDI* tissue Doppler imaging, *TV* tricuspid valve

dysfunction. Patients with combined RV/LV dysfunction had lower LV ejection fractions and higher medial E/e' ratios as compared to the other two groups (Table 2).

Clinical outcomes

Unadjusted 1-year survival was significantly lower in the cohort with isolated RV dysfunction as compared to patients with no RV dysfunction or combined RV/LV dysfunction ($p = 0.003$ by log-rank test) (Fig. 3). Unadjusted in-hospital mortality (30 vs. 16.7 vs. 22.4%; $p = 0.07$), ventilator-free days (9.9 [IQR 5.2–19.1] vs. 5.6 [IQR 4.1–10.4] vs. 6.6 [IQR 4–20.7] days); $p = 0.39$), ICU length of stay (3.2 [IQR 2–6.6] vs. 3 [IQR 1.6–5.4] vs. 2.9 [IQR 1.6–6.6] days; $p = 0.27$), ICU-free days (5 [IQR 1.9–13.6] vs. 4.9 [IQR 2.7–9.2] vs. 4.9 [IQR 2.1–11] days; $p = 0.84$) and hospital length of stay (9.3 [IQR 5.8–19.4] vs. 8.5 [IQR 6–14.4] vs. 9.8 [IQR 6.1–16.6] days; $p = 0.43$) were not different between the patients with isolated RV dysfunction, combined RV/LV dysfunction and no RV dysfunction. In the admission echocardiogram, 1-year survivors had higher tricuspid regurgitant jet velocity (2.9 [IQR 2.5–3.2] vs. 2.7 [IQR 2.4–3] m/s; $p = 0.005$) and RV systolic pressure (45 [IQR 36–56] vs. 41 [IQR 33–51] mmHg; $p = 0.002$), but did not differ in semiquantitative RV size (53.1 vs. 50%; $p = 0.53$), semiquantitative RV function (45.2 vs. 47.3%; $p = 0.66$), TAPSE (17.5 [IQR 14–22.3] vs. 18 [IQR 15–21] mm; $p = 0.90$) and tricuspid annulus peak systolic TDI velocity (0.13 [IQR 0.1–0.15] vs. 0.13 [IQR 0.1–0.13] m/s; $p = 0.76$). A sensitivity

analysis using visually estimated parameters (RV enlargement and RV dysfunction) only to define RV dysfunction did not demonstrate significant differences in in-hospital mortality. None of the measured echocardiographic parameters of RV function were different between hospital survivors and non-survivors.

In a cox-proportional hazards model adjusting for age, comorbidity, severity of illness, septic shock and use of mechanical ventilation, RV dysfunction was not an independent predictor of survival at 1 year in the total cohort (HR 0.9 [95% CI 0.6–1.5]; $p = 0.83$) (Table 3). Isolated RV dysfunction, however, was independently associated with worse long-term survival—HR 1.6 (95 CI 1.2–2.1), $p = 0.002$. Additional sensitivity analysis did not demonstrated combined RV/LV dysfunction to be an independent predictor of 1-year survival in the total cohort (HR 0.9 [95% CI 0.6–1.3]; $p = 0.52$).

Discussion

RV dysfunction was noted in nearly two-thirds of patients with severe sepsis and septic shock who underwent early echocardiography in this study. Patients with RV dysfunction had higher hypercapnia and use of mechanical ventilation. When adjusted for age, comorbidity, severity of illness and use of mechanical ventilation, isolated RV dysfunction was an independent predictor of worse 1-year survival. However, presence of RV dysfunction did not impact short-term mortality and in-hospital outcomes in this study.

Prior studies on RV dysfunction in sepsis and critical illness have conflicted regarding the prognostic impact of RV dysfunction [3, 7, 20, 21]. This is likely due to heterogeneity in the timing of echocardiography, modality of echocardiography and definitions used. Consistent with this study, a recent meta-analysis did not demonstrate any correlation of semiquantitative RV size and function parameters with short-term mortality in sepsis [22]. Interestingly in our study, RV dysfunction was predictive of long-term survival. These results corroborate those by Orde et al. who demonstrated reduced RV longitudinal strain to correlate with 6-month mortality (OR 1.1 [95% CI 1.02–1.26]; $p = 0.02$) in sepsis and septic shock [21]. In this study cohort, tricuspid regurgitant jet velocity and RV systolic pressure were significantly higher in 1-year survivors; however, no difference was noted in short-term survivors. This could potentially be a reflection of the acute loading conditions in sepsis resuscitation that subsequently resolved over long-term follow-up. In addition to semi-quantitative parameters, objective parameters such as TAPSE and tricuspid annulus peak systolic TDI velocity have also been used to define RV dysfunction in patients with sepsis and septic shock. Harmankaya et al. demonstrated lower tricuspid annulus peak systolic TDI

Table 1 Baseline characteristics of cohorts

Parameter	Isolated RV dysfunction ($n = 100$)	RV/LV dysfunction ($n = 114$)	No RV dysfunction ($n = 174$)	p
Age (years)	65.6 (55.2–77.5)	69.3 (55.3–77.4)	64.7 (53.4–74.7)	0.22
Male sex	48 (48)	59 (51.8)	91 (52.3)	0.78
Admitting location				0.13
Emergency room	53 (53)	52 (45.6)	86 (49.4)	
Hospital floors	21 (21)	28 (24.6)	55 (31.6)	
Outside transfer	26 (26)	34 (29.8)	33 (19)	
Source of sepsis				0.22
Respiratory	27 (27)	27 (23.7)	27 (15.5)	
Abdominal	2 (2)	3 (2.6)	8 (4.6)	
Genitourinary	4 (4)	6 (5.3)	18 (10.3)	
Skin/soft tissue	3 (3)	2 (1.8)	9 (5.2)	
Other/unknown	38 (38)	45 (39.5)	69 (39.7)	
Not available	26 (26)	31 (27.2)	43 (24.7)	
Body mass index (kg/m^2)	30.8 (24.6–36.7)	28.6 (25–33.5)	28.7 (24–33.7)	0.29
Body surface area (m^2)	2.0 (1.8–2.3)	1.9 (1.8–2.2)	1.9 (1.8–2.2)	0.27
Hypertension	35 (35)	51 (44.7)	71 (40.8)	0.35
Coronary artery disease	10 (10)	23 (20.2)	23 (13.2)	0.09
Prior myocardial infarction	7 (7)	13 (11.4)	14 (8.1)	0.48
Obstructive sleep apnea	10 (10)	19 (16.7)	22 (12.6)	0.34
Chronic lung disease	24 (24)	27 (23.7)	41 (23.6)	0.99
Charlson comorbidity index	5 (3–7)	6 (4–8)	5 (3–8)	0.40
APACHE-III score	85.5 (68.3–110)	84 (69–104)	81 (66–105)	0.54
SOFA score (day 1)	9 (7–12)	9 (7–11)	8 (5–12)	0.07
Septic shock	80 (80)	82 (71.9)	119 (68.4)	0.11
ARDS	30 (30)	36 (31.6)	49 (28.2)	0.82
Mild (n)	6	10	15	
Moderate (n)	18	18	22	
Severe (n)	6	8	12	
Acute kidney injury	62 (62)	74 (64.9)	110 (63.2)	0.91
Admission troponin-T (ng/mL)	0.06 (0.02–0.17)	0.05 (0.03–0.15)	0.06 (0.02–0.16)	0.90
Highest lactate (mmol/L)	2.8 (1.8–5.8)	3.2 (1.8–5.5)	3 (1.6–5.4)	0.86
pH	7.34 (7.26–7.39)	7.33 (7.26–7.4)	7.36 (7.29–7.42)	0.03
pCO_2 (mmHg)	39 (33–45)	36 (30–44)	36 (31–42)	0.04
PaO_2/FiO_2 ratio (mmHg)	170 (127–287)	196 (129–283)	197 (111–288)	0.87
Mechanical ventilation	67 (67)	58 (50.9)	88 (50.6)	0.03
PEEP (cm H$_2$O)	7.5 (5–10)	8 (5–10)	7.5 (5–10)	0.34
PIP (cm H$_2$O)	25 (18–31)	23 (17–29)	21 (14–27)	0.04
Plateau pressure (cm H$_2$O)	23 (17–30)	20 (16–26)	21 (15–25)	0.17
Mean airway pressure (cm H$_2$O)	14 (10–19)	14 (11–17)	13 (10–17)	0.39
Total norepinephrine (mg)	18.5 (4.7–46.8)	11.6 (3.8–33.5)	14.3 (3.8–44.3)	0.45
Crystalloid 24 h (L)	4.2 (2.4–6.8)	4.2 (2–6.2)	4.2 (2.1–7.2)	0.71

Represented as: total (percentage) or median (interquartile range)

APACHE-III Acute Physiology and Chronic Health Evaluation III therapy, *ARDS* acute respiratory distress syndrome, *FiO₂* fraction of inspired oxygen, *LV* left ventricular, *paO₂* partial pressure of arterial oxygen, *pCO₂* partial pressure of carbon dioxide, *PEEP* positive end-expiratory pressure, *PIP* peak inspiratory pressure, *RV* right ventricular, *SOFA* Sequential Organ Failure Assessment

velocity (11.8 ± 4.2 vs. 13.6 ± 3.3 vs. 15.1 ± 2.1 cm/s; $p = 0.002$) in non-survivors compared to survivors and control groups, respectively [3]. The present study did not demonstrate an association between either TAPSE or tricuspid annulus peak systolic TDI velocity and mortality. TAPSE has high sensitivity in critical illness but poor

Table 2 Echocardiographic parameters of cohorts*

Parameter	Isolated RV dysfunction (n = 100)		RV/LV dysfunction (n = 114)		No RV dysfunction (n = 174)		p
	N	Value	N	Value	N	Value	
RV enlargement	100	82 (82)	113	79 (69.9)	158	0 (0)	<0.001
RV dysfunction	100	58 (58)	114	80 (70.2)	157	0 (0)	<0.001
TR velocity (m/s)	36	2.8 (2.4–3.1)	66	2.7 (2.3–2.9)	33	2.7 (2.4–2.9)	0.22
RV systolic pressure (mmHg)	82	45 (33–58)	107	41 (33–48)	113	39 (32–46)	0.01
Estimated RA pressure (mmHg)	84	10 (5–15)	108	10 (5–14)	122	10 (5–10)	0.006
TAPSE (mm)	10	20 (13.3–23.3)	25	18 (15–19.5)	6	25.5 (21.5–28.5)	0.007
TV systolic velocity TDI (m/s)	35	0.14 (0.12–0.15)	60	0.13 (0.10–0.14)	27	0.17 (0.16–0.18)	<0.001
LV ejection fraction (%)	81	61 (56–67)	81	53 (45–61)	113	60 (55–65)	<0.001
LV end-systolic diameter (mm)	81	28 (24.5–32.5)	100	32 (28–37)	126	47 (43–51)	<0.001
LV end-diastolic diameter (mm)	87	46 (41–50)	109	47 (43–51)	111	30 (26–33)	0.17
LV mass index (g/m^2)	73	83 (67–101.5)	100	88 (70–100)	108	90 (74–102)	0.26
LV stroke volume index (mL/m^2)	73	42 (34.5–50)	104	37.5 (30.3–46)	116	41 (36–48)	0.009
Cardiac index (L/min/m^2)	73	3.7 (3.1–4.5)	104	3.3 (2.8–4.1)	116	3.8 (3.2–4.4)	<0.001
Left atrial volume index (mL/m^2)	39	21 (23–37)	63	35 (28–43)	61	33 (29–38.5)	0.16
LV peak systolic velocity (m/s)	66	0.13 (0.11–0.15)	85	0.12 (0.1–0.14)	70	0.15 (0.13–0.17)	<0.001
Mitral E velocity (m/s)	70	0.8 (0.6–1.0)	88	0.8 (0.7–1.0)	108	0.9 (0.8–1.1)	0.001
Mitral A velocity (m/s)	63	0.8 (0.6–0.9)	69	0.8 (0.6–0.9)	99	0.8 (0.7–1.0)	0.04
Mitral E/A ratio	63	1.0 (0.8–1.3)	69	1.0 (0.8–1.5)	99	1.0 (0.8–1.4)	0.44
Mitral e' velocity (medial) (m/s)	68	0.08 (0.06–0.09)	91	0.07 (0.05–0.08)	105	0.07 (0.06–0.1)	0.02
Mitral e' velocity (lateral) (m/s)	52	0.10 (0.08–0.13)	67	0.09 (0.08–0.10)	76	0.1 (0.08–0.12)	0.01
Mitral E/e' ratio (medial)	65	10 (8.3–13.8)	84	12.5 (10–15)	100	12.1 (9.2–15)	0.04
Mitral E/e' ratio (lateral)	49	7.9 (5.7–10)	61	9 (7.6–11.6)	72	9.2 (7.2–12)	0.01

Represented as: total (percentage) or median (interquartile range)

LV left ventricle, *RA*, right atrial, *RV* right ventricular, *TAPSE* tricuspid annular plane systolic excursion, *TDI* tissue Doppler imaging, *TR* tricuspid regurgitation, *TV* tricuspid valve

*Not all parameters were measured in all patients. Individual *n* for each cohort is presented in the table

specificity [23]. This could potentially be explained by the role of ventricular interdependence, the lack of control for acute right ventricular afterload that can influence the biventricular relationship and the concomitant improvement in right and left ventricular ejection fractions [4, 24]. In this current study, TAPSE showed a strong linear relationship with mitral valve lateral annulus velocity highlighting the influence of LV systolic dysfunction on TAPSE. In this study, the median LVEF in the cohort with combined RV and LV dysfunction was 53% (IQR 45–61%), representing a low incidence of isolated LV systolic dysfunction that could influence RV function.

Isolated RV dysfunction, and not biventricular dysfunction, was an independent predictor of higher long-term mortality. This was an unexpected finding that could be explained by multiple hypotheses. The RV is exquisitely sensitive to increase in afterload from lung disease, and isolated RV dysfunction could reflect cor-pulmonale from severe respiratory failure. This is consistent with the higher use of mechanical ventilation, elevated pCO_2

and lower pH in this cohort from this study. However, mechanical ventilation was not a significant predictor for outcomes after adjustment for other factors in multivariate analysis. These data do not allow RV dysfunction induced or aggravated by respiratory failure to be distinguished from direct effects of sepsis on the RV itself. Alternately, prior literature has suggested that LV dysfunction is an adaptive mechanism in patients with sepsis [25, 26]. Hence, combined biventricular dysfunction might be a benign adaptive response in sepsis, whereas isolated RV dysfunction could reflect the inability of the RV to respond appropriately to stress and physiological demand [27]. Furthermore, the definitions of LV systolic dysfunction and diastolic dysfunction need further validation in the sepsis population that could influence clinical outcomes [2, 28].

This study has various limitations. Echocardiography was only performed in 44% of the population, so the prevalence of RV dysfunction among all patients with sepsis could not be evaluated. Patients without prior

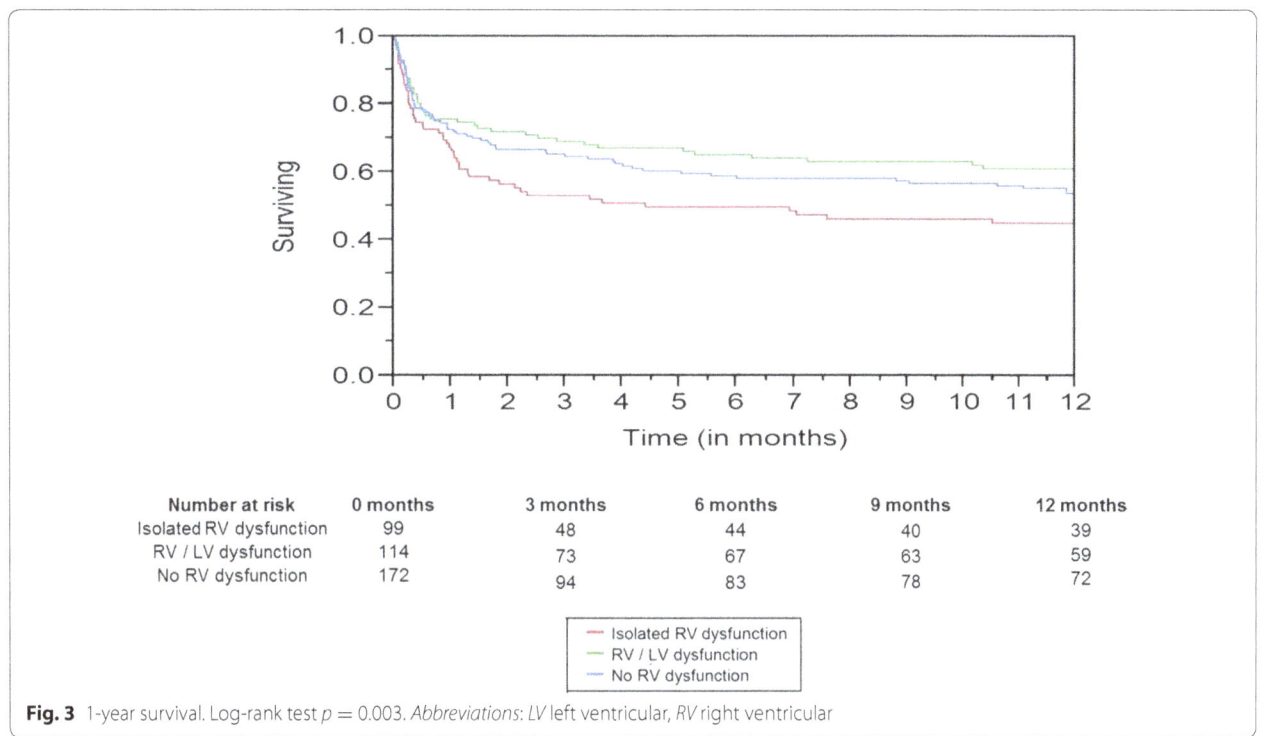

Fig. 3 1-year survival. Log-rank test $p = 0.003$. *Abbreviations*: *LV* left ventricular, *RV* right ventricular

Table 3 Multivariate analysis for 1-year survival with sensitivity analysis

Parameter	Univariate analysis		Multivariate analysis	
	Odds ratio (95% CI)*	p	Hazard ratio (95% CI)	p
RV dysfunction	0.9 (0.6–1.5)	0.83	0.9 (0.7–1.2)	0.40
Isolated RV dysfunction	1.5 (0.9–2.4)	0.11	1.6 (1.2–2.1)	0.002
Age (years)	1.1 (1.1–1.1)	0.007	1.0 (0.9–1.0)	1.11
Charlson comorbidity index	1.1 (1.1–1.2)	0.02	1.1 (1.1–1.1)	0.04
APACHE-III	1.1 (1.1–1.1)	<0.001	1.1 (1.1–1.1)	<0.001
Septic shock	1.9 (1.2–3.2)	0.01	1.2 (0.9–1.7)	0.24
Mechanical ventilation	1.2 (0.8–1.8)	0.58	1.1 (0.8–1.5)	0.69

Represented as: odds ratio (95% confidence interval) or hazard ratio (95% confidence interval)

APACHE-III Acute Physiology and Chronic Health Evaluation III, *CI* confidence interval

*Unit OR are presented for continuous predictors

echocardiography and prior lung disease were included due to the low likelihood of chronic RV dysfunction; however, RV dysfunction could have been 'unmasked' on admission echocardiography. It is likely that patients with abnormal RV function on two-dimensional imaging underwent more detailed assessment of other RV parameters. Additionally, RV dysfunction from sepsis could not reliably be distinguished from RV dysfunction from respiratory failure due to the retrospective nature of the study. The potential influence of echocardiographic results on clinical care and outcomes could not be assessed due to the historical nature of this study. The study duration correlated with the evolution of critical

care ultrasonography and changes in health care delivery at the Mayo Clinic, which conceivably could have influenced the study results. Finally, the single-region, single-institution and referral patient population of the Mayo Clinic could impact the generalizability to other populations.

Future directions for clinical research include systematically evaluating RV function in sepsis with advanced diagnostic techniques such as strain imaging that might have greater yield on homogenizing the definition of RV dysfunction. Complex heart–lung interactions, impact of mechanical ventilation and influence of volume expansion on RV function in septic patients are potential avenues for clinical and translational research. Evaluation of the pulmonary circulation using noninvasive modalities in these patients will aid in a more holistic understanding of fluid, vasopressor and ventilator management during critical illness.

Conclusions

RV dysfunction was common in this contemporary cohort of patients with severe sepsis and septic shock that underwent echocardiography. Isolated RV dysfunction was noted to be associated with worse 1-year survival in the total cohort. These results need further validation in carefully designed prospective studies to understand the long-term significance of RV dysfunction.

Abbreviations
APACHE: Acute Physiology and Chronic Health Evaluation; ASE: American Society of Echocardiography; CI: confidence interval; HR: hazard ratio; ICU: intensive care unit; IQR: interquartile range; LV: left ventricular; OR: odds ratio; RV: right ventricular; SOFA: Sequential Organ Failure Assessment; TAPSE: tricuspid annular plane systolic excursion; TDI: tissue Doppler imaging.

Authors' contributions
SV, AS, OG, JBG and JCJ were involved in study design, literature review, data analysis and statistical analysis. SV, MK, GP, AS, RK and JCJ contributed to data management, data analysis and drafting manuscript. SV, MK, GP, AS, RK, KK, OG, JBG and JCJ had access to the data. KK, OG, JBG and JCJ involved in manuscript revision, intellectual revisions and mentorship. SV, MK, GP, AS, RK, KK, OG, JBG and JCJ provided final approval. All authors read and approved the final manuscript.

Author details
[1] Department of Cardiovascular Medicine, Mayo Clinic, 200 First Street SW, Rochester, MN 55905, USA. [2] Division of Pulmonary and Critical Care Medicine, Department of Medicine, Mayo Clinic, 200 First Street SW, Rochester, MN 55905, USA. [3] Multidisciplinary Epidemiology and Translational Research in Intensive Care (METRIC) Laboratory, Mayo Clinic, 200 First Street SW, Rochester 55905, MN, USA. [4] Center for Clinical and Translational Science, Mayo Clinic Graduate School of Biomedical Sciences, Mayo Clinic, 200 First Street SW, Rochester 55905, MN, USA. [5] Department of Anesthesiology and Perioperative Medicine, Mayo Clinic, 200 First Street SW, Rochester 55905, MN, USA. [6] Division of Nephrology and Hypertension, Department of Medicine, Mayo Clinic, 200 First Street SW, Rochester 55905, MN, USA.

Acknowledgements
METRIC Laboratory, Anesthesia Clinical Research Unit, Echocardiography and Vascular Physiology Research Unit and Cardiac Catheterization Laboratory Interventional Research Database Unit.

Competing interests
All authors report no financial or intellectual conflicts of interest related to this manuscript.

Funding
(1) Supported, in part, by CTSA Grant Number UL1 TR000135 from the National Center for Advancing Translational Sciences (NCATS), a component of the National Institutes of Health (NIH). Its contents are solely the responsibility of the authors and do not necessarily represent the official view of NIH. (2) Supported, in part, by intramural funding from the Critical Care Research Committee, Critical Care Independent Multidisciplinary Program, Mayo Clinic, Rochester MN.

References
1. Sanfilippo F, Corredor C, Fletcher N, Landesberg G, Benedetto U, Foex P, et al. Diastolic dysfunction and mortality in septic patients: a systematic review and meta-analysis. Intensive Care Med. 2015;41(6):1004–13.
2. Sevilla Berrios RA, O'Horo JC, Velagapudi V, Pulido JN. Correlation of left ventricular systolic dysfunction determined by low ejection fraction and 30-day mortality in patients with severe sepsis and septic shock: a systematic review and meta-analysis. J Crit Care. 2014;29(4):495–9.
3. Harmankaya A, Akilli H, Gul M, Akilli NB, Ergin M, Aribas A, et al. Assessment of right ventricular functions in patients with sepsis, severe sepsis and septic shock and its prognostic importance: a tissue Doppler study. J Crit Care. 2013;28(6):1111.e7–11.
4. Chan CM, Klinger JR. The right ventricle in sepsis. Clin Chest Med. 2008;29(4):661–76 (ix).
5. Mekontso Dessap A, Boissier F, Charron C, Begot E, Repesse X, Legras A, et al. Acute cor pulmonale during protective ventilation for acute respiratory distress syndrome: prevalence, predictors, and clinical impact. Intensive Care Med. 2016;42(5):862–70.
6. Pulido JN, Afessa B, Masaki M, Yuasa T, Gillespie S, Herasevich V, et al. Clinical spectrum, frequency, and significance of myocardial dysfunction in severe sepsis and septic shock. Mayo Clin Proc. 2012;87(7):620–8.
7. Landesberg G, Jaffe AS, Gilon D, Levin PD, Goodman S, Abu-Baih A, et al. Troponin elevation in severe sepsis and septic shock: the role of left ventricular diastolic dysfunction and right ventricular dilatation. Crit Care Med. 2014;42(4):790–800.
8. Afessa B, Keegan MT, Hubmayr RD, Naessens JM, Gajic O, Long KH, et al. Evaluating the performance of an institution using an intensive care unit benchmark. Mayo Clin Proc. 2005;80(2):174–80.
9. Herasevich V, Pickering BW, Dong Y, Peters SG, Gajic O. Informatics infrastructure for syndrome surveillance, decision support, reporting, and modeling of critical illness. Mayo Clin Proc. 2010;85(3):247–54.
10. Levy MM, Fink MP, Marshall JC, Abraham E, Angus D, Cook D, et al. 2001 SCCM/ESICM/ACCP/ATS/SIS international sepsis definitions conference. Crit Care Med. 2003;31(4):1250–6.
11. Harrison AM, Thongprayoon C, Kashyap R, Chute CG, Gajic O, Pickering BW, et al. Developing the surveillance algorithm for detection of failure to recognize and treat severe sepsis. Mayo Clin Proc. 2015;90(2):166–75.
12. Schramm GE, Kashyap R, Mullon JJ, Gajic O, Afessa B. Septic shock: a multidisciplinary response team and weekly feedback to clinicians improve the process of care and mortality. Crit Care Med. 2011;39(2):252–8.
13. Herasevich V, Pieper MS, Pulido J, Gajic O. Enrollment into a time sensitive clinical study in the critical care setting: results from computerized septic shock sniffer implementation. J Am Med Inform Assoc. 2011;18(5):639–44.
14. Singh B, Singh A, Ahmed A, Wilson GA, Pickering BW, Herasevich V, et al. Derivation and validation of automated electronic search strategies to extract Charlson comorbidities from electronic medical records. Mayo Clin Proc. 2012;87(9):817–24.
15. Siontis B, Elmer J, Dannielson R, Brown C, Park J, Surani S, et al. Multifaceted interventions to decrease mortality in patients with severe sepsis/septic shock-a quality improvement project. PeerJ. 2015;3:e1290.
16. Lang RM, Badano LP, Mor-Avi V, Afilalo J, Armstrong A, Ernande L, et al. Recommendations for cardiac chamber quantification by echocardiography in adults: an update from the American Society of Echocardiography and the European Association of Cardiovascular Imaging. J Am Soc Echocardiogr. 2015;28(1):1–39.e14.
17. Rudski LG, Lai WW, Afilalo J, Hua L, Handschumacher MD, Chandrasekaran K, et al. Guidelines for the echocardiographic assessment of the right heart in adults: a report from the American Society of Echocardiography endorsed by the European Association of Echocardiography, a registered branch of the European Society of Cardiology, and the Canadian Society of Echocardiography. J Am Soc Echocardiogr. 2010;23(7):685–713 (quiz 86–8).
18. Nagueh SF, Smiseth OA, Appleton CP, Byrd BF 3rd, Dokainish H, Edvardsen T, et al. Recommendations for the evaluation of left ventricular diastolic function by echocardiography: an update from the American Society of Echocardiography and the European Association of Cardiovascular Imaging. J Am Soc Echocardiogr. 2016;29(4):277–314.
19. Rocca WA, Yawn BP, St Sauver JL, Grossardt BR, Melton LJ 3rd. History of the Rochester epidemiology project: half a century of medical records linkage in a US population. Mayo Clin Proc. 2012;87(12):1202–13.

20. Furian T, Aguiar C, Prado K, Ribeiro RV, Becker L, Martinelli N, et al. Ventricular dysfunction and dilation in severe sepsis and septic shock: relation to endothelial function and mortality. J Crit Care. 2012;27(3):319. e9–15.

21. Orde SR, Pulido JN, Masaki M, Gillespie S, Spoon JN, Kane GC, et al. Outcome prediction in sepsis: speckle tracking echocardiography based assessment of myocardial function. Crit Care. 2014;18(4):R149.

22. Huang SJ, Nalos M, McLean AS. Is early ventricular dysfunction or dilation associated with lower mortality rate in adult severe sepsis and septic shock? A meta-analysis. Crit Care. 2013;17(3):R96.

23. Lamia B, Teboul JL, Monnet X, Richard C, Chemla D. Relationship between the tricuspid annular plane systolic excursion and right and left ventricular function in critically ill patients. Intensive Care Med. 2007;33(12):2143–9.

24. Liu D, Du B, Long Y, Zhao C, Hou B. Right ventricular function of patients with septic shock: clinical significance. Zhonghua Wai Ke Za Zhi. 2000;38(7):488–92.

25. Antonucci E, Fiaccadori E, Donadello K, Taccone FS, Franchi F, Scolletta S. Myocardial depression in sepsis: from pathogenesis to clinical manifestations and treatment. J Crit Care. 2014;29(4):500–11.

26. Jardin F, Fourme T, Page B, Loubieres Y, Vieillard-Baron A, Beauchet A, et al. Persistent preload defect in severe sepsis despite fluid loading: a longitudinal echocardiographic study in patients with septic shock. Chest. 1999;116(5):1354–9.

27. Vieillard-Baron A. Septic cardiomyopathy. Ann Intensive Care. 2011;1(1):6.

28. Lanspa MJ, Gutsche AR, Wilson EL, Olsen TD, Hirshberg EL, Knox DB, et al. Application of a simplified definition of diastolic function in severe sepsis and septic shock. Crit Care. 2016;20(1):243.

12

Effect of inspiratory synchronization during pressure-controlled ventilation on lung distension and inspiratory effort

Nuttapol Rittayamai[1,2,3], François Beloncle[1,2,4], Ewan C. Goligher[1,5,6,7], Lu Chen[1,2], Jordi Mancebo[8,9], Jean-Christophe M. Richard[10,11] and Laurent Brochard[1,2]*

Abstract

Background: In pressure-controlled (PC) ventilation, tidal volume (V_T) and transpulmonary pressure (P_L) result from the addition of ventilator pressure and the patient's inspiratory effort. PC modes can be classified into fully, partially, and non-synchronized modes, and the degree of synchronization may result in different V_T and P_L despite identical ventilator settings. This study assessed the effects of three PC modes on V_T, P_L, inspiratory effort (esophageal pressure–time product, PTP_{es}), and airway occlusion pressure, $P_{0.1}$. We also assessed whether $P_{0.1}$ can be used for evaluating patient effort.

Methods: Prospective, randomized, crossover physiologic study performed in 14 spontaneously breathing mechanically ventilated patients recovering from acute respiratory failure (1 subsequently withdrew). PC modes were fully (PC-CMV), partially (PC-SIMV), and non-synchronized (PC-IMV using airway pressure release ventilation) and were applied randomly; driving pressure, inspiratory time, and set respiratory rate being similar for all modes. Airway, esophageal pressure, $P_{0.1}$, airflow, gas exchange, and hemodynamics were recorded.

Results: V_T was significantly lower during PC-IMV as compared with PC-SIMV and PC-CMV (387 ± 105 vs 458 ± 134 vs 482 ± 108 mL, respectively; $p < 0.05$). Maximal P_L was also significantly lower (13.3 ± 4.9 vs 15.3 ± 5.7 vs 15.5 ± 5.2 cmH$_2$O, respectively; $p < 0.05$), but PTP_{es} was significantly higher in PC-IMV (215.6 ± 154.3 vs 150.0 ± 102.4 vs 130.9 ± 101.8 cmH$_2$O $\times$ s $\times$ min^{-1}, respectively; $p < 0.05$), with no differences in gas exchange and hemodynamic variables. PTP_{es} increased by more than 15% in 10 patients and by more than 50% in 5 patients. An increased $P_{0.1}$ could identify high levels of PTP_{es}.

Conclusions: Non-synchronized PC mode lowers V_T and P_L in comparison with more synchronized modes in spontaneously breathing patients but can increase patient effort and may need specific adjustments.

Clinical Trial Registration Clinicaltrial.gov # NCT02071277

Keywords: Airway pressure release ventilation, Lung-protective ventilation, Spontaneous ventilation, Transpulmonary pressure, Ventilator-induced lung injury

Background

To date, volume-controlled ventilation is the most commonly employed mode during the first few days of mechanical ventilation [1]. The use of pressure-controlled

*Correspondence: BrochardL@smh.ca
[2] Keenan Research Centre and Li Ka Shing Knowledge Institute, St. Michael's Hospital, 30 Bond St, Toronto, ON M5B 1W8, Canada
Full list of author information is available at the end of the article

(PC) modes has steadily increased, and they are now preferentially used. Under passive conditions in PC mode, the ventilator is the only respiratory pump and V_T depends entirely on the set pressure, inspiratory time, and the respiratory system mechanics [2]. Inactivity of the respiratory muscles results in rapid muscle weakness [3, 4], whereas allowing spontaneous breathing improves gas exchange [5] and might prevent ventilator-induced diaphragm dysfunction (VIDD) [6, 7]. When patients make spontaneous breathing efforts, however, the total driving pressure will be the sum of the pressure generated by the ventilator (P_{aw}) and the patient's respiratory muscles. Therefore, transpulmonary pressure (P_L) and V_T are more difficult to control and may exceed safe limits in patients who require lung-protective ventilation, such as acute respiratory distress syndrome (ARDS).

Pressure-controlled modes can be classified according to the degree of inspiratory synchronization as fully, partially, and non-synchronized modes (Fig. 1). The nomenclature of each mode, however, varies with ventilator brand making sometimes difficult for the clinician to appreciate this distinction (Additional file 1: Table S1). In fully synchronized mode or PC continuous mandatory ventilation (PC-CMV), mechanically assisted breaths are triggered every time the patient generates spontaneous efforts. In partially synchronized mode or PC synchronized intermittent mandatory ventilation (PC-SIMV), there is a synchronization time window allowing the patient to trigger an assisted breath within the time window or to take a breath without assistance if efforts occur outside the synchronization window. Finally, in non-synchronized mode or PC intermittent mandatory

ventilation (PC-IMV), low and high pressure levels are alternately delivered for fixed intervals and patient inspiratory efforts are possible but do not trigger any additional assistance and are not intentionally synchronized. Several breath types can be observed during PC-IMV, which will result in different breathing patterns (Additional file 1: Fig. S1) [8]. A study by Richard and colleagues comparing three PC types of modes in a bench model suggested that non-synchronized modes resulted in lower P_L and V_T than the two other modes despite identical settings and simulated effort [9]. Though these effects are potentially attractive for offering a better lung-protective strategy, using a non-synchronized mode may also lead to unpredictable effects on patient's inspiratory effort. Because we don't know if the risk of having large V_T and P_L is better represented by the average values, the variability of the values needs to be also examined.

The pressure–time product (PTP) and work of breathing using Campbell's diagram are the standard methods for assessing patient inspiratory effort during mechanical ventilation [10]. However, these techniques need complex calculations based on esophageal manometry. The airway occlusion pressure at 0.1 s ($P_{0.1}$), an index of

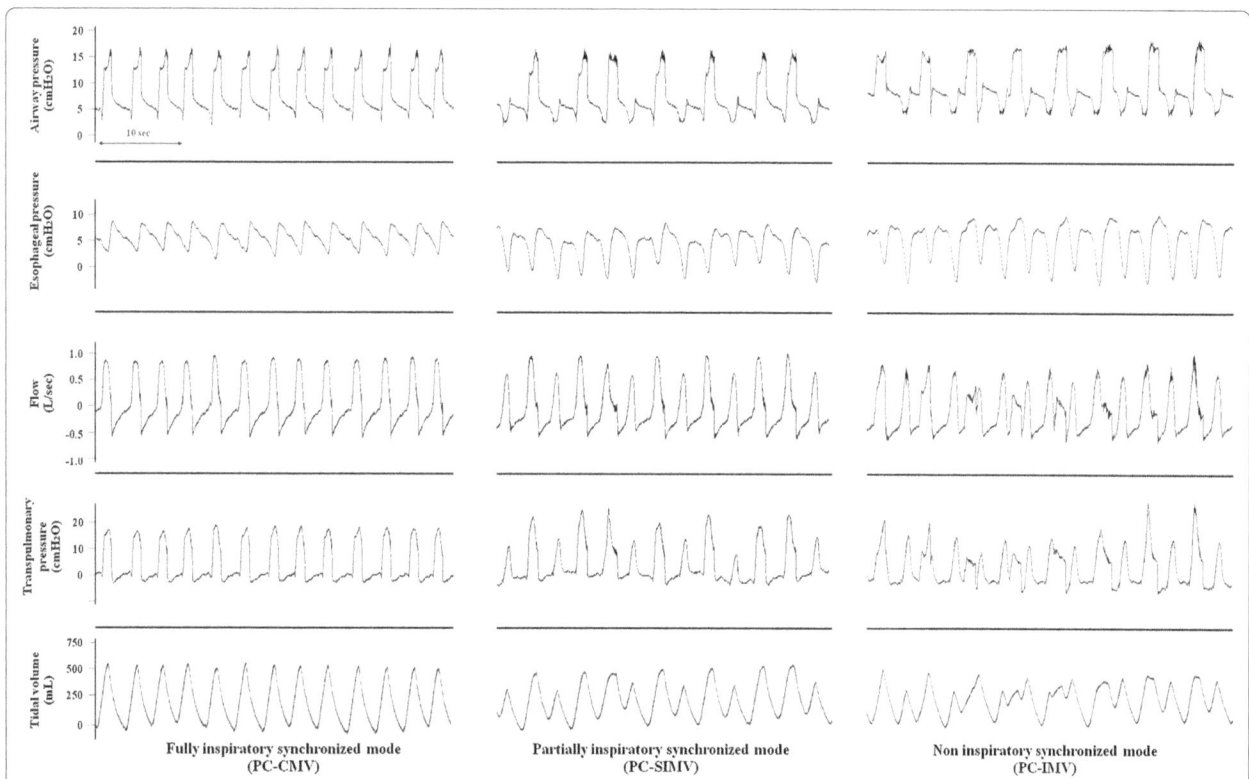

Fig. 1 Tracings of airway pressure, esophageal pressure, flow, transpulmonary pressure, and tidal volume during each pressure-controlled mode of ventilation. The degree of inspiratory synchronization leads to varying in transpulmonary pressure and tidal volume. *PC-CMV* pressure-controlled continuous mandatory ventilation, *PC-SIMV* pressure-controlled synchronized intermittent mandatory ventilation, *PC-IMV* pressure-controlled intermittent mandatory ventilation

respiratory drive available on modern ventilators, could be an alternative method for assessing inspiratory effort.

The primary objective of this study was to assess whether non-synchronized modes of ventilation result in more protective ventilation strategy over the two other PC modes as evaluated by V_T and P_L; secondary objectives included the effect of different degree of inspiratory synchronization on inspiratory effort determined by esophageal pressure–time product (PTP_{es}) and by $P_{0.1}$.

Methods

Study population and settings

The study was conducted in Medical–Surgical Intensive Care Units at two academic hospitals in Toronto, Canada (Clinicaltrial.gov # NCT02071277). The Research Ethics Board at St. Michael's Hospital and Mt. Sinai Hospital approved the study protocol, and informed consent was obtained from patients or their substitute decision makers prior to enrollment.

Patients were eligible for enrollment if they were spontaneously breathing under mechanical ventilation with a pressure assist-control mode or pressure support ventilation (PSV) with a ventilator driving pressure level of at least 10 cmH$_2$O (to ensure that patients were not yet on minimal support). Patients were not included if they had hemodynamic instability (> 20% variation of mean arterial pressure and/or heart rate or need doses of norepinephrine higher than 0.2 mcg/kg/min), a set positive end-expiratory pressure (PEEP) above 12 cmH$_2$O, a fractional oxygen concentration (FiO$_2$) above 0.6, a severe acid–base disturbance (arterial pH < 7.30 or > 7.55). There should be no contraindication to insert esophageal balloon catheter, chronic neuromuscular disease, intracranial hypertension, or pregnancy.

Ventilators and equipment

A Dräger Evita-XL or a Dräger V500 ventilator (Dräger, Lubeck, Germany) which provided the three different synchronized PC modes was used. We used PCV+ assist, PCV+, and APRV modes on the Evita-XL and PC-AC, PC-SIMV+, and APRV on the V500 ventilator to represent PC-CMV, PC-SIMV, and PC-IMV, respectively. Of note, we used the mode called APRV as the only available non-synchronized mode, but the settings were similar to other classical PC-CMV modes and not to "usual" approaches using APRV with prolonged high pressure–time.

Airflow was measured with a Fleisch No. 2 pneumotachograph placed between the endotracheal tube and the Y-piece of the ventilator, connected to a differential pressure transducer (MP 150, Biopac Systems, Goleta, California, USA). Airway pressure (P_{aw}) was measured between the endotracheal tube and the

pneumotachograph via a pressure transducer (MP 150). Esophageal pressure (P_{es}) was measured using a Nutrivent catheter (Sidam, Mirandola, Italy) connected to pressure transducers (MP 150). The correct position of the esophageal balloon was assessed by an occlusion test [11, 12].

The analog signals of airflow, P_{aw}, and P_{es} were digitized at a sampling rate of 100 Hz and stored in a laptop for subsequent calculations and analyzes using AcqKnowledge software (Biopac Systems). Volume was obtained by integration of airflow signal over time, regardless of the mode. Tidal volume variability was assessed by the coefficients of variation of tidal volume (calculated as the standard deviation divided by the mean value). P_L was calculated by subtraction of P_{aw} from P_{es} and presented as the maximal and minimal values; mean P_L was calculated as the quotient of the area under the P_L-time tracing divided by total cycle duration. ΔP_L was measured as the difference between maximal and minimal P_L at the end of inspiration. PTP_{es} was calculated as the surface enclosed within the P_{es} and the relaxation line of the chest wall over inspiratory time [13, 14] and expressed in cmH$_2$O × s × min^{-1} using a dedicated software (Sistema Respiratorio, Barcelona, Spain). Algorithm to calculate PTP_{es} is detailed in Additional file 1: Fig. S2.

$P_{0.1}$ was measured using AcqKnowledge software from the fall in P_{aw} during the first 100 ms of an occluded (zero flow) spontaneous inspiration using the end-expiratory hold function.

Study protocol

Patients were studied in a semi-recumbent position. Three different PC modes were applied for 20 min each in random order as determined by a blind envelope pull. The ventilator settings (inspiratory pressure, PEEP, set respiratory rate, FiO$_2$, and inspiratory time) were kept unchanged and similar across all modes. These settings were as close as possible to those previously chosen by the responsible clinician, using the same driving pressure; if the patient was put on PSV mode, then the set respiratory rate during the study was set to reach the same total minute ventilation. No pressure support was added during PC-SIMV and PC-IMV. The first 15 min was devoted to ensure patient's full adaptation to the mode, and signal acquisition was done during the following 5 min. The last 2 min of the recording was analyzed offline and presented as the average values over the selected period. Sedation assessed by RASS was left to the discretion of the attended physician and not modified for the duration of the study. The occlusions to measure $P_{0.1}$ were performed and recorded every minute during 5 min of data acquisition. Arterial blood gases were collected before starting the protocol and at the end of the three studied periods. Hemodynamic variables (mean arterial pressure and heart rate) were also recorded during the study.

Statistical analysis

Statistical analysis was performed with Statistical Package for the Social Sciences (version 20.0, IBM SPSS, Chicago, IL, USA). Continuous variables are reported as mean ± SD, and categorical variables are reported as number and percentage. We used an analysis of variance with repeated measures followed by a post hoc pairwise test to compare the difference between the three modes.

We also performed a correlation analysis between the individual changes in $P_{0.1}$ and the individual changes in PTP_{es} in order to determine whether $P_{0.1}$ could reliably indicate the direction of the changes in patients' effort. Receiver operating characteristic (ROC) curve was used to evaluate a cutoff point for $P_{0.1}$ in predicting excess patient's inspiratory effort determined as $PTP_{es} > 200$ cmH$_2$O × s × min^{-1}. This value was chosen as the upper value, i.e., mean value plus one standard deviation, tolerated by patients passing a successful spontaneous breathing trial [14]. A p value < 0.05 was considered as statistically significant.

Results

We enrolled 14 patients from March 2014 to July 2015. Mean age was 58 ± 12 years, and APACHE II score was 18.0 ± 5.1. Other baseline characteristics are shown in Table 1. The majority of patients (62%) had been ventilated for ARDS, and 46% were still under light levels of continuous intravenous sedation at the time of the measurements. (Average RASS score of these patients was −2 ± 1.) All but one patient tolerated the three PC modes. The latter patient was in respiratory acidosis before the study, worsened just after starting the study, and was secondarily excluded.

Effect on breathing pattern and transpulmonary pressure

The main results are shown in Table 2 and Figs. 2 and 3. The percentage of spontaneous breathing during PC-SIMV and PC-IMV was 6.8 and 17.4% of total minute ventilation. We found that average V_T and V_T per predicted body weight were significantly lower during PC-IMV in comparison with the two other modes (PC-IMV vs PC-CMV, $p < 0.001$; PC-IMV vs PC-SIMV, $p = 0.049$). Tidal volume variability was significantly higher during PC-IMV as compared with the other modes (PC-IMV vs PC-CMV, p = 0.001; PC-IMV vs PC-SIMV, $p = 0.028$) (Fig. 2). Total respiratory rate also significantly increased during PC-IMV in comparison with PC-SIMV and PC-CMV (PC-IMV vs PC-CMV, $p = 0.007$; PC-IMV vs PC-SIMV, $p = 0.025$).

Average values of maximal P_L and the mean P_L during PC-IMV were significantly lower when compared to PC-CMV ($p = 0.006$) and PC-SIMV ($p = 0.004$), but no difference in minimum P_L during each mode of ventilation was found (Fig. 3). There was a nonsignificant trend toward a decreased ΔP_L at the end of inspiration with decreasing degree of inspiratory synchronization (PC-IMV vs PC-CMV, $p = 0.144$; PC-IMV vs PC-SIMV, $p = 0.152$). No difference in minute ventilation, PaO$_2$/FiO$_2$, PaCO$_2$, and arterial pH was found between modes. In addition, no significant differences in mean arterial pressure and heart rate were found between the three PC modes (Table 2).

Effect on patient's inspiratory effort

Patient's inspiratory effort determined by PTP_{es} was higher during PC-IMV in comparison with the two other modes (PC-IMV vs PC-CMV, $p = 0.005$; PC-IMV vs PC-SIMV, $p = 0.023$), as shown in Table 3. Compared to the two other modes, PTP_{es} increased by more than 15% in 10 patients and by more than 50% in 5 patients.

We found that $P_{0.1}$, measured during manual occlusions, significantly increased from 2.6 ± 1.7 cmH$_2$O during PC-CMV to 3.7 ± 2.3 cmH$_2$O during PC-IMV ($p = 0.048$) (Additional file 1: Fig. S3). We observed a strong correlation between $P_{0.1}$ and PTP_{es} with a correlation coefficient of 0.754 ($p < 0.001$). In addition, the area under the ROC curve for $P_{0.1}$ to predict excess patient's inspiratory effort was 0.93 (95% confidence interval, 0.85–1.00) (Additional file 1: Fig. S4). A cutoff value for $P_{0.1}$ above 3.5 cmH$_2$O had a sensitivity of 92% and specificity of 89% in predicting $PTP_{es} > 200$ cmH$_2$O × s × min^{-1}.

Discussion

We found that spontaneous efforts during different PC modes with identical ventilator settings have very different effects on V_T and P_L. PC-IMV has no synchronization and provides less V_T and P_L and more V_T variability than either PC-CMV or PC-SIMV, which have full or partial synchronization. No differences in terms of gas exchange and hemodynamics were found between the modes in this short-term study. The non-synchronized mode was, however, often associated with higher levels of patients' effort. Inspiratory effort was strongly correlated with $P_{0.1}$. In this context, $P_{0.1}$ might be used to detect excessive inspiratory effort.

Patients with acute respiratory failure, in particular ARDS, should be ventilated with a lung-protective strategy to reduce the risk of ventilator-induced lung injury (VILI) and to improve survival [15–17]. Using low V_T and optimum PEEP to minimize P_L can mitigate VILI [18]. Although neuromuscular blocking agents can be used initially, allowing spontaneous breathing can reduce

Table 1 Patient characteristics and ventilator settings

Patient	Gender	Age (years)	Cause of acute respiratory failure	Intubation days	APACHE II score	RASS score	Inspiratory pressure above PEEP (cmH$_2$O)	PEEP (cmH$_2$O)	Inspiratory time (s)	Set rate (breath/min)	FiO$_2$	Discharge status
1	M	62	Sepsis, ARDS	14	12	−2	10	8	1	15	0.5	Alive
2*	F	65	COPD with exacerbation	2	13	0	12	5	0.9	26	0.45	Alive
3	M	80	COPD with exacerbation	15	13	0	10	8	1.1	19	0.3	Alive
4	M	66	Sepsis, ARDS	3	16	−2	16	8	1	20	0.4	Alive
5	M	68	Congestive heart failure	4	16	−2	12	10	1	20	0.5	Alive
6	M	48	Pneumonia, ARDS	13	17	−2	10	10	0.9	14	0.4	Dead
7	M	38	Multiple trauma	7	11	−3	12	8	1	16	0.4	Alive
8	F	41	Seizure, ARDS	7	20	−3	10	8	1	18	0.4	Alive
9	M	69	Sepsis, ARDS	9	18	−3	18	10	0.8	25	0.5	Dead
10	M	46	IPF exacerbation, ARDS	10	19	−3	20	8	0.8	24	0.5	Alive
11	F	67	Cardiac arrest	7	19	−3	14	12	1	20	0.5	Alive
12	M	49	Sepsis, ARDS	8	24	−3	14	12	1	22	0.4	Alive
13	M	63	Pneumonia, ARDS	2	25	−1	16	10	0.9	13	0.4	Dead
14	F	51	Pneumonia	11	29	−3	16	10	1.2	14	0.45	Dead

ARDS acute respiratory distress syndrome, COPD chronic obstructive pulmonary disease, IPF idiopathic pulmonary fibrosis, PEEP positive end-expiratory pressure, RASS Richmond Agitation Sedation Scale

* Patient #2 was excluded from the data analysis due to termination of the study

Table 2 Breathing pattern, respiratory and hemodynamic variables during three pressure-controlled modes

	PC-CMV	PC-SIMV	PC-IMV
Tidal volume (mL)	482 ± 107	457 ± 133	387 ± 104*,#
Tidal volume per predicted body weight (mL/kg)	7.3 ± 1.4	7.0 ± 2.1	5.9 ± 1.5*,#
Tidal volume variability (%)	13.7 ± 13.7	21.6 ± 13.1	36.0 ± 18.0*,#
Maximal P_L (cmH$_2$O)	15.5 ± 5.2	15.3 ± 5.7	13.3 ± 4.9*,#
Mean P_L (cmH$_2$O)	9.8 ± 3.0	8.8 ± 3.3ᵛ	7.0 ± 3.0*,#
Minimum P_L (cmH$_2$O)	-3.2 ± 2.8	-3.5 ± 3.4	-3.5 ± 3.2
ΔP_L (cmH$_2$O)	12.0 ± 6.9	11.9 ± 7.0	10.3 ± 4.6
Total respiratory rate (breaths/min)	22 ± 4	23 ± 6	27 ± 7*,#
Minute ventilation (L/min)	10.2 ± 2.1	9.8 ± 1.9	9.9 ± 2.0
PaO$_2$/FiO$_2$ ratio	216 ± 60	223 ± 55	218 ± 63
PaCO$_2$ (mmHg)	48 ± 10	49 ± 11	50 ± 10
Arterial pH	7.37 ± 0.06	7.37 ± 0.07	7.36 ± 0.07
Mean arterial pressure (mmHg)	80 ± 10	80 ± 11	85 ± 14
Heart rate (beats/min)	96 ± 14	95 ± 13	96 ± 15

PC-CMV pressure-controlled continuous mandatory ventilation, *PC-SIMV* pressure-controlled synchronized intermittent mandatory ventilation, *PC-IMV* pressure-controlled intermittent mandatory ventilation

* $p < 0.05$, PC-CMV versus PC-IMV; # $p < 0.05$, PC-SIMV versus PC-IMV; ᵛ $p < 0.05$, PC-CMV versus PC-SIMV

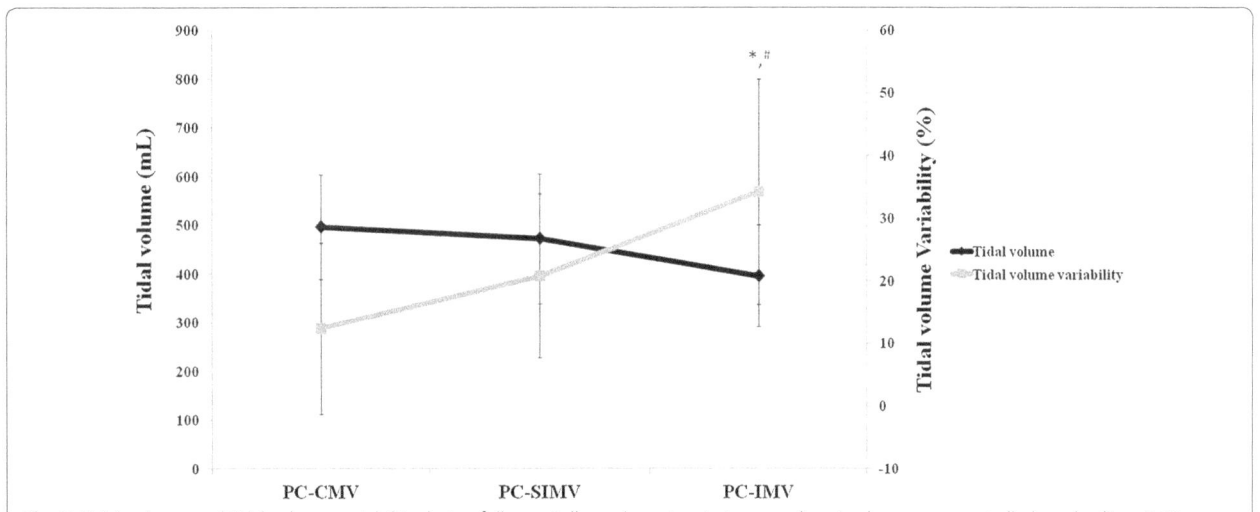

Fig. 2 Tidal volume and tidal volume variability during fully, partially, and non inspiratory synchronized pressure-controlled modes (* $p < 0.05$; PC-IMV vs PC-CMV and # $p < 0.05$; PC-IMV vs PC-SIMV). *PC-CMV* pressure-controlled continuous mandatory ventilation, *PC-SIMV* pressure-controlled synchronized intermittent mandatory ventilation, *PC-IMV* pressure-controlled intermittent mandatory ventilation

VIDD [6, 7, 19], improves lung aeration and oxygenation [5, 20–22], and may attenuate VILI especially when the degree of lung injury is moderate [23, 24]. PC modes have been increasingly used, in particular, after 48 h of mechanical ventilation [1] because it provides a variable flow rate and may well respond to patient's demand and reduce work of breathing [2]. However, when patients breathe spontaneously during PC modes, the patient's inspiratory effort can increase P_L and V_T which has the potential to worsen lung injury [25, 26].

Our study shows that the level of inspiratory synchronization should be considered when using a PC mode and probably individualized. Richard et al. [9] demonstrated on a bench that V_T and P_L significantly increased when the degree of synchronization increased. These findings are confirmed by the present study in that non-synchronized mode lowers the average V_T and P_L in comparison with synchronized mode. Variation in V_T and P_L may occur because of different breath types during PC-IMV, and higher distending pressure may develop during some breath types such as type B breath (Additional file 1: Fig.

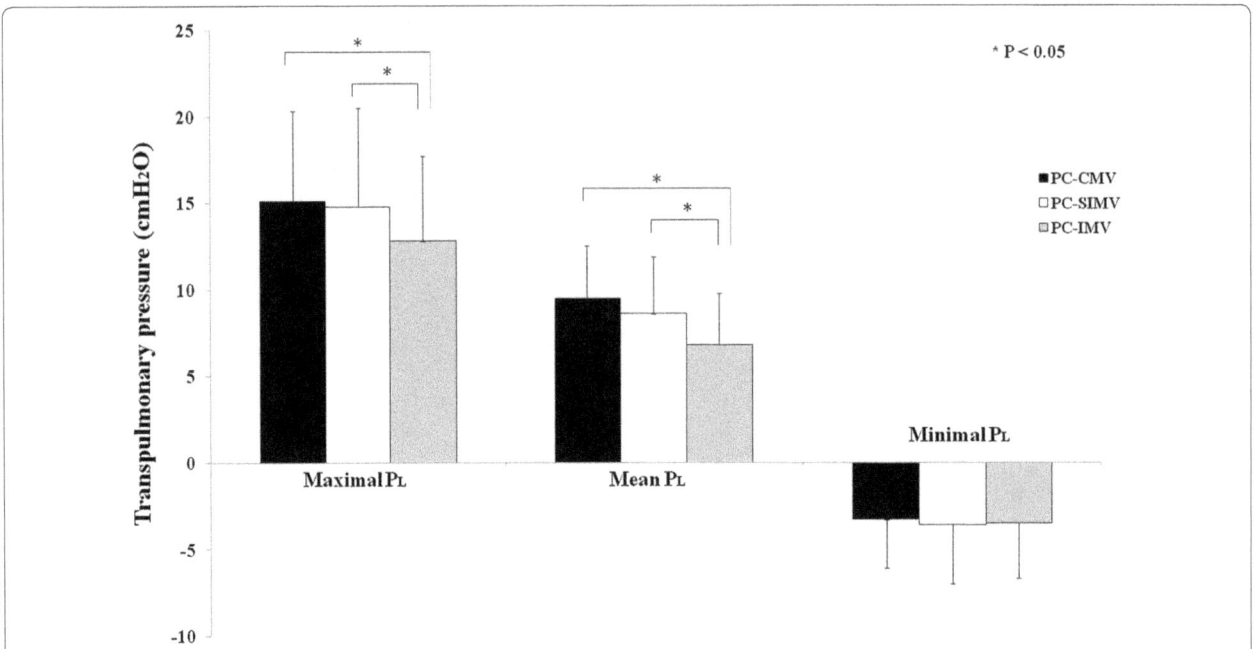

Fig. 3 Maximal, mean, and minimum transpulmonary pressure (P_L) during the three pressure-controlled modes of ventilation. *PC-CMV* pressure-controlled continuous mandatory ventilation, *PC-SIMV* pressure-controlled synchronized intermittent mandatory ventilation, *PC-IMV* pressure-controlled intermittent mandatory ventilation

Table 3 Patient inspiratory effort [esophageal pressure–time product (PTP_{es})] and respiratory drive [airway occlusion pressure at 0.1 s ($P_{0.1}$)] during three pressure-controlled modes

	PC-CMV	PC-SIMV	PC-IMV
PTP_{es} (cmH$_2$O × s × min^{-1})	130 ± 101	150 ± 102	215 ± 154*,#
$P_{0.1}$ (cmH$_2$O)	2.6 ± 1.7	2.9 ± 1.9	3.7 ± 2.3*

PC-CMV pressure-controlled continuous mandatory ventilation, *PC-SIMV* pressure-controlled synchronized intermittent mandatory ventilation, *PC-IMV* pressure-controlled intermittent mandatory ventilation

* $p < 0.05$, PC-CMV versus PC-IMV; # $p < 0.05$, PC-SIMV versus PC-IMV

S1). However, the average inspiratory time in our study was around 1 s and patients had little chances to breathe at high pressure level. Furthermore, we did not add pressure support during PC-SIMV and PC-IMV limiting the chance of higher V_T and P_L. In addition, variable V_T during non-synchronized modes may mimic a more natural breathing pattern and higher variability has been associated with improved respiratory mechanics and outcomes [27–30]. Calzia et al. [31] compared PC-SIMV with PSV in 19 patients after coronary artery bypass grafting. The results showed that V_T was lower during PC-SIMV (called "biphasic CPAP") than during PSV (which could be considered as fully synchronized PC mode). Gama de Abreu and colleagues [32] also compared PC-SIMV to PSV in 10 anesthetized pigs with acute lung injury. They

found that average V_T was higher during PSV compared to PC-SIMV, with no differences in terms of gas exchange and hemodynamics. These findings are in line with the results of our study. In contrast, a study by Yoshida et al. [33] conducted in 18 patients with ARDS compared a non-synchronized mode with PSV set to deliver equal mean Paw. Authors showed that lung aeration and oxygenation improved during the non-synchronized mode and no differences in hemodynamics were found between modes. Our results suggest that a non-synchronized mode may be considered to be used as a transition mode between fully controlled ventilation and the resumption of spontaneous efforts in order to reduce the risk of VILI in patients with ARDS or at high risk of ARDS.

PC-IMV provided less V_T and P_L than the other modes, but patient inspiratory effort frequently increased either because of the lack of synchronization between the patient and the ventilator or, more likely in some patients, because insufficient setting of mechanical ventilation was provided, increasing the drive to breathe [34, 35]. Calzia et al. [31] also found that PTP_{es} increased during PC-SIMV in comparison with PSV. Appropriate titration of sedative/analgesic drugs and/or adaptation of the level of ventilation (i.e. using higher respiratory rate) may alleviate the patient's high inspiratory drive. This strategy should be considered when using partially or non-synchronized modes. Other approaches for alleviating patient inspiratory effort such as using higher PEEP, extracorporeal carbon dioxide removal, or partial neuro-muscular blockade [36] may need to be explored in the future. In our study, we did not modify the backup respiratory rate, which was probably insufficient during this mode in some patients. Strong spontaneous efforts may worsen lung injury and overstretch the dependent lung zones because of a pendelluft phenomenon, especially when severe lung injury is present [25, 37]. A study by Güldner et al. [38] demonstrated that spontaneous ventilation during APRV improved oxygenation and reduced lung stress and strain regardless of the level of spontaneous effort. This latter finding may be explained by lowering V_T and P_L with non-synchronized mode. Spontaneous breathing during non-synchronized mode is recommended to be in the range of 10–30% of total minute ventilation to improve ventilation/perfusion matching and gas exchange and to avoid excessive work of breathing [39, 40]. In our study 16.7% of spontaneous breathing during PC-IMV is consistent with this suggestion to keep spontaneous breathing less than 30%. Thus, maintaining the advantages of non-synchronized modes while avoiding high respiratory effort merits to be attempted.

Of note, calculations of work of breathing using Campbell's diagram and PTP_{es} are the gold standard for evaluating patient's inspiratory effort but these techniques are not available at the bedside. $P_{0.1}$ is a simple and noninvasive method, available on most modern ventilators, which evaluates the respiratory center drive [41]. Our study showed a good correlation between $P_{0.1}$ and PTP_{es}, confirming the results of previous studies conducted in different populations and with various ventilator modes [42–44]. We need to confirm that $P_{0.1}$ can be a good surrogate marker of patient's excessive inspiratory effort but it shows promising results to be used by clinicians to indicate when excessive levels of effort occur.

Our study is a short-term physiologic study and clinical outcomes were not evaluated, which limit the clinical conclusions that can be inferred from the study. The APRV mode used in this study was set to mimic the conventional ventilator setting. We did not measure respiratory mechanics to avoid sedation that may affect spontaneous breathing. We also did not measure biomarkers to assess the effect of inspiratory synchronization on lung injury. We need investigation in larger clinical studies and for longer periods of time to evaluate the impact of different types of PC mode, but we believe these data are useful to better understand how these modes can be used.

Conclusions

Non-synchronized PC ventilation provides less V_T, lower P_L and more breath to breath variability than partially and fully synchronized modes, despite identical ventilator settings. In this regard, this mode may help to protect the lungs and its use as a transition mode, between fully controlled ventilation and the resumption of spontaneous efforts. The risk is to increase patient's effort, and therefore, a close monitoring of respiratory drive as well as acid–base and ventilation status is needed.

Abbreviations
ARDS: acute respiratory distress syndrome; APRV: airway pressure release ventilation; P_{aw}: airway pressure; PC: pressure-controlled; PC-CMV: PC continuous mandatory ventilation; PC-IMV: PC intermittent mandatory ventilation; PC-SIMV: PC synchronized intermittent mandatory ventilation; PEEP: positive end-expiratory pressure; P_{es}: esophageal pressure; P_L: transpulmonary pressure; PSV: pressure support ventilation; PTP_{es}: esophageal pressure–time product; $P_{0.1}$: airway occlusion pressure at 0.1 s; ROC: receiver operating characteristic; VIDD: ventilator-induced diaphragmatic dysfunction; VILI: ventilator-induced lung injury; V_T: tidal volume.

Authors' contributions
NR, FB, ECG, JCMR, and LB contributed to the study conception and design. NR, FB, ECG, and LC contributed to data collection. NR, JM, and LB contributed to the data analysis and interpretation and prepared the first draft of the manuscript. All authors contributed to the critical revision and final approval of the manuscript. LB had full access to all the data in the study and takes responsibility for the content of the manuscript. All authors read and approved the final manuscript.

Author details
[1] Interdepartmental Division of Critical Care Medicine, University of Toronto, Toronto, ON, Canada. [2] Keenan Research Centre and Li Ka Shing Knowledge Institute, St. Michael's Hospital, 30 Bond St, Toronto, ON M5B 1W8, Canada. [3] Division of Respiratory Diseases and Tuberculosis, Department of Medicine, Faculty of Medicine Siriraj Hospital, Bangkok, Thailand. [4] Medical Intensive Care Unit, Hospital of Angers, University of Angers, Angers, France. [5] Department of Medicine, University of Toronto, Toronto, Canada. [6] Department of Physiology, University of Toronto, Toronto, Canada. [7] Division of Respirology, Department of Medicine, University Health Network and Mount Sinai Hospital, Toronto, Canada. [8] Centre de recherche du Centre Hospitalier de l, Université de Montréal (CRCHUM), University of Montreal', Montreal, Canada. [9] Servei de Medicina Intensiva, Hospital Sant Pau, Barcelona, Spain. [10] Emergency Department, General Hospital of Annecy, Annecy, France. [11] INSERM UMR 955 eq 13, Créteil, France.

Acknowledgements
The authors thank Dr. RabiaWaheed for considerable help with the measurements.
    Funding was provided by Keenan Chair in Critical Care and Acute respiratory Failure.
    This study was presented as an oral presentation at the 28th Annual Congress of the European Society of Intensive Care Medicine (October 3–7, 2015) in Berlin, Germany.

Competing interests
NR was receiving a grant from his home institution in Thailand. FB was receiving a grant from his home institution in France. LB's laboratory has received research grants and/or equipment from the following companies: Covidien (PAV), General Electric (lung volume measurement), Fisher Paykel (Optiflow), Philips (sleep), Air Liquide (Helium, CPR). LB has received consultant fees from Covidien and Air Liquide. JM research institute has received research grants from Covidien (PAV), General Electric (lung volume measurement). JM has received speaker's honoraria from Covidien and Hamilton. JCMR has received speaker's honoraria from Covidien and Vygon. JCMR received consultant salary from Air Liquide Medical Systems. ECG and LC declare that they have no competing interests.

References

1. Esteban A, Frutos-Vivar F, Muriel A, Ferguson ND, Peñuelas O, Abraira V, et al. Evolution of mortality over time in patients receiving mechanical ventilation. Am J Respir Crit Care Med. 2013;188(2):220–30.

2. Rittayamai N, Katsios CM, Beloncle F, Friedrich JO, Mancebo J, Brochard L. Pressure-controlled vs volume-controlled ventilation in acute respiratory failure: a physiology-based narrative and systematic review. Chest. 2015;148(2):340–55.

3. Levine S, Nguyen T, Taylor N, Friscia ME, Budak MT, Rothenberg P, et al. Rapid disuse atrophy of diaphragm fibers in mechanically ventilated humans. N Engl J Med. 2008;358(13):1327–35.

4. Jaber S, Petrof BJ, Jung B, Chanques G, Berthet J-P, Rabuel C, et al. Rapidly progressive diaphragmatic weakness and injury during mechanical ventilation in humans. Am J Respir Crit Care Med. 2011;183(3):364–71.

5. Putensen C, Mutz NJ, Putensen-Himmer G, Zinserling J. Spontaneous breathing during ventilatory support improves ventilation–perfusion distributions in patients with acute respiratory distress syndrome. Am J Respir Crit Care Med. 1999;159(4 Pt 1):1241–8.

6. Sassoon CSH, Zhu E, Caiozzo VJ. Assist-control mechanical ventilation attenuates ventilator-induced diaphragmatic dysfunction. Am J Respir Crit Care Med. 2004;170(6):626–32.

7. Futier E, Constantin J-M, Combaret L, Mosoni L, Roszyk L, Sapin V, et al. Pressure support ventilation attenuates ventilator-induced protein modifications in the diaphragm. Crit Care Lond Engl. 2008;12(5):R116.

8. Kallet RH. Patient-ventilator interaction during acute lung injury, and the role of spontaneous breathing: part 2: airway pressure release ventilation. Respir Care. 2011;56(2):190–203 **(discussion 203–206)**.

9. Richard JCM, Lyazidi A, Akoumianaki E, Mortaza S, Cordioli RL, Lefebvre JC, et al. Potentially harmful effects of inspiratory synchronization during pressure preset ventilation. Intensive Care Med. 2013;39(11):2003–10.

10. Brochard L, Martin GS, Blanch L, Pelosi P, Belda FJ, Jubran A, et al. Clinical review: respiratory monitoring in the ICU—a consensus of 16. Crit Care Lond Engl. 2012;16(2):219.

11. Baydur A, Behrakis PK, Zin WA, Jaeger M, Milic-Emili J. A simple method for assessing the validity of the esophageal balloon technique. Am Rev Respir Dis. 1982;126(5):788–91.

12. Akoumianaki E, Maggiore SM, Valenza F, Bellani G, Jubran A, Loring SH, et al. The application of esophageal pressure measurement in patients with respiratory failure. Am J Respir Crit Care Med. 2014;189(5):520–31.

13. Sassoon CS, Light RW, Lodia R, Sieck GC, Mahutte CK. Pressure–time product during continuous positive airway pressure, pressure support ventilation, and T-piece during weaning from mechanical ventilation. Am Rev Respir Dis. 1991;143(3):469–75.

14. Jubran A, Tobin MJ. Pathophysiologic basis of acute respiratory distress in patients who fail a trial of weaning from mechanical ventilation. Am J Respir Crit Care Med. 1997;155(3):906–15.

15. Acute Respiratory Distress Syndrome Network, Brower RG, Matthay MA, Morris A, Schoenfeld D, Thompson BT, et al. Ventilation with lower tidal volumes as compared with traditional tidal volumes for acute lung injury and the acute respiratory distress syndrome. N Engl J Med. 2000;342(18):1301–8.

16. Determann RM, Royakkers A, Wolthuis EK, Vlaar AP, Choi G, Paulus F, et al. Ventilation with lower tidal volumes as compared with conventional tidal volumes for patients without acute lung injury: a preventive randomized controlled trial. Crit Care Lond Engl. 2010;14(1):R1.

17. Serpa Neto A, Simonis FD, Barbas CSV, Biehl M, Determann RM, Elmer J, et al. Association between tidal volume size, duration of ventilation, and sedation needs in patients without acute respiratory distress syndrome: an individual patient data meta-analysis. Intensive Care Med. 2014;40(7):950–7.

18. Samary CS, Santos RS, Santos CL, Felix NS, Bentes M, Barboza T, et al. Biological impact of transpulmonary driving pressure in experimental acute respiratory distress syndrome. Anesthesiology. 2015;123(2):423–33.

19. Gayan-Ramirez G, Testelmans D, Maes K, Rácz GZ, Cadot P, Zádor E, et al. Intermittent spontaneous breathing protects the rat diaphragm from mechanical ventilation effects. Crit Care Med. 2005;33(12):2804–9.

20. Varelmann D, Muders T, Zinserling J, Guenther U, Magnusson A, Hedenstierna G, et al. Cardiorespiratory effects of spontaneous breathing in two different models of experimental lung injury: a randomized controlled trial. Crit Care Lond Engl. 2008;12(6):R135.

21. Wrigge H, Zinserling J, Neumann P, Defosse J, Magnusson A, Putensen C, et al. Spontaneous breathing improves lung aeration in oleic acid-induced lung injury. Anesthesiology. 2003;99(2):376–84.

22. McMullen SM, Meade M, Rose L, Burns K, Mehta S, Doyle R, et al. Partial ventilatory support modalities in acute lung injury and acute respiratory distress syndrome—a systematic review. PLoS ONE. 2012;7(8):e40190.

23. Xia J, Zhang H, Sun B, Yang R, He H, Zhan Q. Spontaneous breathing with biphasic positive airway pressure attenuates lung injury in hydrochloric acid-induced acute respiratory distress syndrome. Anesthesiology. 2014;120(6):1441–9.

24. Xia J, Sun B, He H, Zhang H, Wang C, Zhan Q. Effect of spontaneous breathing on ventilator-induced lung injury in mechanically ventilated healthy rabbits: a randomized, controlled, experimental study. Crit Care Lond Engl. 2011;15(5):R244.

25. Yoshida T, Uchiyama A, Matsuura N, Mashimo T, Fujino Y. Spontaneous breathing during lung-protective ventilation in an experimental acute lung injury model: high transpulmonary pressure associated with strong spontaneous breathing effort may worsen lung injury. Crit Care Med. 2012;40(5):1578–85.

26. Yoshida T, Uchiyama A, Matsuura N, Mashimo T, Fujino Y. The comparison of spontaneous breathing and muscle paralysis in two different severities of experimental lung injury. Crit Care Med. 2013;41(2):536–45.

27. Ma B, Suki B, Bates JHT. Effects of recruitment/derecruitment dynamics on the efficacy of variable ventilation. J Appl Physiol Bethesda Md 1985. 2011;110(5):1319–26.

28. Lefevre GR, Kowalski SE, Girling LG, Thiessen DB, Mutch WA. Improved arterial oxygenation after oleic acid lung injury in the pig using a computer-controlled mechanical ventilator. Am J Respir Crit Care Med. 1996;154(5):1567–72.

29. Suki B, Alencar AM, Sujeer MK, Lutchen KR, Collins JJ, Andrade JS, et al. Life-support system benefits from noise. Nature. 1998;393(6681):127–8.

30. Kiss T, Silva PL, Huhle R, Moraes L, Santos RS, Felix NS, et al. Comparison of different degrees of variability in tidal volume to prevent deterioration of respiratory system elastance in experimental acute lung inflammation. Br J Anaesth. 2016;116(5):708–15.

31. Calzia E, Lindner KH, Witt S, Schirmer U, Lange H, Stenz R, et al. Pressure–time product and work of breathing during biphasic continuous positive airway pressure and assisted spontaneous breathing. Am J Respir Crit Care Med. 1994;150(4):904–10.

32. de Abreu MD, Cuevas M, Spieth PM, Carvalho AR, Hietschold V, Stroszczynski C, et al. Regional lung aeration and ventilation during pressure support and biphasic positive airway pressure ventilation in experimental lung injury. Crit Care Lond Engl. 2010;14(2):R34.

33. Yoshida T, Rinka H, Kaji A, Yoshimoto A, Arimoto H, Miyaichi T, et al. The impact of spontaneous ventilation on distribution of lung aeration in patients with acute respiratory distress syndrome: airway pressure release ventilation versus pressure support ventilation. Anesth Analg. 2009;109(6):1892–900.

34. Marini JJ, Smith TC, Lamb VJ. External work output and force generation during synchronized intermittent mechanical ventilation. Effect of machine assistance on breathing effort. Am Rev Respir Dis. 1988;138(5):1169–79.

35. Viale JP, Duperret S, Mahul P, Delafosse B, Delpuech C, Weismann D, et al. Time course evolution of ventilatory responses to inspiratory unloading in patients. Am J Respir Crit Care Med. 1998;157(2):428–34.

36. Doorduin J, Nollet JL, Roesthuis LH, van Hees HWH, Brochard LJ, Sinderby CA, et al. Partial neuromuscular blockade during partial ventilatory support in sedated patients with high tidal volumes. Am J Respir Crit Care Med. 2017;195(8):1033–42.

37. Yoshida T, Torsani V, Gomes S, De Santis RR, Beraldo MA, Costa ELV, et al. Spontaneous effort causes occult pendelluft during mechanical ventilation. Am J Respir Crit Care Med. 2013;188(12):1420–7.

38. Güldner A, Braune A, Carvalho N, Beda A, Zeidler S, Wiedemann B, et al. Higher levels of spontaneous breathing induce lung recruitment and

reduce global stress/strain in experimental lung injury. Anesthesiology. 2014;120(3):673–82.

39. Carvalho NC, Güldner A, Beda A, Rentzsch I, Uhlig C, Dittrich S, et al. Higher levels of spontaneous breathing reduce lung injury in experimental moderate acute respiratory distress syndrome. Crit Care Med. 2014;42(11):e702–15.

40. Putensen C, Zech S, Wrigge H, Zinserling J, Stüber F, Von Spiegel T, et al. Long-term effects of spontaneous breathing during ventilatory support in patients with acute lung injury. Am J Respir Crit Care Med. 2001;164(1):43–9.

41. Conti G, Antonelli M, Arzano S, Gasparetto A. Measurement of occlusion pressures in critically ill patients. Crit Care Lond Engl. 1997;1(3):89–93.

42. Mancebo J, Albaladejo P, Touchard D, Bak E, Subirana M, Lemaire F, et al. Airway occlusion pressure to titrate positive end-expiratory pressure in patients with dynamic hyperinflation. Anesthesiology. 2000;93(1):81–90.

43. Alberti A, Gallo F, Fongaro A, Valenti S, Rossi A. P0.1 is a useful parameter in setting the level of pressure support ventilation. Intensive Care Med. 1995;21(7):547–53.

44. Berger KI, Sorkin IB, Norman RG, Rapoport DM, Goldring RM. Mechanism of relief of tachypnea during pressure support ventilation. Chest. 1996;109(5):1320–7.

13

Nebulized heparin for patients under mechanical ventilation

Gerie J. Glas[1*], Ary Serpa Neto[2,3,4], Janneke Horn[1], Amalia Cochran[5], Barry Dixon[6], Elamin M. Elamin[7], Iris Faraklas[5], Sharmila Dissanaike[8], Andrew C. Miller[9,10] and Marcus J. Schultz[1]

Abstract

Pulmonary coagulopathy is a characteristic feature of lung injury including ventilator-induced lung injury. The aim of this individual patient data meta-analysis is to assess the effects of nebulized anticoagulants on outcome of ventilated intensive care unit (ICU) patients. A systematic search of PubMed (1966–2014), Scopus, EMBASE, and Web of Science was conducted to identify relevant publications. Studies evaluating nebulization of anticoagulants in ventilated patients were screened for inclusion, and corresponding authors of included studies were contacted to provide individual patient data. The primary endpoint was the number of ventilator-free days and alive at day 28. Secondary endpoints included hospital mortality, ICU- and hospital-free days at day 28, and lung injury scores at day seven. We constructed a propensity score-matched cohort for comparisons between patients treated with nebulized anticoagulants and controls. Data from five studies (one randomized controlled trial, one open label study, and three studies using historical controls) were included in the meta-analysis, compassing 286 patients. In all studies unfractionated heparin was used as anticoagulant. The number of ventilator-free days and alive at day 28 was higher in patients treated with nebulized heparin compared to patients in the control group (14 [IQR 0–23] vs. 6 [IQR 0–22]), though the difference did not reach statistical significance ($P = 0.459$). The number of ICU-free days and alive at day 28 was significantly higher, and the lung injury scores at day seven were significantly lower in patients treated with nebulized heparin. In the propensity score-matched analysis, there were no differences in any of the endpoints. This individual patient data meta-analysis provides no convincing evidence for benefit of heparin nebulization in intubated and ventilated ICU patients. The small patient numbers and methodological shortcomings of included studies underline the need for high-quality well-powered randomized controlled trials.

Keywords: Anticoagulants, Administration, Inhalation, Mechanical ventilation, Humans, Heparin, Intensive care

Background

Pulmonary coagulopathy is a characteristic feature of various forms of lung injury, including acute respiratory distress syndrome (ARDS) [1–4], pneumonia [1, 5, 6], and inhalation trauma [7]. Recently, it was even demonstrated that mechanical ventilation has the potential to alter the pulmonary hemostatic balance [8], with remarkably similar changes in coagulation and fibrinolysis as found in ARDS, pneumonia, or inhalation trauma [1, 4, 7, 9].

Fibrin deposition and hyaline membrane formation are considered important early features in diffuse alveolar damage, the hallmark of ARDS [1, 10–12]. Pulmonary activation of coagulation is likely to be involved in containing inflammation or infection to the site of injury and may have evolved as a host-protective mechanism [13, 14]. However, these local hemostatic disturbances could also be deleterious, as excessive or persistent fibrin deposition has been associated with alveolar collapse due to impaired surfactant function [15], pulmonary edema and impaired gas exchange [16], and eventually pulmonary fibrosis [17].

*Correspondence: g.j.glas@amc.uva.nl
[1] Laboratory of Experimental Intensive Care and Anesthesiology (L·E·I·C·A), Department of Intensive Care, Academic Medical Center, Meibergdreef 9, 1105 AZ Amsterdam, The Netherlands
Full list of author information is available at the end of the article

While preclinical studies provided support for the use of nebulized or systemic anticoagulants to prevent lung injury in animals [18, 19], clinical studies in ventilated patients thus far showed conflicting results [19, 20]. Clinical trials have been performed in patients with (mild) ARDS or sepsis, focusing on *systemic* treatment with anticoagulants such as recombinant human (rh)-activated protein C, antithrombin, rh-tissue factor pathway inhibitor, and unfractionated heparin. All but one trial were unsuccessful in improving patient outcomes [21–32]. It has been suggested that higher concentrations of an anticoagulant in the pulmonary compartment may be necessary to affect pulmonary disturbances [19]. Thus, *local* administration of anticoagulants to the pulmonary compartment could be considered a more effective anticoagulant intervention.

Over the last decades, nebulized heparin has been safely administered in a number of pulmonary conditions [33–35]. Studies in healthy volunteers showed nebulized heparin to reach the lower respiratory tract [36], distribute uniformly in the lungs [36], and exert local anticoagulant effects [35]. In line herewith, nebulized heparin attenuated pulmonary coagulopathy in critically ill patients with acute lung injury [37]. Intrapulmonary administered heparin crosses the alveolar membrane into the circulation, being absorbed rapidly and released gradually into the blood [38]. Indeed, there is evidence of a dose-dependent effect of heparin nebulization on plasma levels of aPTT [35, 39], with a threshold dose of 150,000 IU of heparin resulting in a measurable increase in aPTT [35]. This effect on systemic coagulation does not seem to potentiate the risk of bleedings [39–41], suggesting heparin nebulizations to be safe. Nevertheless, data on the feasibility and safety of heparin nebulizations in ventilated patients are scarce [19], and there are very limited data on the use of nebulized anticoagulants in ventilated patients. A systematic review recently showed conflicting effects of nebulized anticoagulation in burn patients with inhalation injury, a patient population in which this intervention is frequently applied [20]. It remains unclear whether nebulized anticoagulation is beneficial for all ventilated intensive care unit (ICU) patients. We performed an individual patient data meta-analysis to determine the association between nebulized anticoagulants and outcomes of intubated and ventilated ICU patients to test the hypothesis that nebulization of anticoagulants improves outcome.

Methods
Systematic search
Publications were identified through a systematic search of PubMed (1966–2014), Scopus, EMBASE, and Web of Science. Search terms referred to the

intervention (nebulized, vaporized, aerosolized) and anticoagulant agents (anticoagulants, anticoagulation, antithrombins, heparin), as well as conditions of the patient population (acute lung injury, ARDS, critical illness, burn, smoke, inhalation injury) and mechanical ventilation. Searches were not limited by date or language. The detailed search strategy is shown in Additional file 1: Appendix 1.

Titles and available abstracts of the articles identified were screened. Studies were eligible for inclusion if they evaluated nebulized or aerosolized anticoagulants, including heparins, heparinoids, antithrombins, and/or fibrinolytics, in ventilated ICU patients. There were no restrictions regarding age of patients. Case reports and ongoing studies were excluded. Retrieved articles were screened for pertinent information, and reference lists of eligible articles were screened for potentially important papers. Quality of evidence for randomized and nonrandomized studies were assessed with use of, respectively, the Cochrane Collaboration's tool for assessing risk of bias [42] and the Newcastle Ottawa Scale [43], see Additional file 1: Appendix 5.

Collection of individual patient data
The corresponding author of each included study was contacted and asked for individual patient data. This included demographic and baseline characteristics, dose and duration of nebulized anticoagulants, duration of ventilation, occurrence of pneumonia, length of stay in the ICU and hospital, and mortality. Ventilatory parameters and lung injury scores (LIS) [44] were collected up to 7 days from admission. Data were accepted in any kind of electronic format.

Primary outcome
The primary outcome was the number of ventilator-free days and alive at day 28, defined as the number of days alive and without ventilation until day 28.

Secondary outcomes
Secondary outcomes included mortality during hospital stay, ICU-free days at day 28, defined as the number alive and outside the ICU at day 28, and hospital-free days and alive at day 28, defined as the number of days alive and outside hospital at day 28. PaO_2/FiO_2 and LIS at day seven, calculated from the available data, and occurrence of pneumonia during hospital stay.

Statistical analysis
Continuous variables were presented as median and interquartile range (median [IQR]). Binary and categorical variables were presented as frequencies and percentages [n (%)].

Patients were analyzed according to use or not of nebulized anticoagulants. Time-to-event was defined as time from the day of inclusion in the study to the event of interest. We used a Cox proportional-hazards regression model to examine simultaneous effects of multiple covariates on outcomes, censoring patient data at the time of death, or hospital discharge. In all models, the categorical variables were tested for trend with the nonuse of nebulized anticoagulants as reference. The proportional-hazards assumption was assessed plotting partial residuals against survival time. A test for interaction between pairs of variables in the final model was performed. The effect of each variable in these models was assessed with the use of the Wald test and described by the hazard ratio with 95 % confidence interval (CI). The initial model included age and baseline PaO_2/FiO_2. The final model was developed by dropping each variable in turn from the model and by conducting likelihood-ratio tests to compare the full and the nested models. We used a significance level of 0.05 as the cutoff to exclude a variable from the model. Finally, use of nebulized anticoagulants (no vs. yes) was added to the model. Kaplan–Meier curves and log-rank test were used to determine the univariate significance of the study variables.

A linear mixed model was used to analyze time-course variables. A repeated-measures generalized linear model (GLM) was used to assess the time interaction for ventilatory and oxygenation parameters during mechanical ventilation. The model includes two factors: (1) study group (fixed factor), each level of the study group factor had a different linear effect on the value of the dependent variable; (2) time as covariate, time was considered to be a random sample from a larger population of values, and the effect was not limited to the chosen times.

Subgroup analyses were used to assess the effect of tidal volume size in the following prespecified subgroups: (1) age (<18 vs. ≥18 years); (2) dose of nebulized anticoagulant (low dose, defined as 30,000 U/day versus high dose, defined as ≥60,000 U/day); and (3) patient population (burn vs. non-burn). Propensity scores were estimated for each patient with logistic regression using two clinically relevant baseline characteristics (age and baseline PaO_2/FiO_2). Propensity score matching is described in detail in the supplemental material (Appendix file 1: Appendix 4). We conducted a post hoc sensitivity analysis in the matched cohort, including age (<18 vs. ≥18 years), dose of nebulized anticoagulant (low dose, defined as 30,000 U/day vs. high dose, defined as 60,000 U/day or higher), patient population (burn vs. non-burn), and tidal volume size (low, defined as ≤560 ml vs. high, defined as >560 ml by using the median as a cutoff value). All analyses were conducted with Review Manager v.5.1.1 (The Nordic Cochrane Centre, The Cochrane Collaboration,

Copenhagen, Denmark), SPSS v.20 (IBM Corporation, New York, USA), and R v.2.12.0 (R Foundation for Statistical Computing, Vienna, Austria). For all analyses two-sided P values <0.05 were considered significant.

Results
Systematic search
The search yielded 216 potentially relevant publications (Fig. 1). Based on the titles or abstracts, 202 publications were excluded. The remaining 14 publications reported on ten clinical studies, all on nebulized heparin [39–41, 45–55]. One publication reported on an ongoing trial [49]. Nine studies were eligible for inclusion in our individual patient data meta-analysis (521 patients). However, the corresponding authors of three studies did not provide the individual patient data [41, 45, 48], and one could not be contacted [53]. Therefore, data from five studies (286 patients) were available for the meta-analysis [39, 40, 50–52].

Table 1 summarizes the study characteristics of the included studies. All three studies conducted in burn patients with inhalation injury were retrospective studies with historical controls [50–52]. One open label phase I study and one randomized controlled trial were conducted in critically ill patients [39, 40]. One study had a mixed population with both pediatric and adult patients [50], and all other studies were performed in adult patients. Dosage of heparin varied from 30,000 to 400,000 U/day.

Of note, patients treated with nebulized heparin were ventilated with lower tidal volumes during the first 7 days of ventilation (Additional file 1: Appendix 3: Tables S1

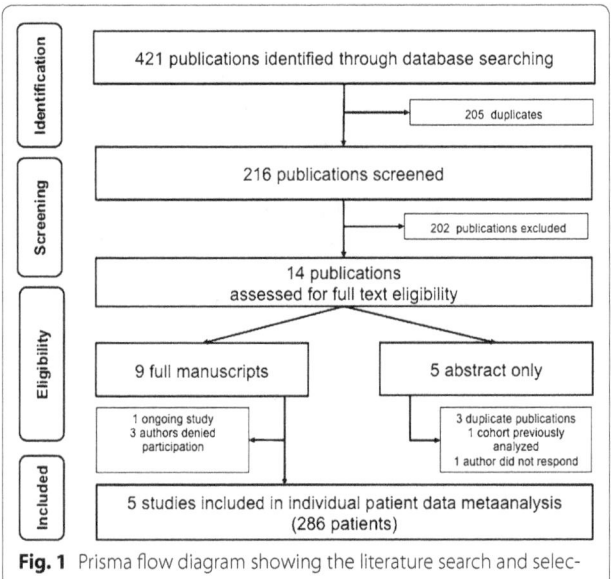

Fig. 1 Prisma flow diagram showing the literature search and selection strategy

Table 1 Characteristics of studies included in the individual patient data meta-analysis

Authors (year)	Design	Population (adult/pediatric)	Number of patients		Dose of heparin	Outcomes included in IPD meta-analysis	References
			Heparin	Control			
Holt (2008)	Retrospective with historical control	Smoke inhalation (adult and pediatric)	62	88	30,000	VFD-28; hospital mortality; pneumonia; PaO$_2$/FiO$_2$ at day 7; hospital-free days and alive at day 28	[50]
Dixon (2008)	Open label phase 1 trial	Critically ill (adult)	16	–	50,000–400,000	VFD-28; ICU mortality; ICU and hospital-free days and alive at day 28	[39]
Miller (2009)	Retrospective with historical control	Smoke inhalation (adult)	16	14	60,000	VFD-28; hospital mortality; PaO$_2$/FiO$_2$ and LIS at day 7; ICU and hospital-free days and alive at day 28; pneumonia	[52]
Dixon (2010)	Randomized controlled trial	Critically ill (adult)	25	25	150,000	VFD-28; hospital mortality; PaO$_2$/FiO$_2$ and LIS at day 7; ICU and hospital-free days and alive at day 28	[40]
Kashefi (2014)	Retrospective with historical control	Smoke inhalation (adult)	20	20	30,000	VFD-28; hospital mortality; pneumonia; PaO$_2$/FiO$_2$; and hospital-free days and alive at day 28	[51]

VFD-28 ventilator-free days and alive at day 28, *IPD* individual patient data meta-analysis, *LIS* Lung injury scores

and Appendix 4: Table S5). All other ventilatory parameters were similar between the two study groups (Additional file 1: Appendix 2: Figures S2 and S3; Appendix 3: Table S1).

Table 2 summarizes the demographic data of the included patients. For the propensity score-matched cohort, 248 patients could be analyzed (Additional file 1: Appendix 4: Table S3).

Effects of heparin on outcome

The median number of ventilator-free days and alive at day 28 did not differ in patients treated with nebulized heparin compared to patients in the control group (14, IQR 0–23 vs. 6, IQR 0–22 days, $P = 0.459$). A statistically significant difference was found for ICU-free days at day 28 (3 [0–19] vs. 0 [0–14] days, $P = 0.035$). The LIS at day seven were also significantly lower in patients treated with nebulized heparin (2.0 [1.0–2.5] vs. 2.2 [1.7–3.0] days, $P = 0.027$). There was no difference in hospital mortality (Table 3 and Additional file 1: Appendix 2: Figure S1), hospital-free days and alive at day 28 or occurrence of pneumonia during hospital stay (Table 3).

In subgroup analyses, there was no difference in number of ventilator-free days at day 28, overall mortality nor number of hospital-free days and alive at day 28, according to age (<18 vs. ≥18 years), dose of heparin, type of population and tidal volume size (Additional file 1: Appendix 3: Table S2).

Propensity score-matched cohort

Results of the meta-analysis in the propensity score-matched cohort are presented in the online supplement (Additional file 1: Appendix 4: Tables S3–S6).

The median number of ventilator-free days at day 28 in patients treated with nebulized heparin was higher than that in control patients (16 [0–23] vs. 5 [0–20] days), but again this difference did not reach statistical significance ($P = 0.133$). Also, no statistical differences were found for the number of ICU-free days and alive at day 28 and LIS at day seven and other secondary endpoints (Additional file 1: Appendix 2: Figure S1 and Appendix 4: Table S4).

Also in this part of the analysis, it was found that patients treated with nebulized heparin were ventilated with lower tidal volumes than control patients during the first 7 days of ventilation (Additional file 1: Appendix 4: Table S5). In the post hoc sensitivity analysis on age, dose of heparin, type of population and tidal volume size, no differences were found for ventilator-free days and hospital-free days at day 28 (Additional file 1: Appendix 4: Table S6).

Discussion

Nebulization of heparin, alone or combined with other agents, did not improve the outcome of mechanically ventilated patients in this individual patient data meta-analysis. Even though patients who received nebulization with heparin demonstrated higher numbers of ventilator-free days and alive at day 28, differences

Table 2 Characteristics of the patients included in the individual patient data analysis

Variables	Overall cohort ($N = 286$)		
	Nebulized heparin ($N = 139$)	Control ($N = 147$)	SD (%), P
Age, years	50.0 (36.0–69.0)	45.0 (31.0–63.0)	17.6, 0.09
	($N = 139$)	($N = 147$)	
Gender, male (%)	81 (65.9)	107 (72.8)	−19.0, 0.14
APACHE III	22.0 (17.0–31.0)	24.0 (15.0–32.0)	5.1, 0.74
	($N = 57$)	($N = 39$)	
% TBSA	25.5 (12.9–52.2)	31.2 (16.5–52.2)	−5.1, 0.51
	($N = 90$)	($N = 110$)	
Dosage of heparin (U/day)	30,000	0.0	–
	(30,000–100,000)	(0.0–0.0)	
Dosage of NAC (mg/day)	3600 (3600–3600)	0.0 (0.0–0.0)	–
Duration of treatment	7.0 (3.0–12.0)	0.0 (0.0–0.0)	–
Baseline LIS	2.0 (0.7–2.5)	2.0 (1.2–3.0)	−26.2, 0.29
	($N = 41$)	($N = 39$)	
Baseline PaO_2/FiO_2	219.5 (158.2–316.5)	270.0 (163.5–366.5)	−18.3, 0.09
	($N = 136$)	($N = 141$)	

Values are median (IQR) or no./total no. (%). Not all requested data were available for each study

SD standardized difference, *TBSA* total burn surface area, *NAC* N-acetylcysteine, *LIS* lung injury scores, *N* number of patients

Table 3 Primary and secondary outcomes

Variables	Nebulized heparin ($N = 139$)	Control ($N = 147$)	Odds ratio[a] (95 % CI)	P
Primary outcome				
Ventilator-free days at day 28	14.0 (0.0–23.0)	6.0 (0.0–22.0)		0.459
	($N = 139$)	($N = 144$)		
Secondary outcomes				
Overall mortality	34/139 (24.5)	35/147 (23.8)	0.65 (0.50–1.56)[b]	0.653
	($N = 139$)	($N = 147$)		
PaO_2/FiO_2 at day seven (mmHg)	242.5 (206.0–300.0)	220.2 (179.4–297.7)		0.098
	($N = 61$)	($N = 78$)		
LIS at day seven	2.0 (1.0–2.5)	2.2 (1.7–3.0)		0.027
	($N = 40$)	($N = 48$)		
Pneumonia during hospital stay	48/82 (58.5)	48/106 (45.3)	1.49 (0.79–2.80)	0.219
	($N = 82$)	($N = 106$)		
ICU-free days at day 28	2.9 (0.0–19.0)	0.0 (0.0–14.2)		0.035
	($N = 78$)	($N = 62$)		
Hospital-free days at day 28	0.0 (0.0–12.0)	0.0 (0.0–14.0)		0.951
	($N = 139$)	($N = 147$)		

Values are median (IQR), and others are no./total no. (%)

Not all requested data were available for each study

LIS lung injury scores, *CI* confidence interval, *N* number of patients

[a] Adjusted by: age and baseline PaO_2/FiO_2

[b] Presented as hazard ratio adjusted by: age, %TBSA, and baseline PaO_2/FiO_2

were not statistically significant. We did find a higher number of ICU-free days and alive at day 28 and lower LIS at day seven in patients treated with nebulized heparin. A propensity score-matched cohort analysis, however, showed no beneficial effects of heparin nebulization.

The aim of this individual patient data meta-analysis was to investigate the effectiveness of nebulized anticoagulants in intubated and ventilated ICU patients. Since heparin was the only anticoagulant agent used in the included studies, we are unable to ascertain the potential efficacy of any other anticoagulant, due to paucity of available evidence. Also, the majority of patients included were patients with inhalation injury (220 of 286). Thus, conclusions on the effects of nebulized heparin for intubated and ventilated ICU patients in general cannot be made. As adverse effects of mechanical ventilation may be more severe in burn patients, it is possible that these patients benefit more from nebulized anticoagulants compared to non-burn or smoke inhalation patients [19].

Reported effects of nebulized heparin on duration of mechanical ventilation and other outcomes such as mortality in patients with inhalation injury have been conflicting. Beneficial effects of heparin nebulization could have been confounded by improvements in ICU care in general as they were conducted around a change in institutional protocol [45, 52]. In two other before–after studies no beneficial effects of heparin nebulizations were seen [50, 51]. Furthermore, in three of the included studies [50–52], nebulized heparin was combined with the use of mucolytic agents and bronchodilators. This highlights the difficulty to distinguish between the effects of heparin nebulization and other parts of treatment on patient outcome in retrospective studies with historical controls.

One important finding of our individual patient data meta-analysis was that patients receiving heparin nebulization were ventilated with lower tidal volumes compared to control patients. While in theory improved clinical outcomes could have been caused by nebulization of heparin, it could also function as an important confounder, since low tidal volume ventilation is associated with a better outcome, also in patients without ARDS [56–60]. Still, relatively high tidal volumes were used in all included studies which may hamper extrapolation to current ventilation practices. On the other hand, while lower tidal volumes are increasingly being used [61, 62], guidelines inconsistently advise on tidal volume size in ICU patients without ARDS and current ventilation practice is uncertain [63].

Dosage of heparin varied from 30,000 to 400,000 U/day. Several studies suggested a dose-dependent effect of heparin nebulization in which dosages of 30,000 U/day improved outcomes in pediatric patients [45] but failed to improve outcomes in adults [50, 51], while higher dosages did improve outcome of adult patients

[48, 52]. The present meta-analysis could not confirm this. Types of nebulizers and its position in the circuit may affect the delivery of nebulized drugs in ventilated patients [64–66]. Furthermore, aerosol particle size distribution and heparin concentrations may also influence the amount of heparin delivered to the lower respiratory tract [67]. The method of nebulization differed between studies. Three studies used mesh nebulizers [39, 40, 50], and two studies used jet nebulizers [51, 52]. Thus, the delivered amount of nebulized drugs may have varied.

Our results contradict the conclusion of a previous systematic review concluding that inhaled anticoagulation regimens improve survival and decrease morbidity in smoke inhalation patients [20]. This may be due to some major differences between the two studies. First, as our aim was to investigate the effect of heparin nebulization in any critically ill patient, we included different studies. Second, the use of individual patient data allowed standardization of the analyses across studies irrespective of how the data were reported [68].

One major limitation of this meta-analysis is that we were only able to analyze the individual data of 286 patients out of 521 potentially eligible patients as the authors of four studies did not provide individual patient data. Other limitations are caused by the methodological shortcomings of included studies. Only one of the included studies was a small, but properly conducted randomized controlled trial [40]. The other studies, mostly small in size, used an open label design or were retrospective cohort studies with use of historical controls. Due to these limitations, the results from this meta-analysis should be interpreted with great caution. To account for some of those limitations we used propensity score matching correcting for relevant baseline characteristics. However, imbalances such as the presence of unmeasured confounders are likely to remain [69]. Nevertheless, the post hoc sensitivity analysis indicates that the results of this meta-analysis were affected neither by factors such as age, presence of burn, or inhalation injury nor by differences in tidal volume size and heparin dosages.

Conclusion

No beneficial effects of heparin nebulization on the outcome of ventilated patients were observed in this individual patient data meta-analysis. The small patient numbers and methodological shortcomings of included studies underline the need for high-quality well-powered randomized controlled trials to determine the effect of heparin nebulization on outcome of intubated and ventilated ICU patients.

Abbreviations

ARDS: acute respiratory distress syndrome; CI: confidence interval; GLM: generalized linear model; GRADE: grading of recommendations assessment, development and evaluation; ICU: intensive care unit; IQR: interquartile range; LEICA: Laboratory of Experimental Intensive Care and Anesthesiology; LIS: lung injury scores; SD: standard deviation.

Authors' contributions

GJG, MJS, JH, and ASN contributed to the conception and design of the study, drafted, and revised the manuscript. ASN acquired and analyzed the data. AC, BD, EME, IF, SD, and ACM provided the individual patient data and critically revised the article. All authors read and approved the final manuscript.

Author details

[1] Laboratory of Experimental Intensive Care and Anesthesiology (L·E·I·C·A), Department of Intensive Care, Academic Medical Center, Meibergdreef 9, 1105 AZ Amsterdam, The Netherlands. [2] Department of Critical Care Medicine, Hospital Israelita Albert Einstein, São Paulo, Brazil. [3] Department of Critical Care Medicine, Faculdade de Medicina do ABC, Santo André, Brazil. [4] Program of Post-Graduation, Research and Innovation, Faculdade de Medicina do ABC, Santo André, Brazil. [5] Department of Surgery, University of Utah Health Sciences Center, Salt Lake City, UT, USA. [6] Department of Intensive Care, St. Vincent's Hospital, Melbourne, Australia. [7] Division of Pulmonary, Critical Care, and Sleep Medicine, Department of Internal Medicine, James A. Haley Veteran's Hospital, University of South Florida, Tampa, FL, USA. [8] Department of Surgery, Texas Tech University Health Sciences Center, Lubbock, TX, USA. [9] Department of Critical Care Medicine, Clinical Center, National Institutes of Health, Bethesda, MD, USA. [10] Department of Emergency Medicine, West Virginia University, Morgantown, WV, USA.

Acknowledgements

This study was funded by 'de Nederlandse Brandwondenstichting' (the Dutch Burn Association, Beverwijk, the Netherlands).

Competing interests

The authors declare that they have no competing interests.

References

1. Gunther A, Mosavi P, Heinemann S, Ruppert C, Muth H, Markart P, et al. Alveolar fibrin formation caused by enhanced procoagulant and depressed fibrinolytic capacities in severe pneumonia. Comparison with the acute respiratory distress syndrome. Am J Respir Crit Care Med. 2000;161(2 Pt 1):454–62.
2. Idell S. Coagulation, fibrinolysis, and fibrin deposition in acute lung injury. Crit Care Med. 2003;31(4 Suppl):S213–20. doi:10.1097/01.CCM.0000057846.21303.AB.
3. Idell S, James KK, Levin EG, Schwartz BS, Manchanda N, Maunder RJ, et al. Local abnormalities in coagulation and fibrinolytic pathways predispose to alveolar fibrin deposition in the adult respiratory distress syndrome. J Clin Invest. 1989;84(2):695–705. doi:10.1172/JCI114217.
4. Vervloet MG, Thijs LG, Hack CE. Derangements of coagulation and fibrinolysis in critically ill patients with sepsis and septic shock. Semin Thromb Hemost. 1998;24(1):33–44. doi:10.1055/s-2007-995821.
5. Levi M, Schultz MJ, Rijneveld AW, Van Der Poll T. Bronchoalveolar coagulation and fibrinolysis in endotoxemia and pneumonia. Crit Care Med. 2003;31(4 Suppl):S238–42. doi:10.1097/01.CCM.0000057849.53689.65.
6. Schultz MJ, Millo J, Levi M, Hack CE, Weverling GJ, Garrard CS, et al. Local activation of coagulation and inhibition of fibrinolysis in the lung during ventilator associated pneumonia. Thorax. 2004;59(2):130–5.
7. Hofstra JJ, Vlaar AP, Knape P, Mackie DP, Determann RM, Choi G, et al. Pulmonary activation of coagulation and inhibition of fibrinolysis after burn injuries and inhalation trauma. J Trauma. 2011;70(6):1389–97. doi:10.1097/TA.0b013e31820f85a7.
8. Schultz MJ, Determann RM, Royakkers AA, Wolthuis EK, Korevaar JC, Levi MM. Bronchoalveolar activation of coagulation and inhibition of fibrinolysis during ventilator-associated lung injury. Crit Care Res Pract. 2012;2012:961784. doi:10.1155/2012/961784.
9. Hofstra JJ, Haitsma JJ, Juffermans NP, Levi M, Schultz MJ. The role of bronchoalveolar hemostasis in the pathogenesis of acute lung injury. Semin Thromb Hemost. 2008;34(5):475–84. doi:10.1055/s-0028-1092878

10. International Consensus Conferences in Intensive Care Medicine. Ventilator-associated Lung Injury in ARDS. This official conference report was cosponsored by the American Thoracic Society, The European Society of Intensive Care Medicine, and The Societe de Reanimation de Langue Francaise, and was approved by the ATS Board of Directors, July 1999. Am J Respir Crit Care Med. 1999;160(6):2118–24.
11. Bastarache JA, Ware LB, Bernard GR. The role of the coagulation cascade in the continuum of sepsis and acute lung injury and acute respiratory distress syndrome. Semin Respir Crit Care Med. 2006;27(4):365–76. doi:10.1055/s-2006-948290.
12. Castro CY. ARDS and diffuse alveolar damage: a pathologist's perspective. Semin Thorac Cardiovasc Surg. 2006;18(1):13–9. doi:10.1053/j.semtcvs.2006.02.001.
13. Opal SM. Phylogenetic and functional relationships between coagulation and the innate immune response. Crit Care Med. 2000;28(9 Suppl):S77–80.
14. Schultz MJ, Dixon B. A breathtaking and bloodcurdling story of coagulation and inflammation in acute lung injury. J Thromb Haemost. 2009;7(12):2050–2. doi:10.1111/j.1538-7836.2009.03639.x.
15. Seeger W, Stohr G, Wolf HR, Neuhof H. Alteration of surfactant function due to protein leakage: special interaction with fibrin monomer. J Appl Physiol. 1985;58(2):326–38.
16. Laterre PF, Wittebole X, Dhainaut JF. Anticoagulant therapy in acute lung injury. Crit Care Med. 2003;31(4 Suppl):S329–36. doi:10.1097/01.CCM.0000057912.71499.A5.
17. Marshall R, Bellingan G, Laurent G. The acute respiratory distress syndrome: fibrosis in the fast lane. Thorax. 1998;53(10):815–7.
18. Idell S. Anticoagulants for acute respiratory distress syndrome: can they work? Am J Respir Crit Care Med. 2001;164(4):517–20.
19. Tuinman PR, Dixon B, Levi M, Juffermans NP, Schultz MJ. Nebulized anticoagulants for acute lung injury—a systematic review of pre-clinical and clinical investigations. Crit Care. 2012;16(2):R70. doi:10.1186/cc11325.
20. Miller AC, Elamin EM, Suffredini AF. Inhaled anticoagulation regimens for the treatment of smoke inhalation-associated acute lung injury: a systematic review. Crit Care Med. 2014;42(2):413–9.
21. Abraham E, Reinhart K, Opal S, Demeyer I, Doig C, Rodriguez AL, et al. Efficacy and safety of tifacogin (recombinant tissue factor pathway inhibitor) in severe sepsis: a randomized controlled trial. JAMA. 2003;290(2):238–47. doi:10.1001/jama.290.2.238.
22. Afshari A, Wetterslev J, Brok J, Moller AM. Antithrombin III for critically ill patients. Cochrane Database Syst Rev. 2008;3:CD005370. doi:10.1002/14651858.CD005370.pub2.
23. Bernard GR, Vincent JL, Laterre PF, LaRosa SP, Dhainaut JF, Lopez-Rodriguez A, et al. Efficacy and safety of recombinant human activated protein C for severe sepsis. N Engl J Med. 2001;344(10):699–709. doi:10.1056/NEJM200103083441001.
24. Dhainaut JF, Laterre PF, Janes JM, Bernard GR, Artigas A, Bakker J, et al. Drotrecogin alfa (activated) in the treatment of severe sepsis patients with multiple-organ dysfunction: data from the PROWESS trial. Intensive Care Med. 2003;29(6):894–903. doi:10.1007/s00134-003-1731-1.
25. Eisele B, Lamy M, Thijs LG, Keinecke HO, Schuster HP, Matthias FR, et al. Antithrombin III in patients with severe sepsis. A randomized, placebo-controlled, double-blind multicenter trial plus a meta-analysis on all randomized, placebo-controlled, double-blind trials with antithrombin III in severe sepsis. Intensive Care Med. 1998;24(7):663–72.
26. Jaimes F, De La Rosa G, Morales C, Fortich F, Arango C, Aguirre D, et al. Unfractionated heparin for treatment of sepsis: a randomized clinical trial (The HETRASE Study). Crit Care Med. 2009;37(4):1185–96. doi:10.1097/CCM.0b013e31819c06bc.
27. Laterre PF, Opal SM, Abraham E, LaRosa SP, Creasey AA, Xie F, et al. A clinical evaluation committee assessment of recombinant human tissue factor pathway inhibitor (tifacogin) in patients with severe community-acquired pneumonia. Crit Care. 2009;13(2):R36. doi:10.1186/cc7747.
28. Liu KD, Levitt J, Zhuo H, Kallet RH, Brady S, Steingrub J, et al. Randomized clinical trial of activated protein C for the treatment of acute lung injury. Am J Respir Crit Care Med. 2008;178(6):618–23. doi:10.1164/rccm.200803-419OC.
29. Marti-Carvajal AJ, Sola I, Gluud C, Lathyris D, Cardona AF. Human recombinant protein C for severe sepsis and septic shock in adult and paediatric patients. Cochrane Database Syst Rev. 2012;12:CD004388. doi:10.1002/14651858.CD004388.pub6.

30. Ranieri VM, Thompson BT, Barie PS, Dhainaut JF, Douglas IS, Finfer S, et al. Drotrecogin alfa (activated) in adults with septic shock. N Engl J Med. 2012;366(22):2055–64. doi:10.1056/NEJMoa1202290.

31. Warren BL, Eid A, Singer P, Pillay SS, Carl P, Novak I, et al. Caring for the critically ill patient. High-dose antithrombin III in severe sepsis: a randomized controlled trial. JAMA. 2001;286(15):1869–78.

32. Wunderink RG, Laterre PF, Francois B, Perrotin D, Artigas A, Vidal LO, et al. Recombinant tissue factor pathway inhibitor in severe community-acquired pneumonia: a randomized trial. Am J Respir Crit Care Med. 2011;183(11):1561–8. doi:10.1164/rccm.201007-1167OC.

33. Bendstrup KE, Jensen JI. Inhaled heparin is effective in exacerbations of asthma. Respir Med. 2000;94(2):174–5. doi:10.1053/rmed.1999.0677.

34. Monagle K, Ryan A, Hepponstall M, Mertyn E, Monagle P, Ignjatovic V, et al. Inhalational use of antithrombotics in humans: review of the literature. Thromb Res. 2015;136(6):1059–66. doi:10.1016/j.thromres.2015.10.011.

35. Markart P, Nass R, Ruppert C, Hundack L, Wygrecka M, Korfei M, et al. Safety and tolerability of inhaled heparin in idiopathic pulmonary fibrosis. J Aerosol Med Pulm Drug Deliv. 2010;23(3):161–72. doi:10.1089/jamp.2009.0780.

36. Bendstrup KE, Chambers CB, Jensen JI, Newhouse MT. Lung deposition and clearance of inhaled (99 m)Tc-heparin in healthy volunteers. Am J Respir Crit Care Med. 1999;160(5 Pt 1):1653–8.

37. Dixon B, Schultz MJ, Hofstra JJ, Campbell DJ, Santamaria JD. Nebulized heparin reduces levels of pulmonary coagulation activation in acute lung injury. Crit Care. 2010;14(5):445. doi:10.1186/cc9269.

38. Jaques LB, Mahadoo J, Kavanagh LW. Intrapulmonary heparin. A new procedure for anticoagulant therapy. Lancet. 1976;2(7996):1157–61.

39. Dixon B, Santamaria JD, Campbell DJ. A phase 1 trial of nebulised heparin in acute lung injury. Crit Care. 2008;12(3):R64. doi:10.1186/cc6894.

40. Dixon B, Schultz MJ, Smith R, Fink JB, Santamaria JD, Campbell DJ. Nebulized heparin is associated with fewer days of mechanical ventilation in critically ill patients: a randomized controlled trial. Crit Care. 2010;14(5):R180. doi:10.1186/cc9286.

41. Yip LY, Lim YF, Chan HN. Safety and potential anticoagulant effects of nebulised heparin in burns patients with inhalational injury at Singapore General Hospital Burns Centre. Burns. 2011;37(7):1154–60. doi:10.1016/j.burns.2011.07.006.

42. Higgins JP, Altman DG, Gotzsche PC, Juni P, Moher D, Oxman AD, et al. The Cochrane Collaboration's tool for assessing risk of bias in randomised trials. BMJ. 2011;343:d5928. doi:10.1136/bmj.d5928.

43. Stang A. Critical evaluation of the Newcastle–Ottawa scale for the assessment of the quality of nonrandomized studies in meta-analyses. Eur J Epidemiol. 2010;25(9):603–5. doi:10.1007/s10654-010-9491-z.

44. Murray JF, Matthay MA, Luce JM, Flick MR. An expanded definition of the adult respiratory distress syndrome. Am Rev Respir Dis. 1988;138(3):720–3.

45. Desai MH, Mlcak R, Richardson J, Nichols R, Herndon DN. Reduction in mortality in pediatric patients with inhalation injury with aerosolized heparin/acetylcystine therapy. J Burn Care Rehabil. 1998;19(3):210–2.

46. Dixon B, Santamaria D, Campbell J. Nebulized heparin in acute lung injury. J Aerosol Med Pulm Drug Deliv. 2009;22(2):203.

47. Dixon B, Schultz M, Fink JB, Campbell D, Santamaria JD. Nebulised heparin is associated with fewer days of mechanical ventilation in critically ill patients: a randomised controlled trial. Am J Respir Crit Care Med. 2011;183. **(1 Meeting Abstracts)**

48. Elsharnouby NM, Eid HEA, Abou Elezz NF, Aboelatta YA. Heparin/N-acetylcysteine: an adjuvant in the management of burn inhalation injury. A study of different doses. J Crit Care. 2014;29(1):182.e1–4.

49. Glas GJ, Muller J, Binnekade JM, Cleffken B, Colpaert K, Dixon B, et al. HEPBURN—investigating the efficacy and safety of nebulized heparin versus placebo in burn patients with inhalation trauma: study protocol for a multi-center randomized controlled trial. Trials. 2014;15:91. doi:10.1186/1745-6215-15-91.

50. Holt J, Saffle JR, Morris SE, Cochran A. Use of inhaled heparin/N-acetylcystine in inhalation injury: does it help? J Burn Care Res. 2008;29(1):192–5.

51. Kashefi NS, Nathan JI, Dissanaike S. Does a nebulized heparin/N-acetylcysteine protocol improve outcomes in adult smoke inhalation? Plast Reconstr Surg Glob Open. 2014;2(6):e165. doi:10.1097/gox.0000000000000121.

52. Miller AC, Rivero A, Ziad S, Smith DJ, Elamin EM. Influence of nebulized unfractionated heparin and N-acetylcysteine in acute lung injury after smoke inhalation injury. J Burn Care Res. 2009;30(2):249–56.

53. Otremba S, Faris J. Hall Zimmerman L, Barbat S, White M. Inhaled heparin in critically ill patients with smoke inhalation injury. Crit Care Med. 2013;1:A231–2.

54. Rivero A, Elamin E, Nguyen V, Cruse W, Smith D. Can nebulized heparin and N-acetylcysteine reduce acute lung injury after inhalation lung insult? Chest. 2007;132(4):565S.

55. Kashefi N, Dissanaike S. Does a nebulized heparin/N-acetylcysteine protocol improve clinical outcomes in adult patients with inhalation injury? J Burn Care Res. 2013;1:S82.

56. Determann RM, Royakkers A, Wolthuis EK, Vlaar AP, Choi G, Paulus F, et al. Ventilation with lower tidal volumes as compared with conventional tidal volumes for patients without acute lung injury: a preventive randomized controlled trial. Crit Care. 2010;14(1):R1. doi:10.1186/cc8230.

57. Gajic O, Dara SI, Mendez JL, Adesanya AO, Festic E, Caples SM, et al. Ventilator-associated lung injury in patients without acute lung injury at the onset of mechanical ventilation. Crit Care Med. 2004;32(9):1817–24.

58. Gajic O, Frutos-Vivar F, Esteban A, Hubmayr RD, Anzueto A. Ventilator settings as a risk factor for acute respiratory distress syndrome in mechanically ventilated patients. Intensive Care Med. 2005;31(7):922–6. doi:10.1007/s00134-005-2625-1.

59. Serpa NA, Cardoso SO, Manetta JA, Pereira VG, Esposito DC, Pasqualucci MO, et al. Association between use of lung-protective ventilation with lower tidal volumes and clinical outcomes among patients without acute respiratory distress syndrome: a meta-analysis. JAMA. 2012;308(16):1651–9. doi:10.1001/jama.2012.13730.

60. Serpa Neto A, Simonis FD, Barbas CS, Biehl M, Determann RM, Elmer J, et al. Association between tidal volume size, duration of ventilation, and sedation needs in patients without acute respiratory distress syndrome: an individual patient data meta-analysis. Intensive Care Med. 2014;40(7):950–7. doi:10.1007/s00134-014-3318-4.

61. Putensen C, Theuerkauf N, Zinserling J, Wrigge H, Pelosi P. Meta-analysis: ventilation strategies and outcomes of the acute respiratory distress syndrome and acute lung injury. Ann Intern Med. 2009;151(8):566–76.

62. Esteban A, Ferguson ND, Meade MO, Frutos-Vivar F, Apezteguia C, Brochard L, et al. Evolution of mechanical ventilation in response to clinical research. Am J Respir Crit Care Med. 2008;177(2):170–7. doi:10.1164/rccm.200706-893OC.

63. Neto A, Barbas C, Raventós A, Canet J, Determann R. Rationale and study design of provent—an international multicenter observational study on practice of ventilation in critically ill patients without ARDS. J Clin Trials. 2013;3:146. doi:10.4172/2167-0870.1000146.

64. Ari A, Areabi H, Fink JB. Evaluation of aerosol generator devices at 3 locations in humidified and non-humidified circuits during adult mechanical ventilation. Respir Care. 2010;55(7):837–44.

65. Ari A, Fink JB, Dhand R. Inhalation therapy in patients receiving mechanical ventilation: an update. J Aerosol Med Pulm Drug Deliv. 2012;25(6):319–32. doi:10.1089/jamp.2011.0936.

66. Dhand R. Aerosol delivery during mechanical ventilation: from basic techniques to new devices. J Aerosol Med Pulm Drug Deliv. 2008;21(1):45–60. doi:10.1089/jamp.2007.0663.

67. Bendstrup KE, Newhouse MT, Pedersen OF, Jensen JI. Characterization of heparin aerosols generated in jet and ultrasonic nebulizers. J Aerosol Med. 1999;12(1):17–25.

68. Riley RD, Lambert PC, Abo-Zaid G. Meta-analysis of individual participant data: rationale, conduct, and reporting. BMJ. 2010;340:c221. doi:10.1136/bmj.c221.

69. Winkelmayer WC, Kurth T. Propensity scores: help or hype? Nephrol Dial Transplant. 2004;19(7):1671–3. doi:10.1093/ndt/gfh104.

14

Reliability of respiratory pressure measurements in ventilated and non-ventilated patients in ICU

Clément Medrinal[1,2,3*], Guillaume Prieur[4], Yann Combret[5,6], Aurora Robledo Quesada[3], Tristan Bonnevie[1,2,7], Francis Edouard Gravier[7], Eric Frenoy[8], Olivier Contal[9] and Bouchra Lamia[1,2,4,10]

Abstract

Background: Assessment of maximum respiratory pressures is a common practice in intensive care because it can predict the success of weaning from ventilation. However, the reliability of measurements through an intubation catheter has not been compared with standard measurements. The aim of this study was to compare maximum respiratory pressures measured through an intubation catheter with the same measurements using a standard mouthpiece in extubated patients.

Methods: A prospective observational study was carried out in adults who had been under ventilation for at least 24 h and for whom extubation was planned. Maximal respiratory pressure measurements were carried out before and 24 h following extubation.

Results: Ninety patients were included in the analyses (median age: 61.5 years, median SAPS2 score: 42.5 and median duration of ventilation: 7 days). Maximum respiratory pressures measured through the intubation catheter were as reliable as measurements through a standard mouthpiece (difference in maximal inspiratory pressure: mean bias $= -2.43 \pm 14.43$ cmH$_2$O and difference in maximal expiratory pressure: mean bias $= 1.54 \pm 23.2$ cmH$_2$O).

Conclusion: Maximum respiratory pressures measured through an intubation catheter were reliable and similar to standard measures.

Keywords: Intensive care unit, Mechanical ventilation, Respiratory muscles

Background

Mechanical ventilation generally results in a loss of respiratory muscle strength [1, 2]. The prevalence of respiratory muscle weakness is high, and the causes are multifactorial [3–5]. Assessment of respiratory muscle strength is becoming common practice in intensive care. Assessment techniques range from diaphragm ultrasound to measurement of maximum respiratory pressures. Respiratory muscle strength has been established as prognostic of successful weaning and mortality [6–8].

Measurement of maximum respiratory pressures is a simple, non-invasive method to quantify the global strength of the inspiratory and expiratory muscles. Pressures can be measured using a manometer with a unidirectional valve or the "Negative Inspiratory Force" (NIF) function available on most ventilators. However, these methods require full patient cooperation. Several protocols have thus been developed for use in intensive care to ensure accurate measurements with or without cooperation from the patient [9]. Several studies have attempted to determine optimal methods to ensure quality measurements that are reliable [10–12].

Respiratory pressure measurements are commonly carried out, while the patient is intubated as part of the evaluation to determine the likely success of extubation [5,

---

*Correspondence: medrinal.clement.mk@gmail.com
[3] Intensive Care Unit Department, Groupe Hospitalier du Havre, Avenue Pierre Mendes France, 76290 Montivilliers, France
Full list of author information is available at the end of the article

7]. It is important to carry out longitudinal evaluations of respiratory muscle strength after mechanical ventilation in order to increase understanding of the relationship between strength and long-term rates of mortality [7]. However, the methods used to measure respiratory pressures differ between intubation and extubation and, along with other factors such as lack of patient cooperation and discomfort, this could lead to different values being recorded. To our knowledge, no, or few, studies have evaluated respiratory pressure measurements in non-ventilated patients in ICU, and the reliability of these measurements has not been compared between intubation and extubation.

The aim of this study was to compare maximum respiratory pressures measured through an intubation catheter (intubated patients) with the same measurement using a standard mouthpiece (extubated patients). The secondary aims were to analyse correlations between the two measurements.

Method

Study design and participants

This study was part of a larger, prospective observational cohort study conducted in an 18-bed intensive care unit (ICU) between January 2014 and December 2014 [7]. The study was approved by our Institutional Review Board (Comité de Protection des Personnes Nord-Ouest 3); NCT02363231 www.clinicaltrials.gov. In conformity with the Declaration of Helsinki, all patients participated voluntarily.

Patients were included if they were over 18 years of age and had undergone a minimum of 24 h of MV. They were not included if they had chronic loss of autonomy (a KATZ score below 6/6 [13], a degenerative neurological pathology with disabling muscle weakness, were agitated prior to the evaluation (Ramsay score of 1 or Richmond Agitation-Sedation Scale (RASS) greater than 1) or a decision to withhold life sustaining treatment had been made. Patients who were included but had to be re-intubated during the first 24 h of extubation were excluded from the analysis.

Study protocol

In our ICU, patients are assessed daily (without sedation) to determine whether they are ready to wean from MV. If a patient fulfils extubation criteria and level of cooperation is satisfactory, a weaning trial is carried out under pressure support (inspiratory positive airway pressure of 7 cmH$_2$O with no expiratory positive airway pressure for 30–120 min) [14]. For the purpose of the study, if the trial was successful and extubation was planned, the patient underwent maximum inspiratory and expiratory pressure measurements (MIPs and MEPs) (intubation condition). Twenty-four hours following extubation, MIPs and MEPs were re-measured, this time using a mouthpiece (mouthpiece condition).

Demographic data, reasons for admission to ICU and comorbidities were collected at the time of inclusion, prior to carrying out the MIP and MEP measurements under MV.

In both conditions, the MIP and MEP measurements were carried out with the patient lying in bed with the backrest inclined to 45°. Respiratory physiotherapy was carried out first to ensure that secretions were evacuated, and endotracheal aspiration was carried out for intubated patients.

An electronic manometer, micro-RPM® (Eolys, PAYS), with a unidirectional valve was used to measure respiratory pressures. In both conditions, MIP was measured at the residual volume and patients were instructed accordingly.

In the intubation condition, the manometer was connected to the endotracheal tube using a catheter mount. The patient was disconnected from the ventilator for a minimum of 20 s [11].

In the mouthpiece condition, it was not possible to leave the manometer in position for 20 s. MIP was measured after a maximal exhalation (at the residual volume).

MEP was measured after a maximal inspiration in both conditions. Three MIP and three MEP measurements were carried out for each patient, and the best result was used for the analysis.

Statistical analysis

Descriptive statistics are reported as counts and percentages for categorical data, and means and standard deviations or medians and 25th–75th percentiles for continuous variables, depending on the normality of the distribution. Differences between values were evaluated using a Wilcoxon matched-pairs signed rank test. Univariate linear regression analysis was performed using the least squares method. The Bland–Altman limits of agreement method was used to calculate bias and precision.

Statistical analyses were performed using GraphPad Prism 5. A two-tailed p value of 0.05 was considered significant for all analyses.

Results

One hundred and twenty-four patients were included in the larger study. Of these, 101 accepted to carry out additional measurements. Eleven patients required re-intubation within 24 h of extubation and were excluded from the analysis. Ninety patients thus underwent MIP and MEP measurements in both conditions.

Patient characteristics are described in Table 1. Briefly, 43% of the patients were women, median age was 61.5 years, median BMI was 28.6 kg/m^2, median SAPS2 score was 42.5 and median duration of MV was 7 days.

Median MIP value was 28 (21.7–40.2) cmH$_2$O in the intubation condition and 27 (19–38) cmH$_2$O in the mouthpiece condition ($p = 0.02$). Linear regression showed a significant correlation between the values in each condition ($r = 0.64$ 95% CI [0.5–0.75]; $p < 0.0001$).

The Bland–Altman analysis showed that the MIP values between intubation and extubation were clinically comparable (mean bias (ΔMIP) $= -2.43 \pm 14.43$ cmH$_2$O). (See Fig. 1).

There was no statistically significant difference in MEP values between conditions [47 (30–74) vs. 53.5 (34–76.2) cmH$_2$O; $p = 0.2$]. There was a strong significant correlation between the MEP values in each condition ($r = 0.71$ 95% CI [0.6–0.8]; $p < 0.0001$).

There was no clinical difference between the values in the two conditions as shown by the Bland–Altman analysis (mean bias (ΔMEP) $= 1.54 \pm 23.2$ cmH$_2$O) (See Fig. 2).

No patient-related factors were found to be associated with the measurement bias (age, BMI, SAPS2, number of days under mechanical ventilation, extubation failure). However, there was a correlation between the ΔMIP and the ΔMEP ($r = 0.49$ 95% CI [0.31–0.64]; $p < 0.0001$).

There was a significant correlation between MIP and MEP values in each condition (respectively $r = 0.61$ 95% CI [0.45–0.72]; $p < 0.0001$ and $r = 0.66$ 95% CI [0.52–0.77]; $p < 0.0001$).

Discussion

This study found [1] that the methods of measuring respiratory pressures in intubated and extubated patients produced clinically similar results for both MIP and MEP, and [2] there were strong correlations between the MIP and MEP values in both conditions.

Assessment of respiratory pressures is common practice in ICU [4, 5, 7, 9–12]. Although other tools may more accurately assess muscle strength, measures of respiratory pressure are used to determine if a patient is ready to wean from MV, as well as the prognosis [7, 15]. For this reason, we believed it was important to evaluate the validity of measurements in intubated patients compared with post-extubation measurements using a mouthpiece in order to longitudinally evaluate changes in respiratory muscle strength.

Measurement of maximal respiratory pressures requires patient cooperation, which can be difficult when patients are intubated; however, similar pressures were recorded during intubation and extubation, with slightly higher pressures during intubation. This could

Table 1 Cohort characteristics

	$N = 90$
Female, n (%)	39 (43)
Age, mean (SD)	61.5 (14)
Body mass index (Kg/m²), median (25th–75th percentile)	28.6 (24.4–32)
SAPS II at ICU admission, median (25th–75th percentile)	42.5 (31–57)
No. of admissions to ICU within the last year, n (%)	4 (4.4)
Main diagnosis	
Pneumonia, n (%)	32 (35)
Sepsis, n (%)	8 (9)
COPD/asthma exacerbation, n (%)	12 (13)
Cardiac failure, n (%)	12 (13)
Drug overdose/acute mental status change, n (%)	11 (12)
Intra-abdominal sepsis with surgery, n (%)	14 (15)
Trauma, n (%)	1 (4)
Co-morbidity	
Chronic pulmonary disease, n (%)	23 (25)
Obesity, n (%)	27 (30)
Chronic cardiac insufficiency, n (%)	13 (14)
Cancer, n (%)	15 (17)
Chronic kidney disease, n (%)	14 (15)
Diabetes mellitus, n (%)	17 (19)
Between admission and awakening	
Septic shock, n (%)	45 (50)
ARDS, n (%)	13 (14)
Renal failure, n (%)	30 (33)
Use of catecholamines, n (%)	58 (64)
Use of neuromuscular blockers, n (%)	58 (64)
No. of days of neuromuscular blockers, median (25–75th percentile)	1 (0–3)
Use of corticosteroids, n (%)	21 (78)
Ventilator use (days), median (25th–75th percentile)	7 (4–9)

SAPS simplified acute physiology score, *ICU* intensive care unit, *No.* number, *COPD* chronic obstructive pulmonary disease, *ARDS* acute respiratory distress syndrome

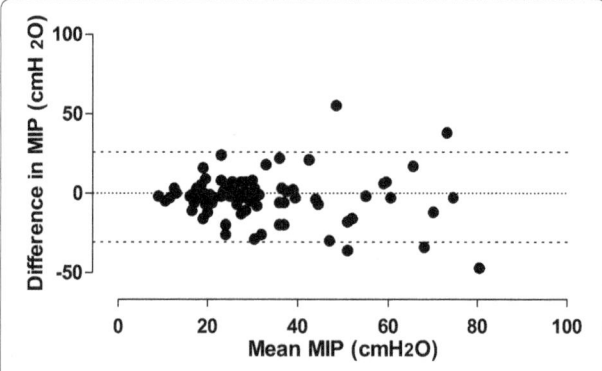

Fig. 1 Bland–Altman analysis of maximal inspiratory pressure correlations: difference versus mean

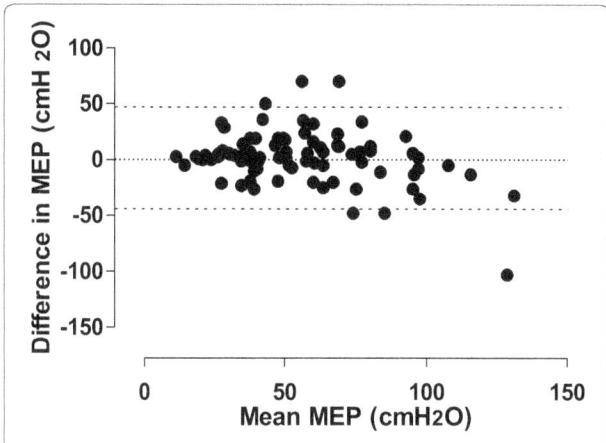

Fig. 2 Bland–Altman analysis of maximal expiratory pressure correlations: difference versus mean

be explained by the fact that mouth leak cannot occur when the patient is intubated with the balloon inflated or because the measurement was carried out over 20 s when the patients were intubated [11]. One study compared the conventional method (values taken at the maximum pressure plateau maintained for at least 1 s) with Marini's method [10] (measurement of inspiratory pressure with a unidirectional valve over 20 s) in 54 patients. MIP was 28% higher using Marini's method with a coefficient of variation of around 10%, indicating good reliability. This procedure can be used for intubated patients but is not reliable in extubated patients. Nevertheless, in the present study, mean MIP variation between the two conditions was -2.43 cmH$_2$O (-8.4%) and for MEP was 1.54 cmH$_2$O (7%), confirming good reliability across conditions and measurements.

The results of this study showed a relationship between MIP and MEP. MEP reflects the patient's capacity to cough, and a low MEP is associated with delayed weaning [15]; however, studies tend to focus on inspiratory muscle strength, neglecting expiratory muscle strength. MIP is reported to be predictive of successful extubation, and we recently showed that low MIP before extubation (MIP ≤ 30 cmH$_2$O) was an independent predictor of an increase in mortality risk 1 year following extubation [7]. However, several authors have stated that values obtained in intubated patients may be underestimated [9, 12, 15]. In the current study, we found that Marini's method (occlusion for 20 s) produced clinically similar values to measurements carried out with a mouthpiece following recommendations [16]. This indicates that if the patient is sufficiently alert, the values are not underestimated and are therefore reliable across different conditions, allowing accurate follow-up of respiratory capacity.

This study has several limitations. Firstly, the observational design comprises several types of inherent bias and we did not perform a sample size calculation. Secondly, it was not possible to evaluate patients who were re-intubated within 24 h. Thirdly, the pressure measurements were not taken in exactly the same conditions. The second measurement 24 h following extubation may have been affected by respiratory muscle fatigue. Finally, we evaluated peak pressure, not pressure maintained over 1 s as recommended [16]. However, the recommendations are more relevant out of ICU where measurements of respiratory pressure differ considerably from the bedside measurements used in ICU [11].

This study has several strengths. The sample size was large and representative of the population of patients in ICU. The test evaluated is simple and easy to carry out at the patient's bedside. Moreover, we showed that the measurements were reliable across two common conditions in ICU (intubated and extubated patients).

Conclusion

Respiratory pressure measurements are reliable in both intubated and non-intubated patients. These results corroborate those of previous studies. Measurements of respiratory pressure can thus be carried out reliably when the patient is intubated and repeated following weaning from MV to carry out longitudinal evaluations of respiratory muscle recovery.

Abbreviations
BMI: body mass index; CI: confidence intervals; ICU: intensive care unit; MIP: maximal inspiratory pressure; MEP: maximal expiratory pressure; MV: mechanical ventilation; NIF: negative inspiratory force; RASS: Richmond Agitation-Sedation Scale; SAPS: simplified acute physiology score.

Author's contributions
C.M., G.P., Y.C., O.C and B.L. designed the study. C.M., B.L. and O.C. coordinated the study. C.M., G.P., E.F., A.R.Q., T.B and F.G. were responsible for patient screening, enrolment, diaphragm assessment, and follow-up. C.M., E.F. O.C. and B.L. analysed the data and wrote the manuscript. All authors contributed to the interpretation of the data and provided comments on the report at various stages of development. All authors approved this manuscript in its final form.

Author details
[1] Normandie Univ, UNIROUEN, EA3830 - GRHV, 76000 Rouen, France. [2] Institute for Research and Innovation in Biomedicine (IRIB), 76000 Rouen, France. [3] Intensive Care Unit Department, Groupe Hospitalier du Havre, Avenue Pierre Mendes France, 76290 Montivilliers, France. [4] Pulmonology Department, Groupe Hospitalier du Havre, Avenue Pierre Mendes France, 76290 Montivilliers, France. [5] Institut de Recherche Expérimentale et Clinique (IREC), Pôle de Pneumologie, ORL et Dermatologie, Université Catholique de Louvain, Brussels 1200, Belgium. [6] Physiotherapy Department, Groupe Hospitalier du Havre, Avenue Pierre Mendes France, 76290 Montivilliers, France. [7] ADIR Association, Bois Guillaume, France. [8] Intensive Care Unit Department, Hôpital Jacques Monod, 76290 Montivilliers, France. [9] University of Applied Sciences and Arts Western Switzerland (HES-SO), Avenue de Beaumont, 1011 Lausanne, Switzerland. [10] Intensive Care Unit, Respiratory Department, Rouen University Hospital, Rouen, France.

Competing interests
The authors declare that they have no competing interests.

Funding
This study was supported by grants from ADIR Association. The funder had no direct influence on the design of the study, the analysis of the data, the data collection, drafting of the manuscript or the decision to publish.

References
1. Levine S, Nguyen T, Taylor N, Friscia ME, Budak MT, Rothenberg P, et al. Rapid disuse atrophy of diaphragm fibers in mechanically ventilated humans. N Engl J Med. 2008;358(13):1327–35.
2. Demoule A, Molinari N, Jung B, Prodanovic H, Chanques G, Matecki S, et al. Patterns of diaphragm function in critically ill patients receiving prolonged mechanical ventilation: a prospective longitudinal study. Ann Intensive Care. 2016;6(1):75.
3. Dres M, Dube BP, Mayaux J, Delemazure J, Reuter D, Brochard L, et al. coexistence and impact of limb muscle and diaphragm weakness at time of liberation from mechanical ventilation in medical intensive care unit patients. Am J Respir Crit Care Med. 2017;195(1):57–66.
4. Medrinal C, Prieur G, Frenoy E, Combret Y, Gravier FE, Bonnevie T, et al. Is overlap of respiratory and limb muscle weakness at weaning from mechanical ventilation associated with poorer outcomes? Intensive Care Med. 2017;43(2):282–3.
5. Jung B, Moury PH, Mahul M, de Jong A, Galia F, Prades A, et al. Diaphragmatic dysfunction in patients with ICU-acquired weakness and its impact on extubation failure. Intensive Care Med. 2016;42(5):853–61.
6. Demoule A, Jung B, Prodanovic H, Molinari N, Chanques G, Coirault C, et al. Diaphragm dysfunction on admission to the intensive care unit. Prevalence, risk factors, and prognostic impact-a prospective study. Am J Respir Crit Care Med. 2013;188(2):213–9.
7. Medrinal C, Prieur G, Frenoy E, Robledo Quesada A, Poncet A, Bonnevie T, et al. Respiratory weakness after mechanical ventilation is associated with one-year mortality—a prospective study. Crit Care. 2016;20(1):231.
8. Zambon M, Greco M, Bocchino S, Cabrini L, Beccaria PF, Zangrillo A. Assessment of diaphragmatic dysfunction in the critically ill patient with ultrasound: a systematic review. Intensive Care Med. 2017;43(1):29–38.
9. Moxham J, Goldstone J. Assessment of respiratory muscle strength in the intensive care unit. Eur Respir J. 1994;7(11):2057–61.
10. Marini JJ, Smith TC, Lamb V. Estimation of inspiratory muscle strength in mechanically ventilated patients: the measurement of maximum inspiratory pressure. J Crit Care. 1986;1(1):32–8.
11. Caruso P, Friedrich C, Denari SD, Ruiz SA, Deheinzelin D. The unidirectional valve is the best method to determine maximum inspiratory pressure during weaning. Chest. 1999;115(4):1096–101.
12. Spadaro S, Marangoni E, Ragazzi R, Mojoli F, Verri M, Longo L, et al. A methodological approach for determination of maximum inspiratory pressure in patients undergoing invasive mechanical ventilation. Minerva Anestesiol. 2015;81(1):33–8.
13. Katz S, Akpom CA. A measure of primary sociobiological functions. Int J Health Serv. 1976;6(3):493–508.
14. Boles JM, Bion J, Connors A, Herridge M, Marsh B, Melot C, et al. Weaning from mechanical ventilation. Eur Respir J. 2007;29(5):1033–56.
15. De Jonghe B, Bastuji-Garin S, Durand MC, Malissin I, Rodrigues P, Cerf C, et al. Respiratory weakness is associated with limb weakness and delayed weaning in critical illness. Crit Care Med. 2007;35(9):2007–15.
16. ATS/ERS Statement on respiratory muscle testing. Am J Respir Crit Care Med. 2002;166(4):518–624.

15

Lung volumes and lung volume recruitment in ARDS: a comparison between supine and prone position

Hernan Aguirre-Bermeo, Marta Turella, Maddalena Bitondo, Juan Grandjean, Stefano Italiano, Olimpia Festa, Indalecio Morán and Jordi Mancebo[*]

Abstract

Background: The use of positive end-expiratory pressure (PEEP) and prone position (PP) is common in the management of severe acute respiratory distress syndrome patients (ARDS). We conducted this study to analyze the variation in lung volumes and PEEP-induced lung volume recruitment with the change from supine position (SP) to PP in ARDS patients.

Methods: The investigation was conducted in a multidisciplinary intensive care unit. Patients who met the clinical criteria of the Berlin definition for ARDS were included. The responsible physician set basal PEEP. To avoid hypoxemia, FiO_2 was increased to 0.8 1 h before starting the protocol. End-expiratory lung volume (EELV) and functional residual capacity (FRC) were measured using the nitrogen washout/washin technique. After the procedures in SP, the patients were turned to PP and 1 h later the same procedures were made in PP.

Results: Twenty-three patients were included in the study, and twenty were analyzed. The change from SP to PP significantly increased FRC (from 965 ± 397 to 1140 ± 490 ml, $p = 0.008$) and EELV (from 1566 ± 476 to 1832 ± 719 ml, $p = 0.008$), but PEEP-induced lung volume recruitment did not significantly change (269 ± 186 ml in SP to 324 ± 188 ml in PP, $p = 0.263$). Dynamic strain at PEEP decreased with the change from SP to PP (0.38 ± 0.14 to 0.33 ± 0.13, $p = 0.040$).

Conclusions: As compared to supine, prone position increases resting lung volumes and decreases dynamic lung strain.

Keywords: ARDS, Lung volumes, Lung strain, Prone, PEEP recruitment, Mechanical ventilation

Background

Acute respiratory distress syndrome (ARDS) is a permeability pulmonary edema, characterized by hypoxemia and a decrease in lung volumes and respiratory system compliance [1, 2]. In patients with ARDS, prone position (PP) produces a more homogeneous distribution of the inspired gas [3] and a better matching between ventilation and perfusion, thereby improving arterial oxygenation [3–5]. Positive end-expiratory pressure (PEEP) and PP have also shown to decrease the percentage of non-aerated and poorly aerated lung tissue and attenuate the regional recruitment–derecruitment phenomena [5–7]. In selected ARDS patients, PP has been proposed to further improve the outcomes [8]. The benefit on survival of PP is not related only to the improvement in gas exchange [9, 10], and the protective effect on ventilator-induced lung injury [3, 9, 11, 12] could also play a role. As compared to supine position (SP), the PP reduces the steep transpulmonary pressure gradient across the vertical axis of the lung, leading to a more homogeneous distribution of pulmonary stress and strain [2, 3, 13].

However, data analyzing the variation in lung volumes with the change from SP to PP in ARDS patients

*Correspondence: jmancebo@santpau.cat
Servei de Medicina Intensiva, Hospital de la Santa Creu i Sant Pau, Universitat Autònoma de Barcelona (UAB), Sant Quintí, 89, 08041 Barcelona, Spain

are scarce and conflicting [4, 14–17]. We hypothesized that in ARDS patients, PP increases lung volumes (i.e., functional residual capacity and end-expiratory lung volume) and might decrease lung strain [16, 18]. Because the measurement of functional residual capacity (FRC) requires to be made at zero end-expiratory pressure (ZEEP), our study included a lung derecruitment maneuver from baseline PEEP to zero PEEP [19–21] subsequently followed by the reinstitution of the basal PEEP level. These allowed to analyze the variation in lung volumes and to estimate lung volume recruitment and lung strain in both supine and prone positions in patients with ARDS.

Methods

The study was performed in the Intensive Care Department at Hospital de la Santa Creu i Sant Pau, Barcelona (Spain). This study was conducted in accordance with the amended Declaration of Helsinki.

Patients

Patients were considered eligible for the study if they met the Berlin definition criteria for ARDS [22] and had an indication for PP in accordance with our department's protocol (PaO_2/FiO_2 ratio of < 150 mm Hg and FiO_2 of $\geq$ 0.6 with PEEP of at least 5 cm H_2O). We recommend to use protective ventilation with individualized low tidal volume (Vt) and moderate PEEP levels. Essentially, PEEP is titrated according to the gas exchange (Sat O_2, measured by pulse oxymeter, around 95%) with end-inspiratory plateau airway pressure (Pplat) not higher than 28 cm H_2O and without hemodynamic instability (mean arterial pressure above 65 mm Hg and no need for fluid replacement). Our detailed ventilatory strategy is included in Additional file 1. Hence, all our patients had been turned in PP before inclusion in the study. To be included, patients had to present an improvement in gas exchange ($FiO_2 \leq$ 0.6 and PEEP $\leq$ 12 cm H_2O) in SP in order to avoid severe hypoxemia because of the derecruitment (induced by PEEP withdrawal and ventilation at ZEEP) during the measurement of FRC. Exclusion criteria were: age < 18 years, tracheostomy, pregnancy, major trauma, barotrauma (presence of extra-alveolar air during mechanical ventilation as assessed by daily chest X ray) and hemodynamic instability (systolic blood pressure < 80 or > 160 mm Hg, heart rate < 50 bpm or > 130 bpm or changes in ± 20% from baseline).

All patients were under continuous sedation and analgesia with intravenous perfusion of midazolam and/or propofol and opioids. During the study period, all patients received neuromuscular blocking agents.

Protocol

The following data were collected: age, height, simplified acute physiology score III at admission, ARDS etiology, days of mechanical ventilation, intensive care unit outcomes, respiratory rate, Vt, PEEP, peak airway pressure, Pplat and arterial blood gases. Respiratory variables were recorded directly from the ventilator.

All patients were ventilated in volume control ventilation using the same ventilator model (Engström Carestation ICU ventilator, General Electric, Madison, WI, USA).

To avoid hypoxemia, defined as oxygen saturation $\leq$ 88% measured through pulse oximetry, we increased the FiO_2 to 0.8 1 h before starting the protocol.

Measurements

Baseline ventilatory and hemodynamic parameters were collected before the protocol to measure lung volumes. The same procedures were carried out in SP and PP and are outlined below (see also Fig. 1):

1. Measurement of end-expiratory lung volume (EELV): EELV is the resting end-expiratory lung volume measured at baseline PEEP.
2. Removal of PEEP and continuation of mechanical ventilation at ZEEP. This derecruitment maneuver

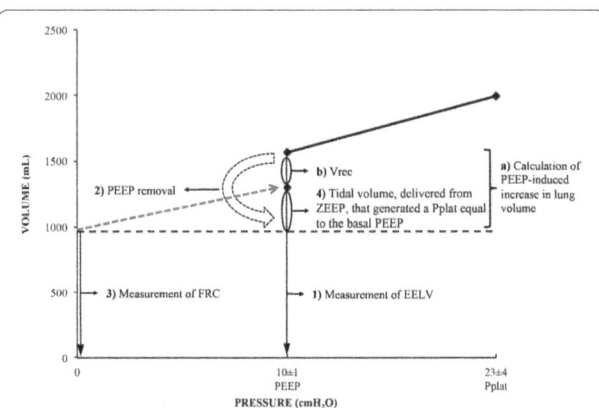

Fig. 1 Lung volumes, measurements and calculations made in the study. The same procedures were carried out in supine and prone positions as follows: (1) measurement of end-expiratory lung volume (EELV): EELV is defined as the resting end-expiratory lung volume at PEEP. (2) Removal of PEEP and continuation of mechanical ventilation at zero end-expiratory pressure (ZEEP). (3) Measurement of functional residual capacity (FRC): FRC is defined as the resting lung volume at ZEEP. (4) Measurement of the tidal volume, delivered from ZEEP, that generated a Pplat equal to the basal PEEP. The same calculations were carried out in supine and prone positions as follows: (a) calculation of PEEP-induced increase in lung volume = EELV minus FRC. (b) Calculation of PEEP-induced lung volume recruitment (Vrec) = PEEP-induced increase in lung volume minus the Vt, delivered from ZEEP, that generated a Pplat equal to the basal PEEP. Blue line represents the compliance at ZEEP

is mandatory to conduct the following step 3, and it is the reason to increase the FiO_2 to 0.8 immediately before starting the protocol (i.e., to avoid hypoxemia).

3. Measurement of functional residual capacity (FRC): FRC is the resting lung volume measured at ZEEP.

4. Measurement of the Vt, delivered from ZEEP, that generated a Pplat equal to the basal PEEP. This step (see Fig. 1) is mandatory to allow a proper estimation of the PEEP-induced lung volume recruitment [19, 20, 23–25].

Once step 4 was completed, the same PEEP that was used at baseline was resumed.

Measurements at ZEEP (FRC and Vt delivered from ZEEP, that generated a Pplat equal to the basal PEEP) included a lung derecruitment maneuver (PEEP removal) that can produce hypoxemia. For the purpose of our investigation, we defined hypoxemia as oxygen saturation $\leq 88\%$ measured through pulse oximetry.

The safety limits and contraindications to remove PEEP were:

1. PEEP removal was contraindicated if $FiO_2 > 0.6$ and PEEP > 12 cm H_2O.

2. We increased the FiO_2 to 0.8 1 h before starting the protocol in order to avoid hypoxemia during PEEP removal.

3. If a patient presented with hypoxemia at any time during the protocol (saturation $\leq 88\%$ measured through pulse oximetry), the measurements were aborted and the patient was excluded.

Lung volumes (EELV and FRC) were measured twice using the nitrogen washout/washin technique available in Engström Carestation ICU ventilator as previously described [24, 26]. Washout/washin technique is a multiple breath maneuver that with a modification of 0.1 in FiO_2 calculates the residual nitrogen in the lung (assuming there is not exchange of nitrogen) by continuous measurements of oxygen and carbon dioxide. The ventilator was carefully calibrated before the measurements according to the manufacturer's specifications. We obtained four values for each lung volume. The mean of the four values was used. As previously suggested [27], patients were excluded if the differences between the four values were more than 20% (cutoff determined by the manufacturer).

After the procedures in SP, the patients were turned to PP and 1 h later the same procedures (from 1 to 4 above) were made in PP. This time span was based in previous data showing that after 1 h in PP gas exchange is stable in the majority of patients [28, 29]. If a patient presented with hypoxemia (oxygen saturation $\leq 88\%$) at any time

during the protocol, the measurements were aborted and the patient was excluded.

The normal reference values for FRC (liters) in the SP were calculated according to the equation described by Ibáñez and Raurich [30], as follows: $5.48 \times$ height-7.05 for men and $1.39 \times$ height-0.424 for women; height units are in meters. Compliance (ml/cm H_2O) was calculated as Vt/(Pplat minus total PEEP), being total PEEP the sum of PEEP plus intrinsic PEEP. Predicted body weight was calculated as follows: $50 + 0.91$(height-152.4) for men and $45.5 + 0.91$(height-152.4) for women; height units are in centimeters. Driving airway pressure was calculated as the difference between Pplat and total PEEP [31].

Calculation of lung volumes and strain

(a) The PEEP-induced increase in lung volume was calculated as EELV minus FRC (see Fig. 1).

(b) PEEP-induced lung volume recruitment (Vrec) was calculated as PEEP-induced increase in lung volume minus the Vt, delivered from ZEEP, that generated a Pplat equal to the basal PEEP (see Fig. 1).

(c) Strain was calculated as previously described [24, 32, 33]:

1. Dynamic strain at ZEEP = Vt/FRC.
2. Dynamic strain at PEEP = Vt/(FRC + Vrec).
3. Static strain at PEEP = (EELV − FRC)/ (FRC + Vrec).
4. Global strain at PEEP = (static strain at PEEP + dynamic strain at PEEP) = (EELV − FRC + Vt)/(FRC + Vrec).

Statistical analysis

Data are expressed as mean $\pm$ SD. We used Wilcoxon test to compare variables between supine and prone positions and U the Mann–Whiney test to compare early and non-early ARDS patients. A p value < 0.05 was considered statistically significant. The SPSS® Statistics (version 20.0, Chicago, IL, USA) statistical software was used for statistical analysis.

Results

The study was conducted from July 2010 to December 2013. Twenty-three patients were included in the study, and twenty were analyzed. One patient was excluded because of hypoxemia during the FRC measurement, and two were excluded because of a technical problem. (The differences between FRC measurements were > 20%.)

Table 1 summarizes the patients' main characteristics at baseline. The mean age of patients was 58 ± 18 years. The main causes of ARDS were pneumonia ($n = 11$) and septic shock ($n = 4$). The study was performed 4 ± 3 days

Table 1 Patients' characteristics at study entry (with FiO_2 0.8)

Patient	Age (years)	Days on MV before study	SAPS III	Vt (ml/kg PBW)	RR (rpm)	PEEP (cm H_2O)	Pplat (cm H_2O)	Δ Paw (cm H_2O)	PaO_2/FiO_2 (mm Hg)	$PaCO_2$ (mm Hg)	Cause of ARDS	Outcome
1	43	6	65	7.4	24	8	28	20	255	40	Pneumonia	S
2	66	1	52	6.1	22	10	20	10	254	60	Pneumonia	S
3	77	5	91	6.7	20	10	22	12	165	44	Pneumonia	S
4	68	4	69	8.4	24	12	21	9	255	44	Pneumonia	S
5	75	4	65	7.8	22	10	18	8	115	38	Pneumonia	S
6	65	7	94	9.2	30	10	21	11	240	53	Pneumonia	S
7	55	2	67	6.8	20	10	22	12	229	35	Peritonitis	S
8	43	2	77	8.1	20	8	26	18	151	48	Peritonitis	D
9	78	3	100	6.3	27	10	29	19	188	41	Peritonitis	D
10	74	2	82	11.0	25	10	28	18	198	43	Pneumonia	D
11	81	4	89	6.7	24	10	20	10	230	34	Septic shock	S
12	30	4	83	6.8	21	10	23	13	265	41	Septic shock	D
13	58	5	71	5.0	30	10	20	10	173	43	Pneumonia	S
14	69	1	101	5.9	28	10	28	18	300	44	Septic shock	D
15	50	14	95	6.0	30	10	25	15	206	42	Septic shock	D
16	55	3	68	7.0	20	8	19	11	129	37	Thoracic Trauma	S
17	30	4	64	6.2	24	12	22	10	104	41	Pneumonia	S
18	37	3	76	5.0	30	12	22	10	299	29	Pneumonia	D
19	80	2	82	6.1	17	12	19	7	230	35	Pneumonia	S
20	31	5	65	6.7	26	12	27	15	218	24	Pancreatitis	D
Mean ± SD	58 ± 18	4 ± 3	78 ± 14	6.9 ± 1.4	24 ± 4	10 ± 1	23 ± 4	13 ± 4	41 ± 8	41 ± 8		

ARDS acute respiratory distress syndrome, *D* died, *PBW* predicted body weight, *MV* mechanical ventilation, *PEEP* positive end-expiratory pressure, *Pplat* end-inspiratory plateau airway pressure, *RR* respiratory rate, *S* survived, *SAPS III* simplified acute physiology score III, *Vt* tidal volume, *Δ Paw* driving airway pressure

after starting mechanical ventilation. At baseline, mean Vt was 6.9 ± 1.4 ml/kg of predicted body weight and mean PEEP was 10 ± 1 cm H_2O.

After assuming the PP, the PaO_2/FiO_2 ratio increased significantly, from 210 ± 57 mm Hg in supine to 281 ± 109 mm Hg in prone ($p = 0.008$) (Table 2).

The mean FRC in SP was significantly lower than its reference value in healthy normal subjects (965 ± 397 vs. 2424 ± 459 ml, $p \leq 0.001$). The change from SP to PP significantly increased both FRC (from 965 ± 397 to 1140 ± 490 ml, $p = 0.008$) and EELV (from 1566 ± 476 to 1832 ± 719 ml, $p = 0.008$) (Figs. 2, 3).

We did not calculate Vrec and derived parameters in four patients because the tidal volume delivered from ZEEP, that generated a Pplat equal to the basal PEEP, was not measured in accordance to the protocol. Vrec ($n = 16$) did not significantly vary with the change of position (269 ± 186 ml in SP to 324 ± 188 ml in PP, $p = 0.263$) (Fig. 2).

We found a significant decrease in the dynamic strain at PEEP with the change from SP to PP from 0.38 ± 0.14 to 0.33 ± 0.13 ($p = 0.040$) (Fig. 4). The dynamic strain at ZEEP also decreased, from 0.52 ± 0.23 in SP to 0.44 ± 0.18 in PP ($p = 0.047$). The remaining variables did not change significantly between supine and prone positions (Table 2) (Additional file 2: Table S1).

In the whole population, the driving pressure in the non-survivor group ($n = 8$) was significantly higher than in the survivor group ($n = 12$) in both SP (16 ± 3 cm H_2O vs. 11 ± 3 cm H_2O, respectively, $p = 0.003$) and

in PP (15 ± 3 cm H_2O vs. 11 ± 3 cm H_2O, respectively, $p = 0.005$). Additional data are also shown (Additional file 2: Table S2).

Discussion

The main findings in this study were that: (1) Prone position significantly increased lung volumes; (2) dynamic strain decreased significantly in prone position compared to supine position; and (3) the change of position from supine to prone did not modify the calculated PEEP-induced lung volume recruitment.

Prone position, oxygenation and lung volumes

In ARDS patients, lung volumes at ZEEP (FRC) and at PEEP (EELV) are typically decreased [18]. Two previous studies have shown that PP significantly increases FRC in ARDS patients [15, 16]. Nevertheless, data about the changes in EELV with the change from SP to PP in ARDS patients are not consistent. Four previous studies have shown that PP increases EELV in ARDS patients as compared to SP [14–17], but another study [4] found that the change of EELV from SP to PP was not significant. These contradictory findings might be explained by differences in lung recruitability, distribution and extension of lung volume alterations, differences in chest wall compliance, the influence of abdominal weight and heart compression, the inclination from the horizontal plane and the use or not of ventral supports [3, 9, 34, 35].

In the present study, we found a 40% decrease in FRC as compared to its reference value in SP, confirming

Table 2 Main characteristics of all patients in each position

Variable	Supine $n = 20$	Prone $n = 20$	p
PaO_2/FiO_2 (mm Hg)	210 ± 57	281 ± 109	0.021
$PaCO_2$ (mm Hg)	41 ± 8	42 ± 9	0.400
Peak airway pressure (cm H_2O)	41 ± 7	41 ± 6	0.284
Pplat (cm H_2O)	23 ± 4	23 ± 4	0.446
Compliance (ml/cm H_2O)	36 ± 11	37 ± 10	0.594
Δ Paw (cm H_2O)	13 ± 4	12 ± 4	0.446
FRC (ml)	965 ± 397	1140 ± 490	0.021
EELV (ml)	1566 ± 476	1832 ± 719	0.009
Vt delivered from ZEEP, that generated a Pplat equal to basal PEEP [ml ($n = 16$)]	333 ± 105	360 ± 127	0.073
Vrec [ml ($n = 16$)]	269 ± 186	324 ± 188	0.501
Dynamic strain at ZEEP	0.52 ± 0.23	0.44 ± 0.18	0.040
Dynamic strain at PEEP ($n = 16$)	0.38 ± 0.14	0.33 ± 0.13	0.020
Static strain at PEEP ($n = 16$)	0.51 ± 0.16	0.48 ± 0.13	0.438
Global strain at PEEP ($n = 16$)	0.89 ± 0.24	0.81 ± 0.18	0.121

Data are presented as mean $\pm$ SD. Dynamic strain at ZEEP = Vt/FRC; dynamic strain at PEEP = Vt/(FRC + Vrec); static strain at PEEP = (EELV − FRC)/(FRC + Vrec); global strain at PEEP = (EELV − FRC + Vt)/(FRC + Vrec)

EELV end-expiratory lung volume, *FRC* functional residual capacity, *PEEP* positive end-expiratory pressure, *Pplat* end-inspiratory plateau airway pressure, *Vrec* PEEP-induced lung volume recruitment, *Vt* tidal volume, *Δ Paw* driving airway pressure

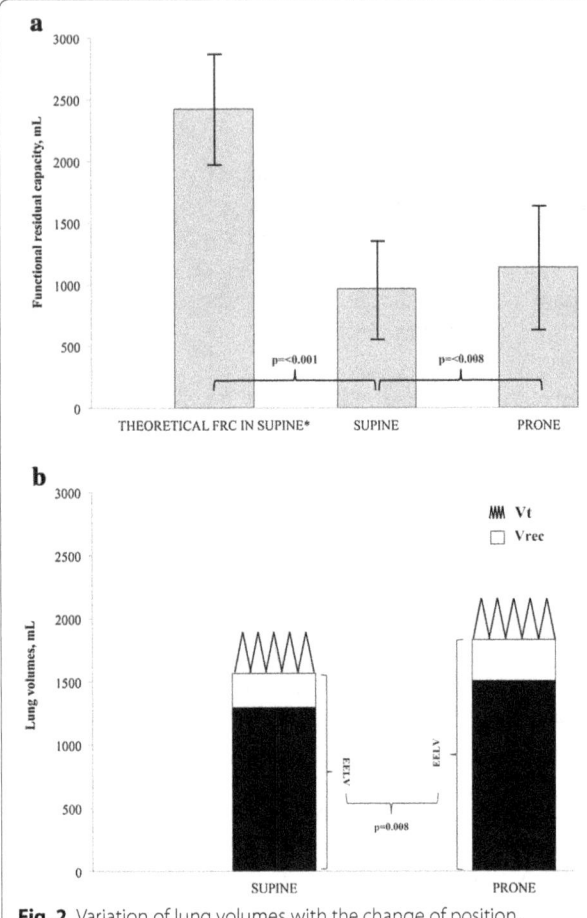

Fig. 2 Variation of lung volumes with the change of position.
a Comparison of different values of functional residual capacity.
b Comparison of EELV and Vrec in supine position and prone position.
EELV, end-expiratory lung volume; Vrec, PEEP-induced lung volume
recruitment; Vt, tidal volume. Data are presented in mean (ml) and SD.
*According to the equation described by Ibañez and Raurich [30]

previous results [18]. We also observed that the FRC and
EELV increased significantly with the change of position
(18% in FRC and 17% in EELV). Santini et al. [7] performed a study in animals with normal lungs, and they
found a significant increase in FRC with the change from
SP to PP. The increase in resting lung volume was mainly
related to a redistribution of aeration: a minor decrease in
non-aerated lung tissue (3%), a major decrease in poorly
aerated tissue (17%) and a major increase (20%) in well-
aerated tissue. Since recruitment, as precisely measured
by thoracic CT scan, refers to tissue recruitment (i.e.,
amount of non-inflated tissue that reinflates at a higher
pressure), the decrease in poorly aerated tissue and the
increase in well-aerated tissue (which contribute to the
end-expiratory lung volume increase induced by PEEP)
are thus considered as better gas distribution within the
lung and not recruitment per se [36].

Prone position and strain

During passive mechanical ventilation, the force applied
by the ventilator generates an internal tension in the fibers of the lung skeleton, called "stress," and the elongation
of these fibers from their resting position is called "strain"
[2]. High values of dynamic lung strain (lung deformation
caused by Vt) and static lung strain (lung deformation
caused by PEEP) are associated with ventilator-induced
lung injury [32, 37].

In an animal model, Protti et al. [33] showed that for
the same global strain, a large static strain is less harmful
than a large dynamic strain. On the same vein, González-
López et al. [38] found that increased strain was associated with a proinflammatory lung response in patients
with acute lung injury. Moreover, Bellani et al. [39] found
in patients with acute lung injury that the intensity of
metabolic activity (a surrogate of inflammation) detected
by positron emission tomography was correlated with
regional strain. Consequently, the significant decrease in
dynamic strain in PP as compared to SP could be another
mechanism of protection of PP against ventilator-
induced lung injury. Therefore, the measurement of lung
volumes at bedside may be an important tool to deliver
a more physiologically based ventilation and encour-
age physicians to increase the use of PP in moderately to
severe ARDS patients [40].

Prone position and PEEP-induced lung volume recruitment

It is still unclear whether the PEEP-induced alveolar
recruitment varies with the change from SP to PP. In an
experimental study in animals with lung injury, Richard
et al. [5] analyzed the variation of alveolar recruitment at
PEEP 10 cm H_2O in SP and PP by means of the positron
emission tomography technique. They found that in PP,
PEEP-induced alveolar recruitment was not higher than
in SP. Interestingly, in this study, the authors observed a
redistribution of densities in PP (recruitment in dorsal
regions with derecruitment in ventral regions). Cornejo
et al. [6] performed another study in ARDS patients to
determine the effects of PEEP and PP on alveolar recruitment. Using the CT scan technique, they found that
increasing PEEP from 5 cm H_2O to 15 cm H_2O significantly increased alveolar recruitment. However, the percentage of recruitment was similar in both positions (36%
in SP and 33% in PP). Using a different methodology,
the data from our study are consistent with these findings, indicating that the effects of PEEP on lung volume
recruitment are similar in both positions (around 17% of
EELV).

A previous study by Grasso et al. [41] found that
alveolar recruitment was higher in the early phase
(1 ± 0.3 days of mechanical ventilation) than in the late
phase of ARDS, but a subsequent study by Gattinoni

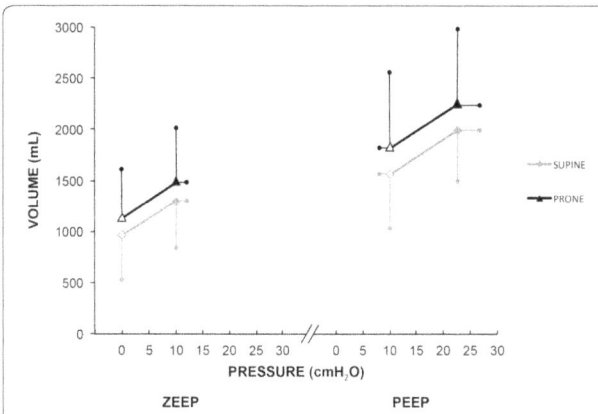

Fig. 3 Variation in lung volumes in supine and prone positions. Clear triangles and clear rhombus are the resting lung volumes at ZEEP and at PEEP. Dark triangles and dark rhombus represent end-inspiratory lung volumes and end-inspiratory lung pressure (Pplat) at ZEEP and at PEEP. PEEP, positive end-expiratory pressure; ZEEP, zero end-expiratory pressure. Data are shown as mean and SD

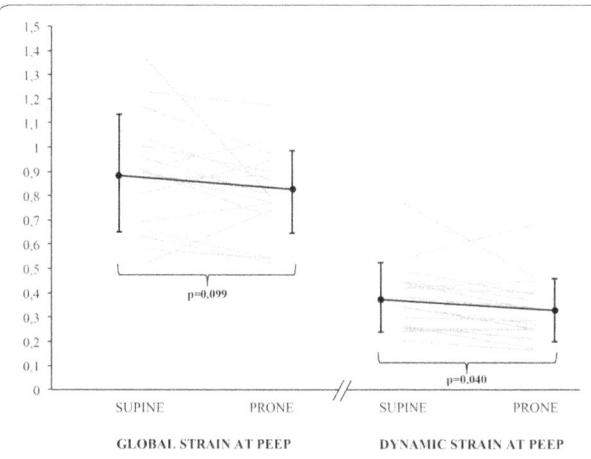

Fig. 4 Variation of individual values of global and dynamic strain at PEEP with the change of position. Dark lines represent mean and SD. PEEP, positive end-expiratory pressure

et al. [42] did not find the same results. In the study of Gattinoni et al. [42], they found that the number of days of mechanical ventilation before the study was similar in patients with a lower percentage of potentially recruitable lung and those with a higher percentage (5 ± 6 vs. 6 ± 6 days, respectively, $p = 0.50$). In our study when we classified ARDS patients in the early phase (< 72 h) and in late phase (> 72 h) (Additional file 2: Table S2), we observed results similar to those of Gattinoni et al. [42]: no statistical differences in lung volume recruitment between the early and late phase group were detected. In our study, however, in the early phase of

ARDS, lung volumes increased and strain decreased with the change from SP to PP, whereas in late phase ARDS we did not observe these findings (Additional file 2: Table S2). These differences could be related to the presence of some degree of hydrostatic pulmonary edema in the early phase of ARDS, and to the presence of fibrosis in the non-early phase of ARDS that predisposes to non-responsiveness to PP in terms of increasing in lung volumes and decreasing strain [43]. Our findings thus suggest that the survival benefit may, in part, be related to the early application of PP as it increases resting lung volumes and decreases lung strain compared to SP. It is also tempting to speculate that the lack of differences in Vrec between supine and prone, and the increase in overall lung volume in prone as compared to supine, can be explained by a decrease of poorly ventilated areas and an increase of well ventilated areas, which in turn might help to decrease lung inhomogeneity. It has been shown that the extent of lung inhomogeneities (as quantified by the amount of poorly ventilated tissue) is associated with worse outcomes in ARDS patients, possibly due to a mechanism of "stress raisers" [44].

Limitations
Like many physiological studies [4, 6, 14–17, 34], our study has a relatively low number of patients. Another limitation is that the measurement of FRC could be subject to the tolerance to PEEP removal and the FiO_2 used. However, when the study was performed, all the patients met the criteria for mild–moderate ARDS according to the Berlin definition [22]. We did not perform a multi-slice spiral lung computed tomography to measure the quantitative changes in alveolar aeration induced by PEEP and PP. Other measurements of lung mechanics (i.e., esophageal pressure and derived variables) and lung biomarkers could help to further explain the effects of PEEP and positioning in ARDS patients, but we did not do these because of lack of adequate equipment at the time of the study. Finally, to confirm the changes, it might have been useful to return the patients from PP to SP and to repeat the same procedures and measurements; this was not done, however, because most patients remained in the PP as per clinical decision after the study had been completed.

Conclusions
As compared to supine, prone position increases resting lung volumes without significantly changing the recruited volume kept by PEEP. Moreover, the change of position from supine to prone decreases dynamic lung strain. These findings help to better understand the beneficial effects of prone position in ARDS patients.

Abbreviations
ARDS: acute respiratory distress syndrome; EELV: end-expiratory lung volume; FRC: functional residual capacity; PEEP: positive end-expiratory pressure; PP: prone position; Pplat: end-inspiratory plateau airway pressure; SP: supine position; Vrec: PEEP-induced lung volume recruitment; Vt: tidal volume; ZEEP: zero end-expiratory pressure.

Authors' contributions
All authors participated in the study design, data collection and analysis, manuscript writing and final approval. All authors read and approved the final manuscript.

Competing interests
General Electric provided the equipment (Engström Carestation ICU ventilator) to conduct this research.

Acknowledgements
Not applicable.

References
1. Ware LB, Matthay MA. The acute respiratory distress syndrome. N Engl J Med. 2000;342:1334–49.
2. Gattinoni L, Pesenti A. The concept of "baby lung". Intensive Care Med. 2005;31:776–84.
3. Gattinoni L, Taccone P, Carlesso E, Marini JJ. Prone position in acute respiratory distress syndrome. Rationale, indications, and limits. Am J Respir Crit Care Med. 2013;188:1286–93.
4. Pelosi P, Tubiolo D, Mascheroni D, Vicardi P, Crotti S, Valenza F, Gattinoni L. Effects of the prone position on respiratory mechanics and gas exchange during acute lung injury. Am J Respir Crit Care Med. 1998;157:387–93.
5. Richard JC, Bregeon F, Costes N, Bars DL, Tourvieille C, Lavenne F, Janier M, Bourdin G, Gimenez G, Guerin C. Effects of prone position and positive end-expiratory pressure on lung perfusion and ventilation. Crit Care Med. 2008;36:2373–80.
6. Cornejo RA, Diaz JC, Tobar EA, Bruhn AR, Ramos CA, Gonzalez RA, Repetto CA, Romero CM, Galvez LR, Llanos O, Arellano DH, Neira WR, Diaz GA, Zamorano AJ, Pereira GL. Effects of prone positioning on lung protection in patients with acute respiratory distress syndrome. Am J Respir Crit Care Med. 2013;188:440–8.
7. Santini A, Protti A, Langer T, Comini B, Monti M, Sparacino CC, Dondossola D, Gattinoni L. Prone position ameliorates lung elastance and increases functional residual capacity independently from lung recruitment. Intensive Care Med Exp. 2015;3:55.
8. Guerin C, Reignier J, Richard JC, Beuret P, Gacouin A, Boulain T, Mercier E, Badet M, Mercat A, Baudin O, Clavel M, Chatellier D, Jaber S, Rosselli S, Mancebo J, Sirodot M, Hilbert G, Bengler C, Richecoeur J, Gainnier M, Bayle F, Bourdin G, Leray V, Girard R, Baboi L, Ayzac L. Prone positioning in severe acute respiratory distress syndrome. N Engl J Med. 2013;368:2159–68.
9. Albert RK, Keniston A, Baboi L, Ayzac L, Guerin C. Prone position-induced improvement in gas exchange does not predict improved survival in the acute respiratory distress syndrome. Am J Respir Crit Care Med. 2014;189:494–6.
10. Guerin C, Baboi L, Richard JC. Mechanisms of the effects of prone positioning in acute respiratory distress syndrome. Intensive Care Med. 2014;40:1634–42.
11. Broccard A, Shapiro RS, Schmitz LL, Adams AB, Nahum A, Marini JJ. Prone positioning attenuates and redistributes ventilator-induced lung injury in dogs. Crit Care Med. 2000;28:295–303.
12. Valenza F, Guglielmi M, Maffioletti M, Tedesco C, Maccagni P, Fossali T, Aletti G, Porro GA, Irace M, Carlesso E, Carboni N, Lazzerini M, Gattinoni L. Prone position delays the progression of ventilator-induced lung injury in rats: does lung strain distribution play a role? Crit Care Med. 2005;33:361–7.
13. Mutoh T, Guest RJ, Lamm WJ, Albert RK. Prone position alters the effect of volume overload on regional pleural pressures and improves hypoxemia in pigs in vivo. Am Rev Respir Dis. 1992;146:300–6.
14. Pelosi P, Bottino N, Chiumello D, Caironi P, Panigada M, Gamberoni C, Colombo G, Bigatello LM, Gattinoni L. Sigh in supine and prone position during acute respiratory distress syndrome. Am J Respir Crit Care Med. 2003;167:521–7.
15. Mentzelopoulos SD, Roussos C, Zakynthinos SG. Static pressure volume curves and body posture in acute respiratory failure. Intensive Care Med. 2005;31:1683–92.
16. Mentzelopoulos SD, Roussos C, Zakynthinos SG. Prone position reduces lung stress and strain in severe acute respiratory distress syndrome. Eur Respir J. 2005;25:534–44.
17. Reutershan J, Schmitt A, Dietz K, Unertl K, Fretschner R. Alveolar recruitment during prone position: time matters. Clin Sci (Lond). 2006;110:655–63.
18. Chiumello D, Carlesso E, Cadringher P, Caironi P, Valenza F, Polli F, Tallarini F, Cozzi P, Cressoni M, Colombo A, Marini JJ, Gattinoni L. Lung stress and strain during mechanical ventilation for acute respiratory distress syndrome. Am J Respir Crit Care Med. 2008;178:346–55.
19. Jonson B, Richard JC, Straus C, Mancebo J, Lemaire F, Brochard L. Pressure-volume curves and compliance in acute lung injury: evidence of recruitment above the lower inflection point. Am J Respir Crit Care Med. 1999;159:1172–8.
20. Maggiore SM, Jonson B, Richard JC, Jaber S, Lemaire F, Brochard L. Alveolar derecruitment at decremental positive end-expiratory pressure levels in acute lung injury: comparison with the lower inflection point, oxygenation, and compliance. Am J Respir Crit Care Med. 2001;164:795–801.
21. Crotti S, Mascheroni D, Caironi P, Pelosi P, Ronzoni G, Mondino M, Marini JJ, Gattinoni L. Recruitment and derecruitment during acute respiratory failure: a clinical study. Am J Respir Crit Care Med. 2001;164:131–40.
22. Ranieri VM, Rubenfeld GD, Thompson BT, Ferguson ND, Caldwell E, Fan E, Camporota L, Slutsky AS. Acute respiratory distress syndrome: the Berlin Definition. JAMA. 2012;307:2526–33.
23. Ranieri VM, Giuliani R, Fiore T, Dambrosio M, Milic-Emili J. Volume-pressure curve of the respiratory system predicts effects of PEEP in ARDS: "occlusion" versus "constant flow" technique. Am J Respir Crit Care Med. 1994;149:19–27.
24. Dellamonica J, Lerolle N, Sargentini C, Beduneau G, Di Marco F, Mercat A, Richard JC, Diehl JL, Mancebo J, Rouby JJ, Lu Q, Bernardin G, Brochard L. PEEP-induced changes in lung volume in acute respiratory distress syndrome. Two methods to estimate alveolar recruitment. Intensive Care Med. 2011;37:1595–604.
25. Richard JC, Brochard L, Vandelet P, Breton L, Maggiore SM, Jonson B, Clabault K, Leroy J, Bonmarchand G. Respective effects of end-expiratory and end-inspiratory pressures on alveolar recruitment in acute lung injury. Crit Care Med. 2003;31:89–92.
26. Olegard C, Sondergaard S, Houltz E, Lundin S, Stenqvist O. Estimation of functional residual capacity at the bedside using standard monitoring equipment: a modified nitrogen washout/washin technique requiring a small change of the inspired oxygen fraction. Anesth Analg. 2005;101:206–12.
27. Dellamonica J, Lerolle N, Sargentini C, Beduneau G, Di Marco F, Mercat A, Richard JC, Diehl JL, Mancebo J, Rouby JJ, Lu Q, Bernardin G, Brochard L. Accuracy and precision of end-expiratory lung-volume measurements by automated nitrogen washout/washin technique in patients with acute respiratory distress syndrome. Crit Care. 2011;15:R294.
28. Chatte G, Sab JM, Dubois JM, Sirodot M, Gaussorgues P, Robert D. Prone position in mechanically ventilated patients with severe acute respiratory failure. Am J Respir Crit Care Med. 1997;155:473–8.
29. Mancebo J, Fernandez R, Blanch L, Rialp G, Gordo F, Ferrer M, Rodriguez F, Garro P, Ricart P, Vallverdu I, Gich I, Castano J, Saura P, Dominguez G, Bonet A, Albert RK. A multicenter trial of prolonged prone ventilation in severe acute respiratory distress syndrome. Am J Respir Crit Care Med. 2006;173:1233–9.
30. Ibanez J, Raurich JM. Normal values of functional residual capacity in the sitting and supine positions. Intensive Care Med. 1982;8:173–7.
31. Amato MB, Meade MO, Slutsky AS, Brochard L, Costa EL, Schoenfeld DA, Stewart TE, Briel M, Talmor D, Mercat A, Richard JC, Carvalho CR, Brower RG. Driving pressure and survival in the acute respiratory distress syndrome. N Engl J Med. 2015;372:747–55.

32. Protti A, Cressoni M, Santini A, Langer T, Mietto C, Febres D, Chierichetti M, Coppola S, Conte G, Gatti S, Leopardi O, Masson S, Lombardi L, Lazzerini M, Rampoldi E, Cadringher P, Gattinoni L. Lung stress and strain during mechanical ventilation: any safe threshold? Am J Respir Crit Care Med. 2011;183:1354–62.

33. Protti A, Andreis DT, Monti M, Santini A, Sparacino CC, Langer T, Votta E, Gatti S, Lombardi L, Leopardi O, Masson S, Cressoni M, Gattinoni L. Lung stress and strain during mechanical ventilation: any difference between statics and dynamics? Crit Care Med. 2013;41:1046–55.

34. Galiatsou E, Kostanti E, Svarna E, Kitsakos A, Koulouras V, Efremidis SC, Nakos G. Prone position augments recruitment and prevents alveolar overinflation in acute lung injury. Am J Respir Crit Care Med. 2006;174:187–97.

35. Nieszkowska A, Lu Q, Vieira S, Elman M, Fetita C, Rouby JJ. Incidence and regional distribution of lung overinflation during mechanical ventilation with positive end-expiratory pressure. Crit Care Med. 2004;32:1496–503.

36. Chiumello D, Marino A, Brioni M, Cigada I, Menga F, Colombo A, Crimella F, Algieri I, Cressoni M, Carlesso E, Gattinoni L. Lung recruitment assessed by respiratory mechanics and computed tomography in patients with acute respiratory distress syndrome. What Is the relationship? Am J Respir Crit Care Med. 2016;193:1254–63.

37. Dreyfuss D, Saumon G. Ventilator-induced lung injury: lessons from experimental studies. Am J Respir Crit Care Med. 1998;157:294–323.

38. Gonzalez-Lopez A, Garcia-Prieto E, Batalla-Solis E, Amado-Rodriguez L, Avello N, Blanch L, Albaiceta GM. Lung strain and biological response in mechanically ventilated patients. Intensive Care Med. 2012;38:240–7.

39. Bellani G, Guerra L, Musch G, Zanella A, Patroniti N, Mauri T, Messa C, Pesenti A. Lung regional metabolic activity and gas volume changes induced by tidal ventilation in patients with acute lung injury. Am J Respir Crit Care Med. 2011;183:1193–9.

40. Guerin C, Beuret P, Constantin JM, Bellani G, Garcia-Olivares P, Roca O, Meertens JH, Maia PA, Becher T, Peterson J, Larsson A, Gurjar M, Hajjej Z, Kovari F, Assiri AH, Mainas E, Hasan MS, Morocho-Tutillo DR, Baboi L, Chretien JM, Francois G, Ayzac L, Chen L, Brochard L, Mercat A, investigators of the APRONET Study Group, the REVA Network, the Réseau recherche de la Société Française d'Anesthésie-Réanimation (SFAR-recherche), the ESICM Trials Group. A prospective international observational prevalence study on prone positioning of ARDS patients: the APRONET (ARDS Prone Position Network) study. Intensive Care Med. 2018;44:22–37. https://doi.org/10.1007/s00134-017-4996-5.

41. Grasso S, Mascia L, Del Turco M, Malacarne P, Giunta F, Brochard L, Slutsky AS, Marco Ranieri V. Effects of recruiting maneuvers in patients with acute respiratory distress syndrome ventilated with protective ventilatory strategy. Anesthesiology. 2002;96:795–802.

42. Gattinoni L, Caironi P, Cressoni M, Chiumello D, Ranieri VM, Quintel M, Russo S, Patroniti N, Cornejo R, Bugedo G. Lung recruitment in patients with the acute respiratory distress syndrome. N Engl J Med. 2006;354:1775–86.

43. Nakos G, Tsangaris I, Kostanti E, Nathanail C, Lachana A, Koulouras V, Kastani D. Effect of the prone position on patients with hydrostatic pulmonary edema compared with patients with acute respiratory distress syndrome and pulmonary fibrosis. Am J Respir Crit Care Med. 2000;161:360–8.

44. Cressoni M, Cadringher P, Chiurazzi C, Amini M, Gallazzi E, Marino A, Brioni M, Carlesso E, Chiumello D, Quintel M, Bugedo G, Gattinoni L. Lung inhomogeneity in patients with acute respiratory distress syndrome. Am J Respir Crit Care Med. 2014;189:149–58.

16

Quality of life and life satisfaction are severely impaired in patients with long-term invasive ventilation following ICU treatment and unsuccessful weaning

Sophie Emilia Huttmann[1], Friederike Sophie Magnet[1], Christian Karagiannidis[1], Jan Hendrik Storre[2,3] and Wolfram Windisch[1*]

Abstract

Background: Health-related quality of life (HRQL), life satisfaction, living conditions, patients' attitudes towards life and death, expectations, beliefs and unmet needs are all poorly understood aspects associated with patients receiving invasive home mechanical ventilation (HMV) following ICU treatment and unsuccessful weaning. Therefore, the present study aimed to assess (1) HRQL, (2) life satisfaction and (3) patients' perspectives on life and death associated with invasive HMV as the consequence of unsuccessful weaning.

Results: Patients undergoing invasive HMV with full technical supply and maximal patient care were screened over a 1-year period and assessed in their home environment. The study comprised the following: (1) detailed information on specific aspects of daily life, (2) self-evaluation of 23 specific daily life aspects, (3) HRQL assessment using the Severe Respiratory Insufficiency Questionnaire, (4) open interviews about the patient's living situation, HRQL, unsolved problems, treatment options, dying and the concept of an afterlife. Out of 112 patients admitted to a specialized weaning centre, 50 were discharged with invasive HMV and 25 out of these (14 COPD and 11 neuromuscular patients) were ultimately enrolled. HRQL and life satisfaction were severely impaired, despite maximal patient care and full supply of technical aids. The most important areas of dissatisfaction identified were mobility, communication, social contact and care dependency. Importantly, 32% of patients would have elected to die in hindsight rather than receive invasive HMV.

Conclusions: Despite maximal patient care and a full supply of technical aids, both HRQL and life satisfaction are severely impaired in many invasive HMV patients who have failed prolonged weaning. These findings raise ethical concerns about the use of long-term invasive HMV following unsuccessful weaning.

Keywords: Health-related quality of life, Home mechanical ventilation, ICU outcome, Respiratory failure, Tracheostomy, End of life

Background

Long-term home mechanical ventilation (HMV) is an increasingly used treatment option for patients with chronic respiratory failure [1, 2]. For this purpose, HMV can be performed either invasively following tracheotomy, or noninvasively using face masks, the latter being the preferred mode [1]. Invasive HMV is only chosen in cases where noninvasive HMV is no longer feasible or sufficient [3]. Here, particularly in patients with neuromuscular disorders (NMDs), invasive HMV should only be electively established after detailed, fully informed consent is given for the procedures involved and their potential consequences [3].

*Correspondence: windischw@kliniken-koeln.de
[1] Department of Pneumology, Cologne-Merheim Hospital, Kliniken der Stadt Köln gGmbH, Witten/Herdecke University Hospital, Ostmerheimer Strasse 200, 51109 Cologne, Germany
Full list of author information is available at the end of the article

In addition, intubation of ICU patients suffering from acute respiratory failure is often accompanied by tracheotomy if mechanical ventilation (MV) has to be applied for a longer period, or if there are foreseeable difficulties with weaning [4]. Even though many patients can eventually be liberated from invasive MV once the acute respiratory failure has been successfully treated, some still require prolonged weaning [4]. In the event that this fails, invasive HMV must once again be implemented [5].

Such patients do not usually have the opportunity during stable phases of their disease to decide whether or not they wish to become tracheotomized. While there is increasing evidence that outcome and health-related quality of life (HRQL) are improved in many patients receiving noninvasive HMV [2, 6], the impact of invasive HMV remains especially unclear in patients receiving invasive HMV after an unsuccessful attempt at weaning.

According to the Severe Respiratory Insufficiency Questionnaire (SRI), a specific HRQL measuring tool [6–8] (https://www.pneumologie.de/service/patienten-information/patienten-fragebogen-zur-befindlichkeit-bei-schwerer-respiratorischer-insuffizienz/), we found that HRQL differed substantially among patients undergoing invasive HMV primarily following weaning failure, with scores ranging from very good to very poor [9]. Older patients with chronic obstructive pulmonary disease (COPD) and more co-morbidities showed a higher tendency for reduced HRQL than patients with NMD. In addition, some patients verbally expressed the severe limitations they faced in daily life [9]. Therefore, it appears that even the most specific questionnaires cannot fully assess the specific and complex living conditions of patients with invasive HMV.

The present study therefore aimed to assess (1) HRQL, (2) life satisfaction and (3) patients' perspectives on life and death associated with invasive HMV following unsuccessful weaning in patients with intubation and subsequent tracheostomy that have become necessary to treat acute-on-chronic respiratory failure by carrying out detailed assessments of the specific living conditions experienced by patients in their respective home environments. The purpose of this was to identify specific problems and undiscovered needs of these patients, as well as the reasons for reduced HRQL and life satisfaction following a new study different from the authors' previous one [9].

Methods

The study protocol was approved by the local ethics committee (Ethikkommission der Ärztekammer Nordrhein, Germany) and performed in accordance with the ethical standards laid down in the Declaration of Helsinki. The study was registered under the German Clinical Trials Register (DRKS00006524) with the Universal Trial Number (UTN): U1111-1159-5354. Informed written consent was obtained from all subjects or legal guardians.

Subjects

The study was performed in adult tracheotomized patients undergoing long-term invasive HMV. All patients were treated on a specialized weaning unit for prolonged weaning (Department of Pneumology, Cologne-Merheim Hospital, University Witten/Herdecke, Germany) following the need for intubation and tracheotomy due to acute respiratory failure prior to the study. Specifically, the weaning unit was accredited by the German Society of Pneumology and Mechanical Ventilation (DGP) and aims for tracheotomized patients who are ready to wean, but who still fit with the category of prolonged weaning according to international criteria while decannulation has not become successful in the external referring hospital [5].

For the purpose of the study, we screened all patients who underwent prolonged weaning (as defined by international and national guidelines [5, 10]) and were treated on the specialized weaning unit between January and December 2014. Eligible patients who died during the recruitment period, as well as those who were successfully weaned from invasive ventilation, with or without the adjunct of NIV, were not included in the final study. Thus, only patients who were discharged to an outpatient environment to continue invasive HMV following unsuccessful weaning were included in the study. A prerequisite for the study was that patients had to be acclimatized to their home environment; therefore, only patients who underwent invasive HMV for at least 2 months were included. Since the patient's ability to perceive his or her own situation was mandatory for the study, severe mental retardation served as an exclusion criterion.

Study design

All patients were visited in their home environment by a physician experienced with ICU medicine and prolonged weaning (first author) who was also experienced in performing interviews in these patients in the home environment according to previous research [9]. Four consecutive steps were performed for each patient:

1. Detailed information about sociodemographics, medical history, living situation, nursing care, medical care, MV, supply of technical aids, treatments (physiotherapy, occupational therapy and speech therapy), nursing dependency and daily living activities, social contacts, daily routine, legal guardianship, and religion/faith was collected. Information from medical documents was also recorded, and inspec-

tion of the home environment as well as interviews with patients, caregivers and relatives was carried out.

2. Based on the collated information, 23 important aspects of living with invasive HMV were defined following discussion and final agreement within the expert panel (all authors). Here, patients were required to indicate whether or not they were satisfied with each of these conditions (yes/no). Care was taken to ensure that the patients' opinion was exclusively assessed, whereby relatives, caregivers or other people were not allowed to answer these questions.

3. Patients completed the original German version of the SRI, an instrument specifically designed to measure HRQL in patients with severe respiratory insufficiency [6–8]. The SRI Questionnaire contains 49 items with seven subscales measuring different aspects of HRQL (Respiratory Complaints, Physical Functioning, Attendant Symptoms and Sleep, Social Relationships, Anxiety, Psychological Well-being, Social Functioning). Each subscale produces a score (0–100), with lower scores indicating poorer health status. The scales can be aggregated to one Summary Score. Answers are given on a 5-point Likert scale ranging from "completely untrue" to "always true". Again, relatives and caregivers were excluded from answering questions.

4. An open interview was performed by posing questions about (1) the living situation, (2) quality of life, (3) unsolved problems regarding the underlying disease, (4) treatment options, (5) dying, and (6) the concept of an afterlife. Again, the six topics for the open interview were determined within the expert group.

Statistical analysis

Demographics, numeric data and SRI values were subjected to normality testing using the Shapiro–Wilk test. All normally distributed data are presented as mean ± standard deviation. Non-normally distributed data (Shapiro–Wilk with P value < 0.05) are provided as median values with minimum and maximum values. Binary data are presented with absolute numbers and percentages [n (%)].

Group comparison of SRI results was performed with respect to (1) the underlying disease (NMD vs. COPD) and (2) the individual's attitude towards tracheostomy and invasive HMV (no regret vs. regret). Therefore, paired t tests were used for normally distributed data. A nonparametric test (Wilcoxon–Mann–Whitney rank-sum test) was used on non-normally distributed data. Group effects were estimated with 95% confidence intervals and tested with a 2-sided level of 0.05.

Results

A flow chart of the study cohort is displayed in Fig. 1.

A total of 25 patients (10 females, median age 64 years, min/max 20;82 years, 14 primarily with COPD, 11 with NMD) were visited in their home environment and intensively studied as outlined in Methods section. Further demographic data, disease classifications, co-morbidities, but also patients' marital statuses and education are listed in Additional file 1: Tables S1 and S2, respectively. Self-evaluation of the relevant daily life aspects is illustrated in Fig. 2.

Overall, 23 different topics were rated by the patients. Data are also provided according to disease categories, showing that COPD patients are more frequently unsatisfied than neuromuscular patients with regard to the 23 listed aspects (Additional file 1: Table S3). Adding to this, detailed information on the underlying circumstances for each of the 23 topics is listed in Additional file 1: Table S4.

As an example, two of the 23 topics (No. 10, Fig. 3 and No. 1, Fig. 4) are illustrated according to the underlying disease.

To this end, the topic most frequently reported as being unsatisfactory was mobility. In particular, a much larger proportion of COPD patients (85.7%) were unsatisfied with their mobility compared to NMD patients (45.5%) (Additional file 1: Table S3). Only one patient (4%) was able to get out of bed without help, 23 patients (92%) were dependent on technical aids and/or personal help and one patient (4%) could not leave the bed at all. However, all patients had individually prescribed technical aids for mobility such as wheel chairs, rollators and lifters (Additional file 1: Table S4). Furthermore, leaving the house with or without help was only possible for 16 patients (64%). Excursions and travelling were possible for 13 (52%) and two patients (8%), respectively.

Regarding the question about "choosing tracheostomy again, in hindsight", 42.9% of COPD patients ($N=6$) and 18.2% of NMD patients ($N=2$; one with amyotrophic lateral sclerosis, one with spinal cord injury) indicated that they would have refused to have a tracheotomy if they had to choose again. Importantly, this question was raised under the assumption that the alternative to tracheotomy was death, as communicated to all patients during the interview. Unfortunately, it remains unclear whether some of these patients eventually asked for withdrawing of mechanical ventilation. Of note, tracheotomy dated back to a median of 23 months (min 6; max 145 months), with no difference between patients who refused and those who didn't. Seven out of eight and 8/8 patients who would have refused a tracheotomy indicated dissatisfaction with MV and mobility, respectively. Finally, 18 patients (72%) had had unplanned hospital

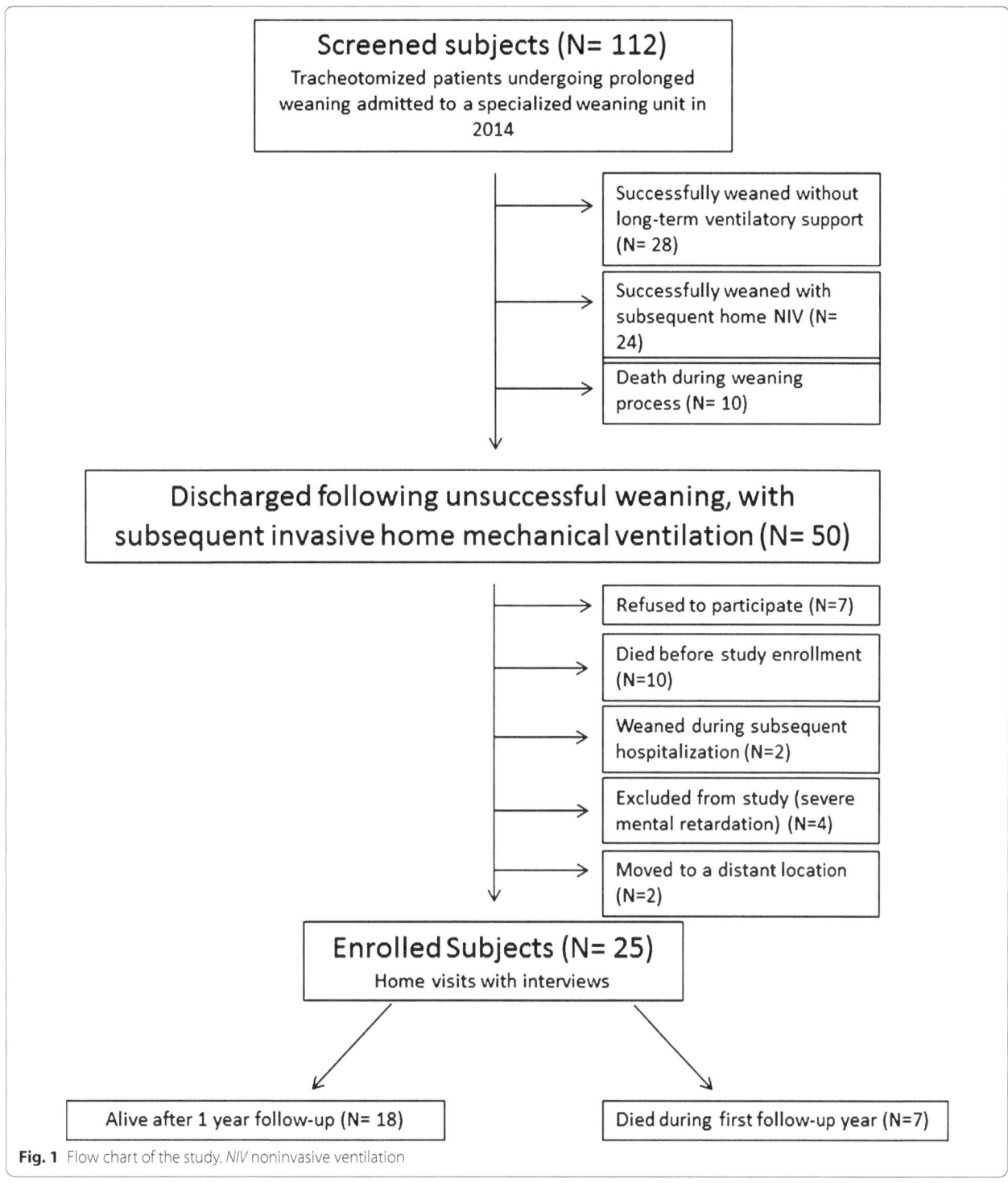

Fig. 1 Flow chart of the study. *NIV* noninvasive ventilation

admissions for the management of acute deteriorations prior to the study.

Another important issue addressed in the interview was communication. In order to communicate, 21 (84%) patients required technical aids (Additional file 1: Table S4). Despite this, the ability to speak was impaired in 48% of patients, to write by hand in 24%, and to write using a computer in 48%. Remarkably, three NMD patients could only communicate with eye movements.

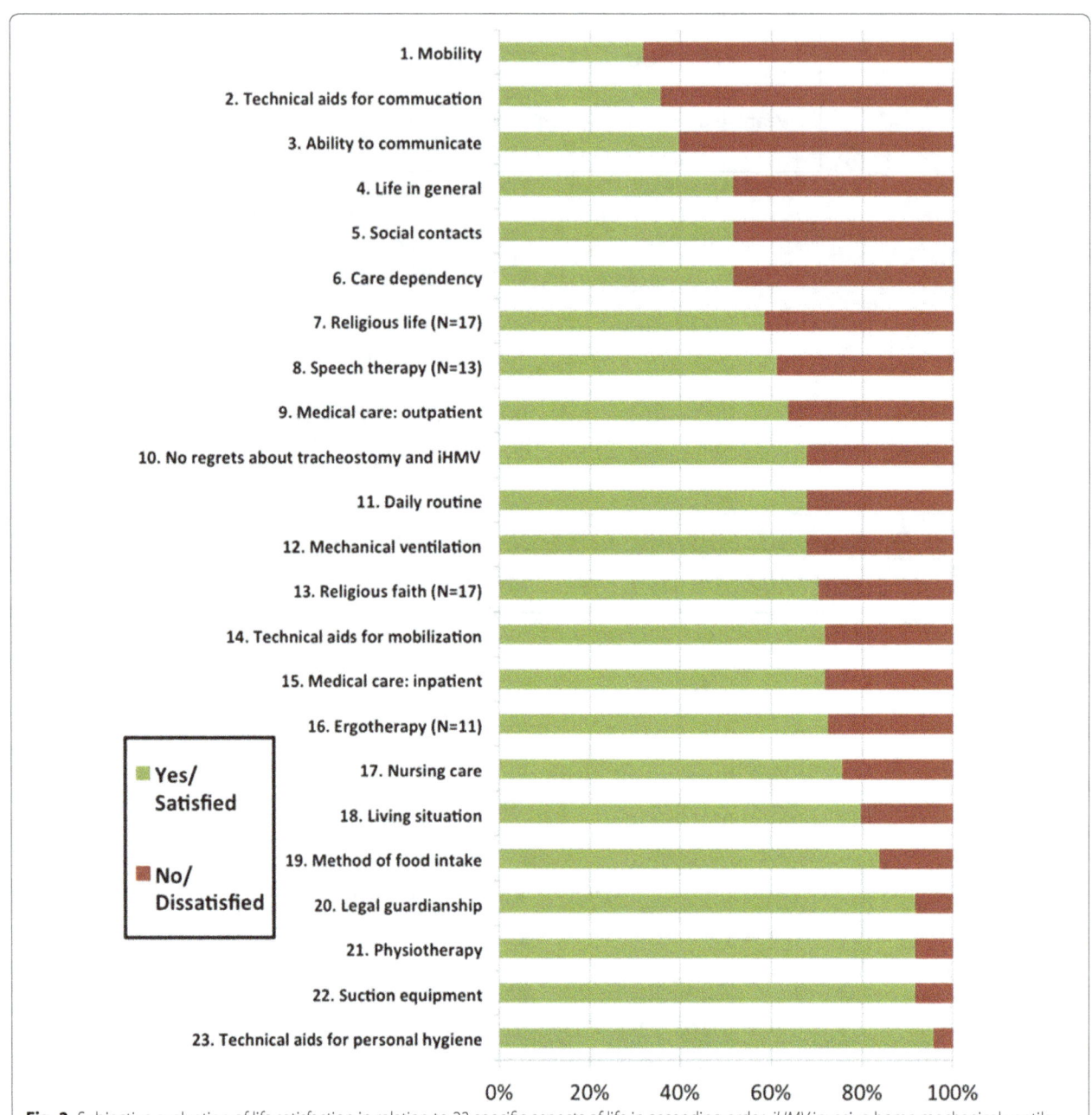

Fig. 2 Subjective evaluation of life satisfaction in relation to 23 specific aspects of life in ascending order. *iHMV* invasive home mechanical ventilation

Most of the patients had family members and/or close friends (Additional file 1: Table S4). Fifteen patients (60%) lived with family members. In contrast, after invasive HMV was established, six (24%) and 14 patients (56%) lost contact with close family members and close friends, respectively. Patients were also highly dependent on nursing care: bathing (100%), dressing (96%), use of the toilet (92%), grooming (76%), feeding (44%).

Regarding outpatient care, 23 patients (92%) received home visits from a general practitioner and four patients (16%) were visited by a specialized respiratory physician. Nevertheless, all patients were assigned to a specialized ventilation centre with a median (min/max) distance of 15 km (0.1/104 km). Outpatient nursing care was provided in 92 of patients. In addition, family members were involved in the nursing care of 48% of patients: primarily in basic care and to a lesser extent in respiratory

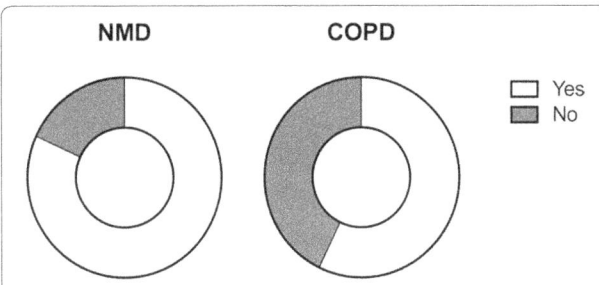

Fig. 3 Degree of satisfaction with history of tracheostomy according to underlying disease—question: In hindsight, would you choose tracheostomy for long-term invasive HMV again? *NMD* neuromuscular disease, *COPD* chronic obstructive pulmonary disease, *HMW* home mechanical ventilation

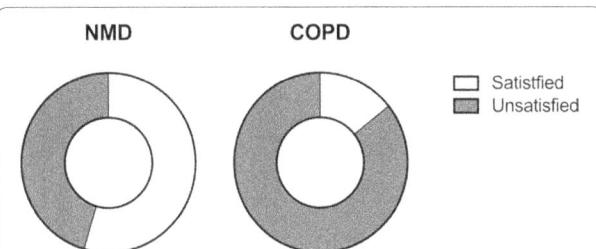

Fig. 4 Degree of satisfaction with mobilization according to underlying disease—question: Are you satisfied with your level of mobility? *NMD* neuromuscular disease, *COPD* chronic obstructive pulmonary disease

care. Eighteen patients (72%) lived in a private home and seven patients (28%) in a nursing facility (Additional file 1: Table S4). Nutrition was provided via percutaneous endoscopic gastrostomy in nine patients (36%).

The daily routine of the 25 patients who underwent invasive HMV is illustrated in Additional file 1: Figure S1 and Table S4. Importantly, patients spent most of their time watching television when they were not asleep (8 h per day). Eleven patients (44%) received continuous ventilation for 24 h per day. In contrast, 14 patients (66%) were intermittently able to breathe spontaneously, with a mean spontaneous breathing period of 8.5 ± 5.7 h per day.

Information on the Subscales and Summary Scale of the SRI is provided in Table 1, with emphasis on the differences between the two patient groups, as well as between those who regretted their tracheostomy and those who didn't. To this end, patients who regretted their tracheostomy had significantly lower SRI results for both the Subscale Anxiety and the Summary Scale, while most of the remaining scales also tended to be lower.

The results of the open interview on the topics of life and death and afterlife are summarized in Table 2. Since the interview was too exhausting for one patient suffering from both COPD and obesity hypoventilation syndrome, detailed interviews are available for 24 patients. With regard to these results, 21 patients (84%) had a religious affiliation: Catholic ($N=13$), Protestant ($N=5$), Muslim ($N=2$) and Hindu ($N=1$). However, only 17 of these patients (68%) reported having an active faith.

Discussion

This is the first study to provide a detailed description of patient characteristics, living conditions, specific aspects of HRQL and attitudes towards life, dying and death in patients with long-term invasive HMV following ICU treatment and unsuccessful weaning. The main finding was that HRQL and life satisfaction are massively impaired in many of these patients, despite maximal patient care and full supply of technical aids. Importantly, one-third of patients indicated that they would not have chosen to have a tracheostomy inserted if they had the chance to decide again, with this decision being based on

Table 1 Sub- and summary scales of the SRI according to underlying disease (NMD vs. COPD) and individual attitudes towards tracheostomy and invasive HMV

$N=25$	Underlying disease			Attitude towards tracheostomy and invasive HMV		
	NMD ($N=11$)	COPD ($N=14$)	P value	No regrets ($N=17$)	Regrets ($N=8$)	P value
Respiratory complaints	52 ± 27	54 ± 27	0.912	56.7 ± 24.9	36.3 ± 21.5	0.059
Physical functioning	27 ± 23	13 (0;58)	0.267	16.7 (0;58,3)	22.9 ± 22.8	0.617
Attendant symptoms and sleep	58 ± 18	66 ± 26	0.393	63.0 ± 21.7	45.1 ± 26.9	0.087
Social relationships	64 ± 19	54 ± 27	0.278	63.9 ± 23.8	47.8 ± 14.5	0.136
Anxiety	58 ± 23	53 ± 35	0.693	58.2 ± 30.3	34.4 ± 24.0	0.063
Psychological well-being	51 ± 26	46 ± 27	0.267	*54.9 $\pm$ 21.0*	*34.0 $\pm$ 24.6*	*0.038*
Social functioning	33 ± 20	42 ± 23	0.320	40.9 ± 24.8	31.0 ± 22.3	0.350
Summary scale	49 ± 16	47 ± 20	0.814	*51.2 $\pm$ 18.3*	*35.9 $\pm$ 13.3*	*0.046*

Data are presented as mean ± standard deviation. For non-normally distributed data, median values with minimum and maximum ranges are given

NMD neuromuscular disorders; *HMV* home mechanical ventilation; *SRI* Severe Respiratory Insufficiency Questionnaire

Table 2 Summary of open interview (N = 24)

Questions 1–6

1. How is your current living situation?
Three patients said that they are able to cope with their respective living conditions
Twenty-one patients felt lousy, stressed and massively impaired. Emotions such as anxiety and sadness, and feelings of being dependent and waiting for death were frequently reported

2. How would you assess your quality of life? What makes your life worth living?
Seventeen patients emphasized that despite their reduced quality of life, the deep relationship with family members and (to a lesser extent) friends, nevertheless, made life worth living. Among these patients, two had the hope of eventually becoming weaned and healed, respectively
Seven patients reported a severely reduced quality of life with nothing available to make it worth living again

3. What are your wishes regarding the treatment of your disease. What are the unresolved problems?
Fourteen patients had wishes that related to their treatment: better ability to speak (N = 1), less pain (N = 2), no further disease progression (N = 1), lung transplantation (N = 1), definitive weaning (N = 2), more awareness (N = 2), technical advances aimed at healing (N = 5)
Ten patients had no wishes relating to their treatment

4. What are your wishes regarding your ventilation therapy? How could this potentially be improved?
Fourteen patients had wishes that related to potential improvements in ventilation therapy: Switching to NIV (N = 1), less dyspnoea (N = 1), no further admissions to hospital (N = 2), longer periods of spontaneous breathing (N = 5), definitive weaning (N = 5)
Ten patients had no wishes relating to potential improvements in ventilation therapy

5. What do you think about dying and death?
Seventeen patients did think about dying and their own death: two patients expressed the wish to die, seven patients had a fear of dying/suffering during dying, and eight patients had no fear of dying
Seven patients thought neither about dying, nor their own death

6. Do you believe in an afterlife? What do you think is going to happen after you die?
Eleven patients believed in an afterlife: two patients had no idea how life after death would be, and nine patients had hopes (being with family members, being free, an eternal life, transmigration of souls, resurrection, being a spirit)
Thirteen patients did not believe in an afterlife

the understanding that refusing a tracheostomy would have led to death. Importantly, based on the SRI scores and interview findings, these patients had the worst HRQL.

Overall, these findings raise ethical concerns about the use of long-term invasive HMV following unsuccessful weaning. In addition, the prognosis of patients with prolonged weaning in the present study was severely impaired. Some patients had already died during the weaning process, others died shortly after they were assigned to invasive HMV prior to study inclusion, and some died in the year following study inclusion. This is in line with recent research that also reported severely impaired prognoses of patients who failed the weaning process [11–13]. In addition, there is increasing evidence to suggest that weaning success rates and patient outcome steadily deteriorate over time, an effect attributed to the observation that more severely ill patients are admitted to weaning centres [12]. This is presumably due to the fact that greater numbers of chronically critical patients are surviving catastrophic illnesses as a result of modern ICU medicine [12]. However, despite the increased success of modern medicine in saving lives, the flipside is that surviving ICU treatment—but remaining dependent on invasive ventilation—is associated with a high risk of extremely poor quality of life. Moreover, there are reportedly many problems and individually raised discomforts and dissatisfactions voiced by HMV

patients in their final months of life [14]. In addition, it has been emphasized that we need to increase our level of consideration for how patients with HMV die [15]. Therefore, ICU medicine should not simply focus on how to best preserve life; it should also consider the long-term living conditions of patients who remain dependent on long-term invasive ventilation. Finally, it remains unclear how many patients regretting getting tracheotomized would eventually asked for withdrawing of mechanical ventilation and how this can be brought to the clinician's attention.

The outcome of the present study is somewhat in contrast to the findings reported by Marchese et al. [13], whereby 90% of patients undergoing invasive HMV would have chosen a tracheostomy again. However, the tracheotomies in the latter study were performed electively, and the patients were younger and had a promising median survival of 49 months. Furthermore, they were cared for primarily by family members, in contrast to our study population, whose primary care was provided by specialized nurses. In addition, the proportion of patients with pulmonary diseases was considerably lower in the Marchese study than the present one [13]. Of note, HRQL and life satisfaction in the present trial were particularly impaired in patients with COPD, in line with the previous observations [9]. Finally, patients in the current study had significant co-morbidities. Therefore, in the light of the evidence presented here and elsewhere, it is most likely that COPD patients in whom weaning has failed after ICU treatment may no longer have a life worth living.

The strength of the present study is that the comprehensive, detailed interview process that took place in the home environment provided meticulous details on how HMV patients live, feel and think. Of note, the two conditions that were associated with the most dissatisfaction were impaired mobility and communication. To this end, 36% of patients could not leave the house and 48% were unable to speak (Additional file 1: Table S3). This is remarkable, especially since aids for mobility and communication were thoroughly provided. Thus, in most cases it is the nature of the maximally advanced disease state that impairs life satisfaction, and this cannot be fully compensated by technical aids and patient care.

Social contact and care dependency were two additional aspects with which patients were dissatisfied. Importantly, patients spent most of their time watching television (median 8 h) during waking hours, with only a median social contact time of 1.5 h. In addition, many patients had lost contact with family members and close friends after the establishment of invasive HMV. However, 71% of the patients emphasized that they had a meaningful relationship with family members, and most were satisfied with their living conditions. To this end, 72% of patients lived in their own private home, and 60% of all patients lived with family members. Based on this finding, it is remarkable that nearly 50% of patients were not satisfied with their social situation. Finally, all patients were extremely dependent on nursing care, and the family members of 48% of patients were involved in patient care, indicating the close interlink between living situation, family contact and patient care. Of note, while there is no information available about how family members would evaluate their level of life satisfaction if a close relative become ventilator dependent in the home environment, previous research has indicated that family members were less satisfied with a relative having a tracheostomy than the patient him/herself [13].

Finally, there was a broad heterogeneity among patients regarding religious life, faith and belief in an afterlife. This was also dependent on different religious affiliations. Some patients had detailed thoughts about their deaths, ranging between positive and negative, and some even verbally expressed their wish to die. In contrast, other patients had no definitive thoughts on this subject and avoided thinking about death. The impact of religious life on HRQL and life satisfaction, however, needs to be further elucidated in future.

As a limitation of the current study and as the prize for the individually detailed investigation, the number of patients was low. In addition, this was a monocentric study. Therefore, it cannot be excluded that patients may respond differently under different conditions, particularly in other countries. Therefore, further studies in different countries are needed to verify the current findings.

Conclusions

In conclusion, despite maximal patient care and a full supply of technical aids, both HRQL and life satisfaction are severely impaired in many invasive HMV patients who have failed prolonged weaning. The most important areas of dissatisfaction are mobility, communication, social contacts and care dependency. Importantly, one-third of patients would have preferred to die rather than receive invasive HMV. This raises ethical concerns about the practice of long-term MV following unsuccessful weaning, even though it still should be taken into account that some patients clearly benefit from long-term invasive HMV. Therefore, to avoid unethical prolongation of life, the disciplines of ICU medicine, prolonged weaning care and long-term outpatient care need to move closer together in order to improve individual decision-making processes that incorporate patients' beliefs, expectations and circumstances.

Abbreviations
COPD: chronic obstructive pulmonary disease; HMV: home mechanical ventilation; iHMV: invasive home mechanical ventilation; MV: mechanical ventilation; HRQL: health-related quality of life; NMD: neuromuscular disorders; SRI: Severe Respiratory Insufficiency Questionnaire.

Authors' contributions
SEH takes responsibility for (is the guarantor of) the content of the manuscript, including the data and analysis. All other authors contributed substantially to the study design, data analysis and interpretation, and the writing of the manuscript, with special contributions as follows: FSM assisted in the collection of data and writing of the manuscript. CK assisted in designing the study and writing the manuscript. JHS assisted in designing the study, collection of data as well as writing the manuscript. WW assisted in designing the study, the collection of the data and writing the manuscript. All authors read and approved the final manuscript.

Author details
[1] Department of Pneumology, Cologne-Merheim Hospital, Kliniken der Stadt Köln gGmbH, Witten/Herdecke University Hospital, Ostmerheimer Strasse 200, 51109 Cologne, Germany. [2] Department of Pneumology, University Medical Hospital, Freiburg, Germany. [3] Department of Intensive Care, Sleep Medicine and Mechanical Ventilation, Asklepios Fachkliniken Munich-Gauting, Gauting, Germany.

Acknowledgements
We acknowledge all participants for the effort they devoted to this study and Dr. Sandra Dieni for proofreading the manuscript prior to submission.

Competing interests
SEH, FSM, CK, JHS and WW received speaking fees from companies dealing with mechanical ventilation outside the presented work.

Funding
All authors state that none of the discussed issues in the present article were dependent on or influenced by financial support or funding. The study was supported by Weinmann Geräte für Medizin GmbH & Co. KG and VIVISOL Deutschland GmbH.

References
1. Lloyd-Owen SJ, Donaldson GC, Ambrosino N, Escarabill J, Farre R, Fauroux B, Robert D, Schoenhofer B, Simonds AK, Wedzicha JA. Patterns of home mechanical ventilation use in Europe: results from the Eurovent survey. Eur Respir J. 2005;25:1025–31.
2. Windisch W. Home mechanical ventilation. In: Tobin MJ, editor. Principles and practice of mechanical ventilation, 3rd edn. p. 683–697. Nex Yoek: Mc Graw Hill Medical; 2012.
3. Windisch W, Walterspacher S, Siemon K, Geiseler J, Sitter H. Guidelines for non-invasive and invasive mechanical ventilation for treatment of chronic respiratory failure. Published by the German Society for Pneumology (DGP). Pneumologie. 2010;64:640–52.
4. Beduneau G, Pham T, Schortgen F, Piquilloud L, Zogheib E, Jonas M, Grelon F, Runge I, Nicolas T, Grange S, et al. Epidemiology of weaning ⁻ outcome according to a new definition. The WIND study. Am J Respir Crit Care Med. 2017;195:772–83.
5. Boles JM, Bion J, Connors A, Herridge M, Marsh B, Melot C, Pearl R, Silverman H, Stanchina M, Vieillard-Baron A, et al. Weaning from mechanical ventilation. Eur Respir J. 2007;29:1033–56.
6. Windisch W. Quality of life in home mechanical ventilation study g: impact of home mechanical ventilation on health-related quality of life. Eur Respir J. 2008;32:1328–36.
7. Windisch W, Freidel K, Schucher B, Baumann H, Wiebel M, Matthys H, Petermann F. The Severe Respiratory Insufficiency (SRI) Questionnaire: a specific measure of health-related quality of life in patients receiving home mechanical ventilation. J Clin Epidemiol. 2003;56:752–9.
8. Windisch W, Budweiser S, Heinemann F, Pfeifer M, Rzehak P. The Severe Respiratory Insufficiency Questionnaire was valid for COPD patients with severe chronic respiratory failure. J Clin Epidemiol. 2008;61:848–53.
9. Huttmann SE, Windisch W, Storre JH. Invasive home mechanical ventilation: living conditions and health-related quality of life. Respiration. 2015;89:312–21.
10. Schönhofer B, Geiseler J, Dellweg D, Moerer O, Barchfeld T, Fuchs H, Karg O, Rosseau S, Sitter H, Weber-Carstens S, et al. S2k-guideline "prolonged weaning". Pneumologie. 2015;69:595–607.
11. Schönhofer B, Euteneuer S, Nava S, Suchi S, Kohler D. Survival of mechanically ventilated patients admitted to a specialised weaning centre. Intensive Care Med. 2002;28:908–16.
12. Polverino E, Nava S, Ferrer M, Ceriana P, Clini E, Spada E, Zanotti E, Trianni L, Barbano L, Fracchia C, et al. Patients' characterization, hospital course and clinical outcomes in five Italian respiratory intensive care units. Intensive Care Med. 2010;36:137–42.
13. Marchese S, Lo Coco D, Lo Coco A. Outcome and attitudes toward home tracheostomy ventilation of consecutive patients: a 10-year experience. Respir Med. 2008;102:430–6.
14. Vitacca M, Grassi M, Barbano L, Galavotti G, Sturani C, Vianello A, Zanotti E, Ballerin L, Potena A, Scala R, et al. Last 3 months of life in home-ventilated patients: the family perception. Eur Respir J. 2010;35:1064–71.
15. Windisch W. Home mechanical ventilation: who cares about how patients die? Eur Respir J. 2010;35:955–7.

17

Pleural effusion during weaning from mechanical ventilation

Keyvan Razazi[1,2,3*] ⊙, Florence Boissier[4,5], Mathilde Neuville[6], Sébastien Jochmans[2,7], Martial Tchir[8], Faten May[1,2], Nicolas de Prost[1,2], Christian Brun-Buisson[1,2], Guillaume Carteaux[1,2] and Armand Mekontso Dessap[1,2,3]

Abstract

Background: Pleural effusion is common during invasive mechanical ventilation, but its role during weaning is unclear. We aimed at assessing the prevalence and risk factors for pleural effusion at initiation of weaning. We also assessed its impact on weaning outcomes and its evolution in patients with difficult weaning.

Methods: We performed a prospective multicenter study in five intensive care units in France. Two hundred and forty-nine patients were explored using ultrasonography. Presence of moderate-to-large pleural effusion (defined as a maximal interpleural distance ≥ 15 mm) was assessed at weaning start and during difficult weaning.

Results: Seventy-three (29%) patients failed weaning, including 46 (18%) who failed the first spontaneous breathing trial (SBT) and 39 (16%) who failed extubation. Moderate-to-large pleural effusion was detected in 81 (33%) patients at weaning start. Moderate-to-large pleural effusion was associated with more failures of the first SBT [27 (33%) vs. 19 (11%), $p < 0.001$], more weaning failures [37 (47%) vs. 36 (22%), $p < 0.001$], less ventilator-free days at day 28 [21 (5–24) vs. 23 (16–26), $p = 0.01$], and a higher mortality at day 28 [14 (17%) vs. 14 (8%), $p = 0.04$]. The association of pleural effusion with weaning failure persisted in multivariable analysis and sensitivity analyses. Short-term (48 h) fluid balance change was not associated with the evolution of interpleural distance in patients with difficult weaning.

Conclusions: In this multicenter observational study, pleural effusion was frequent during the weaning process and was associated with worse weaning outcomes.

Keywords: Mechanical ventilation, Pleural effusion, Weaning, Ultrasonography

Introduction

Several factors may contribute to the occurrence of pleural effusions in critically ill patients, including heart failure, pneumonia, hypoalbuminemia, and fluid overload [1]. Its incidence in mechanically ventilated patients varies depending on the screening method, from approximately 8% with physical examination to more than 60% with routine ultrasonography [1, 2]. Pleural effusion was found in 83% of patients with acute respiratory distress syndrome (ARDS) explored with computed tomography scans [3].

The presence of pleural effusion is associated with a longer duration of mechanical ventilation and intensive care unit (ICU) stay [2]. Although a causal relationship cannot be established, this prolongation may result from altered respiratory mechanics [4] and impeded diaphragmatic contraction [5]. Indeed, pleural effusion increases the total thoracic volume, leading inspiratory muscles to operate in a less advantageous portion of their length–tension curve. Thus, the capacity of the diaphragm to generate pressure decreases when pleural effusion increases [5, 6]. Drainage of large pleural effusions improves oxygenation and respiratory mechanics in mechanically ventilated patients [4, 7].

*Correspondence: keyvan.razazi@aphp.fr
[1] AP-HP, DHU A-TVB, Service de Réanimation Médicale, Hôpitaux Universitaires Henri Mondor, 94010 Créteil, France
Full list of author information is available at the end of the article

Weaning accounts for approximately 40% of the total duration of mechanical ventilation [8], but data on pleural effusion during the weaning process are scarce [9]. The main objective of the present observational multicenter study was to assess the prevalence and risk factors of pleural effusion at initiation of weaning. The second objective was to explore the association of pleural effusion with weaning outcomes, and its evolution during difficult weaning.

Materials and methods

This prospective multicenter observational study recruited patients admitted in five ICUs in France. Inclusion criteria were endotracheal mechanical ventilation for at least 24 h, and the fulfillment of weaning criteria [10] allowing a first spontaneous breathing trial (SBT). Noninclusion criteria were pregnancy or lactation, age less than 18 years, pleural effusion drainage before the first SBT, and a do-not-reintubate decision at time of inclusion.

Weaning protocol and definitions

Weaning initiation was defined as the day of first SBT. The first SBT used a T-piece trial in three centers and a low-level pressure support (7–10 cm H_2O) with zero end-expiratory pressure in two centers, as per usual care. Failure of the SBT was based on predefined criteria (see the online supplement, Additional file 1). Extubation failure was defined as death or reintubation within the 7 days following extubation; this delay was used instead of 48–72 h because prophylactic noninvasive ventilation may postpone reintubation [11]. Indications for prophylactic noninvasive ventilation included patients older than 65 years and those with underlying cardiac or respiratory disease [12]. According to the International Consensus Conference [10], weaning success was defined as a first successful SBT followed by successful extubation. Failure of the weaning process was defined [10] as failure of the first SBT or extubation failure. Because some patients could not be classified with this definition, weaning was also categorized according to the WIND definition [13] as follows: short when the first SBT resulted in a successful termination of the weaning process or death within 1 day after the first SBT; difficult in case of successful weaning or death after more than 1 day but in less than 1 week after the first SBT; prolonged if weaning was still not terminated 7 days after the first SBT. Ventilator-free days at day 28 were computed as days without invasive mechanical ventilation during the 28 days following first SBT; patients who died before day 28 or were dependent on mechanical ventilation for more than 28 days after the first SBT had zero ventilator-free days [14]. Other definitions (e.g., Mac Cabe classification, ARDS, ventilator-associated pneumonia, failure of SBT) and data collection process are reported in the online supplement (Additional file 1).

Lung ultrasonography

Lung ultrasonography was performed on the day of first SBT and repeated on the 2 days following a SBT failure and on the day of extubation, if applicable. Maximal end-expiratory interpleural distance, sonographic patterns of effusion (homogeneously anechoic, complex nonseptated, complex septated, or homogeneously echogenic) [15], and of lung parenchyma (condensation or atelectasis) [16] were assessed on each side with the patient in the semirecumbent position. A moderate-to-large pleural effusion was defined as a maximal interpleural distance ≥ 15 mm (predicting an effusion volume of 300 mL or more) [17]; a large pleural effusion was defined by a maximal interpleural distance ≥ 25 mm [4, 17]. A pleural effusion was deemed drainable if the maximal interpleural distance was ≥ 15 mm, and the effusion was visible over at least three intercostal spaces [18]. When possible, a transthoracic echocardiography was also performed to assess left ventricle ejection fraction (see the online supplement, Additional file 1). In patients with SBT failure, attempts at depletion (by diuretics or ultrafiltration) and fluid balance were collected during the 2 days following the SBT. There was no mandatory depletive strategy for the management of pleural effusion.

Statistical analysis

The primary endpoint was the prevalence of pleural effusion at weaning start. The sample size was calculated by hypothesizing a prevalence of pleural effusion of 40% [1–3], and considering a precision of 8%. The study required a minimum of 170 patients (for an alpha risk of 5%, i.e., a confidence interval of 95%) and a maximum of 260 patients (for an alpha risk of 1%, i.e., a confidence interval of 99%). Continuous data were expressed as medians [25th–75th centiles] unless otherwise specified, and were compared using the Mann–Whitney test. Categorical variables, expressed as percentages, were compared using the Chi-square test or Fisher exact test. To evaluate independent factors associated with the presence of moderate-to-large pleural effusion at weaning start or with failure of the weaning process, significant or marginally significant ($p < 0.10$) bivariate risk factors (using the above mentioned tests) were examined using univariate and multivariable backward stepwise logistic regression analysis. Among related univariate factors, only the most statistically robust (yet clinically relevant) was entered into the regression model in order to minimize the effect of colinearity. The selection process was guided by consistency (less than 5% missing values) and maximal imbalances between groups (as estimated by absolute standardized differences, which are independent of the sample size and variable unit) [19]. Coefficients were computed by the method of maximum likelihood. The calibration of models was assessed by the Hosmer–Lemeshow goodness-of-fit statistic (good fit was defined as p value > 0.05), and discrimination was assessed by the area under the receiver operating characteristics curve (with a value of 1 indicating perfect discrimination, and a value of 0.5 indicating the effects of chance alone). Correlations were tested using the Spearman's method. Two-tailed p values < 0.05 were considered significant. Data were analyzed using the IBM SPSS Statistics for Windows (Version 19.0, IBM Corp Armonk, NY, USA).

Results

Study population

The inclusion period lasted from 2 to 12 months depending on centers, between June 2015 and May 2016. Four hundred seventy-seven patients mechanically ventilated for more than 24 h were screened (Fig. 1). Sixty-seven patients died before weaning start, and 161 patients were excluded because of either a do-not-reintubate decision at time of inclusion ($n = 72$), unavailability of pleural ultrasound ($n = 63$), or drainage of pleural effusion before inclusion ($n = 26$). Thus, the present study comprises 249 patients assessed with lung ultrasonography at weaning initiation. Median duration of mechanical ventilation before weaning was 4 [2–7] days. The weaning trajectories are summarized in Fig. 1. Two hundred and three patients succeeded the first SBT, and 200 of them were extubated (the remainder three patients were not extubated despite the success of the first SBT because of borderline cough, and experienced a novel complication leading to death before any extubation attempt).

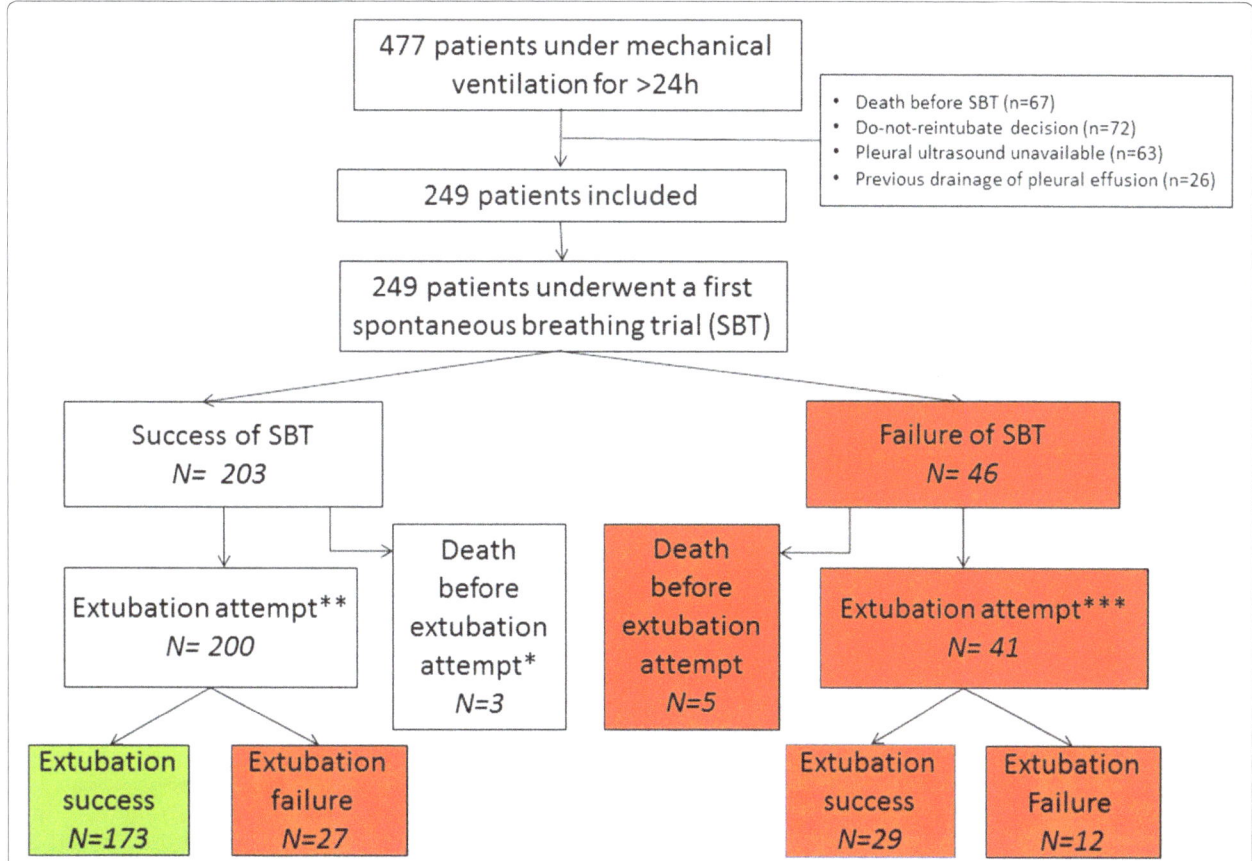

Fig. 1 Study flow chart; green and red squares denote International Consensus Conference classification of weaning success and failure, respectively; *three patients were not extubated despite the success of the first SBT because of borderline cough, and experienced a novel fatal complication leading to death before any extubation attempt; they could not be classified according to the International Consensus Conference **including 192 planned and 7 unplanned. *** Including 39 planned and 2 unplanned

Forty-six patients (18%) failed the first SBT; 41 of them succeeded a subsequent SBT and were extubated latter in the course of weaning, while the remainder five patients died before any extubation attempt. Reasons for SBT failure were respiratory rate > 35 breaths/min with increased accessory muscle activity ($n = 17$), $SpO_2 < 90\%$, while on $FiO_2 \geq 0.5$ ($n = 6$), systolic blood pressure < 90 mmHg or > 180 mmHg ($n = 2$), or a combination of those reasons ($n = 22$).

Overall, 241 patients were extubated during the weaning process, while eight patients died before any extubation attempt. Among the 241 patients extubated, 232 were planned and nine unplanned (including one accidental and eight self-extubations). After extubation, 95 (40%) patients received noninvasive ventilation prophylactically, while twelve (5%) received it for post-extubation acute respiratory failure. A total of 39 (16%) patients failed extubation. The main reason for reintubation was acute respiratory failure ($n = 23$, 73%).

Prevalence and risk factors for pleural effusion

A moderate-to-large pleural effusion was detected in 81 of 249 patients assessed at weaning initiation, for a prevalence of 33%, 95% confidence interval: 27–39%. Most of pleural effusions were homogeneously anechoic ($n = 74$, 93%) and associated with pulmonary condensation or atelectasis ($n = 68$, 85%) (see the online supplement, Table e1, Additional file 1). Seventy-six (31%) patients had a bilateral pleural effusion. The maximal interpleural distance was equally located either on the left ($n = 41$, 51%) or right side ($n = 40$, 49%). Patients with moderate-to-large pleural effusions at weaning initiation were older, had more baseline comorbidities and more organ failures before weaning as compared to their counterparts (see the online supplement, Table e4). In multivariable analysis, older age, McCabe class 2, cardiac disease, acute respiratory failure as cause of intubation, and need for dialysis before the first SBT were the five independent factors associated with a moderate-to-large pleural effusion at initiation of weaning (Table 1).

Outcome of weaning

According to the International Consensus Conference, the 249 patients were classified as follows: 173 (69%) weaning successes (a first successful SBT followed by successful extubation); 76 (31%) weaning failures (including 46 who failed the first SBT and 27 who succeeded the first SBT but failed extubation); three unclassifiable patients (despite the success of the first SBT, they were not extubated because of borderline

Table 1 Univariate and multivariable analysis of factors associated with moderate-to-large pleural effusion

Variables	Missing values, n (%)	Absolute standardized differences	Odd ratio (95% confidence interval), p value by logistic regression	
			Univariate	Multivariable
Age (per year)	0	60.5	1.04 (1.02–1.06), $p < 0.001$	1.03 (1.01–1.05), $p = 0.017$
SAPS II (per point)	0	26.9	1.02 (1.0–1.03), $p = 0.048$	I/NR
Mc Cabe class II (yes vs. no)	0	51.8	4.7 (2.1–10.3), $p < 0.001$	4.2 (1.8–9.9), $p = 0.001$
Cancer or hematological malignancy (yes vs. no)	0	47	3.5 (1.7–7.2), $p = 0.001$	NI
Cardiac disease (yes vs. no)	0	55.1	3.3 (1.1–3.3), $p < 0.001$	2.2 (1.1–4.4), $p = 0.02$
Left ventricle ejection fraction at cardiac ultrasound (%),	44 (18%)	52.9	0.96 (0.93–0.98), $p < 0.001$	NI
Supra-ventricular arrhythmias (yes vs. no)	0	35.8	2.3 (1.3–4.2), $p = 0.007$	NI
Acute respiratory failure as cause of intubation (yes vs. no)	0	31.9	1.9 (1.3–3.9), $p = 0.02$	1.8 (0.98–3.2), $p = 0.059$
Dialysis (yes vs. no)	0	31.5	2.5 (1.2–5.4), $p = 0.02$	2.0 (0.9–4.6), $p = 0.088$
Serum Creatinine (per μmol/L)	0	25.8	1.0 (0.99–1.00), $p = 0.20$	NI
Septic shock (yes vs. no)	0	25.4	1.7 (0.98–2.9), $p = 0.06$	I/NR
ARDS (yes vs. no)	0	22.2	1.7 (0.91–3.1), $p = 0.098$	I/NR
Duration of MV before first SBT (per day)	0	19	1.04 (0.99–1.1), $p = 0.15$	NI

SAPS II simplified acute physiology score, COPD chronic obstructive pulmonary disease, ARDS acute respiratory distress syndrome, SBT spontaneous breathing trial, NI not included, I/NR included, but not retained by the final model

Among related univariate factors, only the most statistically robust (yet clinically relevant) was entered into the regression model in order to minimize the effect of colinearity. The selection process was guided by consistency (less than 5% missing values) and maximal imbalances between groups (as estimated by absolute standardized differences) as follows: Mc Cabe class II was selected among Mc Cabe class II, cancer and hematological malignancy; dialysis was selected among creatininemia and dialysis; cardiac disease was selected among supra-ventricular arrhythmias, left ventricle ejection fraction and cardiac disease; ARDS was selected among duration of mechanical ventilation before the first spontaneous breathing trial and ARDS before inclusion. The multivariable model showed a good calibration as assessed by the Hosmer and Lemeshow goodness-of-fit test [χ^2 (8 df) = 6.42, $p = 0.60$] and a fair discrimination as assessed by the receiver operating characteristics curve [area under the curve of 0.74 (0.67–0.80), $p < 0.001$]

cough, and experienced a novel complication leading to death before any extubation attempt) (Fig. 1). According to the WIND classification, 161 (65%) patients had a short weaning, 60 (24%) had a difficult weaning, and 28 (11%) had a prolonged weaning. The presence of a moderate-to-large pleural effusion at weaning initiation was associated with more failures of the first SBT [27 (33%) vs. 19 (11%), $p < 0.001$], more weaning failures [37 (47%) vs. 36 (22%), $p < 0.001$], less ventilator-free days at day 28 (21 [5–24] vs. 23 [16–26], $p = 0.01$), and a higher mortality at day 28 [14 (17%) vs. 14 (8%), $p = 0.04$] (Table 2, Fig. 2). All variables associated with weaning failure are shown in Table 3 and Table e5. In multivariable analysis, PaO_2/FiO_2 ratio, chronic obstructive pulmonary disease, a longer duration of mechanical ventilation prior to weaning, and the presence of moderate-to-large pleural effusion at weaning initiation were the four independent factors associated with weaning failure (Table 4). In sensitivity analyses, the association of pleural effusion with weaning failure also persisted after adjustment on SAPS II, in selected centers using the T-piece trial, or in those using a low-level pressure support, and when considering pleural effusions deemed drainable (as defined by a maximal interpleural distance ≥ 15 mm with the effusion visible over three intercostal spaces) or those considered large (as defined by a maximal interpleural distance ≥ 25 mm) [4, 17] (Table e3). A moderate-to-large pleural effusion was detected in 60 (28%) of 218 patients assessed on the day of first extubation attempt. The extubation failure rate was higher in patients with a moderate-to-large pleural effusion on the day of extubation as compared to their counterparts [14 (23%) vs. 19 (12%), $p = 0.04$]; of note, this extubation failure rate was similar in patients with or without pleural effusion assessed earlier, at weaning initiation [24 (15%) vs 15 (20%), $p = 0.31$]. As compared to patients without effusion ($n = 168$), those with a unilateral ($n = 21$) or bilateral ($n = 60$) moderate-to-large pleural effusion had similarly altered weaning outcomes, including SBT failure [19 (11.3%) vs. 8 (38.1%) vs. 19 (31.7%), $p < 0.001$] and weaning failure [37 (22.0%) vs. 11 (52.4%) vs. 28 (46.7%), $p < 0.001$].

Evolution of pleural effusion during difficult weaning

Among the 46 patients who failed the first SBT, lung ultrasonography was repeated 24 and 48 h later in 41 and 31 patients, respectively. Patients in whom diuretics and/or ultrafiltration were used had a lower fluid balance as compared with their counterparts (-484 [-1210–330] vs. 858 [205–1806] mL after 24 h, $p < 0.001$), but this depletive strategy did not alter the interpleural distance

(see the online supplement, Table e2, Additional file 1). Fluid balance was not significantly correlated with changes in interpleural distance (ρ 0.13, $p = 0$, 17, see Figure e1 of the online supplement, Additional file 2). Pleural effusion was drained in only four patients during weaning.

Discussion

We herein report the largest study assessing pleural effusion during weaning from mechanical ventilation. A moderate-to-large pleural effusion was detected by ultrasound examination in one-third of 249 patients at initiation of weaning and was associated with weaning failure by multivariable analysis. Depletive strategies did not alter pleural effusion volume on the short term in patients with difficult weaning.

Prevalence and risk factors for pleural effusion

In our study, one-third of patients had a moderate-to-large pleural effusion at the initiation of the weaning process. This prevalence is higher than that of 13% reported by Dres et al. [9]. This discrepancy may be explained by differences in definitions used. Volume of pleural fluid was estimated in our report according to interpleural distance, which may be more sensitive than the classification of the British Thoracic Society [20] used in the latter study; indeed, patients with moderate-to-large pleural effusion in our study had a median interpleural distance inferior to the value found in the Dres' study (27 [20–41] vs. 45 [30–60] mm). Other differences between these two studies include patient's comorbidities (with more patients included with cardiac diseases in our report) and/or timing of inclusion (with less patients excluded because of prior pleural drainage before SBT in our study).

Risk factors for pleural effusion found in our study are in accordance with previous reports [1, 2]. Congestive heart failure is one of the leading factors associated with the occurrence of pleural effusion in ICU [1]. All patients intubated for acute respiratory failure had acute cardiac failure or pneumonia, two common risk factors for pleural effusion [1]. Our study suggests that diastolic dysfunction may be of importance in the association of cardiac failure with pleural effusion. Acute renal failure has also been previously reported as a risk factor for nonmalignant pleural effusions, an association possibly mediated by fluid overload [21]. The association of Mc Cabe class (i.e., a rapidly fatal underlying disease) with pleural effusion may be driven by other comorbidities like liver cirrhosis, cancer, and hypoalbuminemia [22, 23].

Table 2 Characteristics and outcome of 249 mechanically ventilated patients with or without moderate-to-large pleural effusion at first spontaneous breathing trial

Variables	Moderate-to-large pleural effusion		p value
	Absent (n = 168)	Present (n = 81)	
Male gender	98 (58%)	52 (64%)	0.38
Age (years)	61 [50–72]	69 [60–80]	< 0.001
SAPS II score at ICU admission	49 [37–62]	52 [41–67]	0.07
Comorbidities			
Neurological disease	22 (13%)	6 (7%)	0.18
Cardiac disease	93 (55%)	65 (80%)	< 0.001
Cirrhosis	12 (7%)	9 (11%)	0.29
Chronic renal failure	22 (13%)	16 (20%)	0.17
Cancer or hematological malignancy	16 (10%)	22 (27%)	< 0.001
Main reason for intubation			
Coma	54 (32%)	9 (11%)	< 0.001
Acute respiratory failure	51 (30%)	37 (46%)	0.02
Septic shock	22 (13%)	12 (15%)	0.71
Others	41 (24%)	23 (28%)	0.5
From ICU admission to first SBT			
ARDS	32 (19%)	23 (28%)	0.096
Duration of MV before the first SBT	4 [2–7]	4 [3–9]	0.09
Dialysis	15 (9%)	16 (20%)	0.015
Biological and ultrasound data at first SBT			
Serum creatinine (μmol/L)	74 [55–119]	90 [60–164]	0.07
Serum protide (mg/L)	59 [54–66]	59 [51–63]	0.19
Bilateral pleural effusion	16 (10%)	60 (74%)	< 0.001
Maximal interpleural distance (mm)	0 [0–5]	27 [20–41]	< 0.001
Condensation or atelectasis of lung adjacent to the pleural effusion at ultrasound	–	68 (84%)	
Left ventricle ejection fraction (%)	60 [50–60]	50 [39–60]	< 0.001
Outcome			
Pleural effusion drainage during weaning	0	4 (5%)	0.005
Prophylactic NIV post-extubation	62 (38%)	33 (43%)	0.39
Failure of the first SBT	19 (11%)	27 (33%)	< 0.001
Extubation failure	24 (15%)	15 (20%)	0.31
Weaning failure[a]	36 (22%)	37 (47%)	< 0.001
Weaning group[b]			0.03
Short weaning	118 (70%)	43 (53%)	
Difficult weaning	38 (20%)	26 (32%)	
Prolonged weaning	16 (10%)	12 (15%)	
Tracheotomy	4 (2%)	2 (3%)	0.97
VFD from first SBT to day 28 (days)	23 [16–26]	21 [5–24]	0.01
Death in ICU	14 (8%)	13 (16%)	0.07
Death at day 28	14 (8%)	14 (17%)	0.04

Values are indicating number (%) or median [1st–3rd quartile]

[a] According to the international conference consensus (three patients could not be classified)

[b] According to the WIND study classification

SAPS II simplified acute physiology score, *ARDS* acute respiratory distress syndrome, *SBT* spontaneous breathing trial, *NIV* noninvasive ventilation, *ICU* intensive care unit, *VFD* ventilator-free days

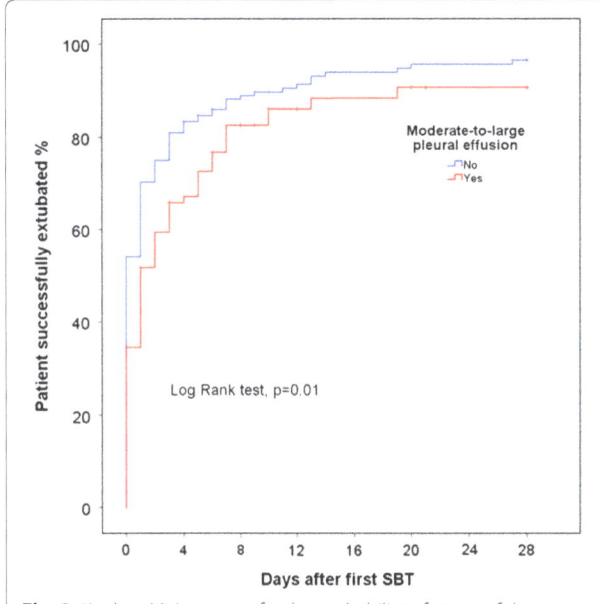

Fig. 2 Kaplan–Meier curves for the probability of successful extubation after the first spontaneous breathing trial in mechanically ventilated patients with (red lines) or without (blue lines) moderate-to-large pleural effusion

our study, most pleural effusions (85%) were associated with condensation or atelectasis.

Clinical implications
There was no significant association between fluid balance and the evolution of pleural effusion during the 48 h following SBT failure. However, the negative fluid balance achieved was modest in the depletive group and this limitation precludes any definite conclusion. Pleural drainage with ultrasonography guidance has a low risk of complication under mechanical ventilator support [7] and may improve oxygenation, respiratory mechanics [4], and diaphragm performance [6, 24]. Removal of pleural fluid may therefore decrease the work of breathing and increase the ability of patients to succeed weaning. Further studies are needed to test whether a strategy of aggressive diuretic management or drainage of pleural effusions, in mechanically ventilated patients entering the weaning process, with others risk factors of weaning failure or a SBT failure, has the potential to decrease its duration [25].

Strengths and limitations
Strengths of our study include the large sample size, the prospective and multicentric design, and the use of ultrasound, which is currently considered the most sensitive method to detect pleural effusion at bedside. Our study has several limitations. First, only 249 of the 477 screened patients were included, a fact that may alter the external validity of our prevalence estimation. Second, the inter- or intra-observer agreement for pleural ultrasonography was not evaluated, but several reports previously demonstrated an excellent agreement for the measurement of left or right maximal interpleural distance [26]. Third, the physicians in charge of the patient were not fully blinded to the ultrasound examination results, and this may have theoretically influenced extubation decision and outcomes. However, criteria for SBT result were defined a priori and independent from ultrasound findings. Fourth, no estimation of respiratory drive (e.g., with airway occlusion pressure) nor respiratory muscle strength (e.g., with maximal inspiratory pressures) was performed. Last, a significant decrease in pleural effusion during difficult weaning may have required more time, and/or more intense depletive fluid management [27].

Conclusion
Moderate-to-large pleural effusion was found in one-third of patients at initiation of weaning and associated with worse outcomes. Depletive strategies did not rapidly alter its evolution. Further studies should test the clinical

Pleural effusion and weaning outcomes
Our study is the first to show an association between moderate-to-large pleural effusion on the one hand and worse weaning outcomes and survival on the other hand. Dres et al. found similar weaning outcomes in patients with or without pleural effusion, but the limited number of patients with pleural effusions in their report ($n = 18$) weakened their conclusions [9]. Our findings are consistent with a previous report by Mattison et al., suggesting an association between pleural effusion and a longer duration of mechanical ventilation [2]. Although pleural effusion in patients with early ARDS do not seem to significantly influence lung physiology and gas exchange [3], its role in the latter stages of mechanical ventilation seems more relevant [4]. Physiological alterations associated with pleural effusion may worsen the respiratory load during the weaning process. Indeed, physiological studies showed that pleural effusion increases chest wall volume and decreases the length of inspiratory muscles and thus their efficiency and power [5, 6]. Umbrello et al. recently showed that during weaning, drainage of a unilateral pleural effusion improves diaphragmatic contractile activity [24]. This improvement could decrease dyspnea and mitigate weaning failure. Pleural fluid accumulation may also result in relaxation atelectasis of the adjacent lung. In

Table 3 Variables associated with weaning failure in 246 mechanically ventilated patients (three patients could not be classified according to the international conference consensus definition)

Variables	Weaning success ($n = 173$)	Weaning failure ($n = 73$)	p value
Male gender	98 (57%)	49 (67%)	0.13
Age (years)	61 [52–73]	69 [60–79]	0.006
Body mass index (kg/m^2)	26 [22–29]	27 [22–32]	0.07
SAPS II at ICU admission	49 [38–62]	49 [39–65]	0.73
Comorbidities			
COPD	23 (13%)	23 (32%)	0.001
Cardiac disease	101 (58%)	55 (75%)	0.01
Main reason for intubation			
Coma	54 (31%)	9 (12%)	0.002
Acute respiratory failure	48 (27%)	39 (53%)	<0.001
Septic shock	24 (14%)	8 (11%)	0.54
Others	47 (27%)	17 (23%)	0.53
From ICU admission to first SBT			
ARDS	28 (16%)	27 (37%)	<0.001
Neuromuscular blockade	26 (15%)	28 (38%)	<0.001
Septic shock	61 (35%)	39 (53%)	0.01
VAP	17 (10%)	16 (22%)	0.01
Supra-ventricular arrhythmias	32 (19%)	22 (30%)	0.04
Duration of MV before first SBT	3 [2–6]	6 [3–12]	<0.001
Dialysis	22 (13%)	8 (11%)	0.70
Fluid balance between ICU admission and first SBT (L)	2.8 [0.9–6.4]	5.7 [0.7–11.4]	0.01
Biological and ultrasound data at first SBT			
PaO$_2$/FiO$_2$ ratio (mmHg)	307 [242–385]	247 [200–299]	<0.001
Moderate-to-large pleural effusion	42 (24%)	37 (51%)	<0.001
Drainable pleural effusion	36 (21%)	29 (40%)	0.002
Large pleural effusion	21 (12%)	25 (34%)	<0.001
Left ventricle ejection fraction (%, $n = 205$)	60 [50–60]	55 [40–60]	0.06
Outcome			
Pleural effusion drainage during weaning	0	4 (6%)	0.01
Prophylactic NIV post-extubation	65 (38%)	30 (44%)	0.35
Tracheotomy	1 (1%)	5 (7%)	0.01
VFD from first SBT to day 28 (days)	23 [20–26]	11 [0–21]	<0.001
Death in ICU	5 (3%)	19 (26%)	<0.001
Death at day 28	8 (5%)	17 (23%)	<0.001

Values are indicating number (%), or median [1st–3rd quartile]

SAPS II simplified acute physiology score, *COPD* chronic obstructive pulmonary disease, *ARDS* acute respiratory distress syndrome, *VAP* ventilator-associated pneumonia, *SBT* spontaneous breathing trial, *NIV* noninvasive ventilation, *ICU* intensive care unit, *VFD* ventilator-free days

usefulness and safety of reducing moderate-to-large pleural effusion at initiation of ventilator weaning, either by aggressive depletion or drainage.

Abbreviations
SBT: spontaneous breathing trial; ARDS: acute respiratory distress syndrome; ICU: intensive care unit.

Authors' contributions
Dr Razazi had full access to all of the data in the study and takes responsibility for the integrity of the data and the accuracy of the data analysis. Dr Razazi, Dr Mekontso Dessap contributed to initial study design, analysis, interpretation of data, drafting of the submitted article, critical revisions for intellectual content. Dr Florence Boissier, Dr Mathilde Neuville, Dr Sébastien Jochmans, Dr Martial Tchir, Dr Faten May, Dr Nicolas de Prost, Dr Christian Brun-Buisson, MD, Dr Guillaume Carteaux contributed to study design and analysis, interpretation of data, drafting of the submitted article, critical revisions for intellectual content. All authors read and approved the final manuscript.

Author details
[1] AP-HP, DHU A-TVB, Service de Réanimation Médicale, Hôpitaux Universitaires Henri Mondor, 94010 Créteil, France. [2] Faculté de Médecine de Créteil, IMRB, GRC CARMAS, Université Paris Est Créteil, 94010 Créteil, France. [3] Unité U955 (Institut Mondor de Recherche Biomédicale), INSERM, Créteil, France.

Table 4 Univariate and multivariable logistic regression of factors associated with weaning failure (n = 246)

Variables	Missing values, n (%)	Absolute standardized differences	Odd ratio (95% confidence interval), p value by logistic regression	
			Univariate	Multivariable
Age (per year)	0	47	1.03 (1.01–1.05), $p = 0.01$	1.02 (0.997–1.05), $p = 0.08$
Body mass index (per kg/m^2)	6 (2%)	32	1.06 (1.01–1.11), $p = 0.02$	I/NR
COPD (yes vs. no)	0	48	3.0 (1.6–5.8), $p = 0.001$	2.2 (1.02–4.7), $p = 0.045$
Cardiac disease (yes vs. no)	0	37	2.2 (1.2–4.0), $p = 0.01$	I/NR
Left ventricle ejection fraction at cardiac ultrasound (%)	44 (18%)	27	0.98 (0.96–1.0), $p = 0.09$	NI
Supra-ventricular arrhythmias (yes vs. no)	0	26	1.9 (1.01–3.6), $p = 0.046$	NI
Septic shock (yes vs. no)	0	37	2.1 (1.2–3.7), $p = 0.01$	I/NR
Fluid balance between ICU admission and first SBT (per L)	15 (6%)	44	1.07 (1.03–1.12), $p = 0.002$	NI
Acute respiratory failure as cause of intubation (yes vs. no)	0	55	3.0 (1.7–5.2), $p < 0.001$	NI
PaO$_2$/FiO$_2$ ratio (per mmHg)	3 (1%)	58	0.994 (0.991–0.997), $p < 0.001$	0.996 (0.993–1.0), $p = 0.03$
Duration of MV before the first SBT (per day)	0	57	1.11 (1.06–1.17), $p < 0.001$	1.11 (1.05–1.17), $p < 0.001$
ARDS before the first SBT (yes vs. no)	0	49	3.0 (1.6–5.7), $p < 0.001$	NI
Neuromuscular blockade before the first SBT (yes vs. no)	0	54	3.5 (1.9–6.6), $p < 0.001$	NI
VAP before the first SBT (yes vs. no)	0	33	2.6 (1.2–5.4), $p = 0.01$	NI
Moderate-to-large pleural effusion (yes vs. no)	0	58	3.2 (1.8–5.7), $p < 0.001$	3.0 (1.5–5.8), $p = 0.001$

SAPS II simplified acute physiology score, *COPD* chronic obstructive pulmonary disease, *ARDS* acute respiratory distress syndrome, *VAP* ventilator-associated pneumonia, *SBT* spontaneous breathing trial, *NI* not included, *I/NR* included, but not retained by the final model

Among related univariate factors, only the most statistically robust (yet clinically relevant) was entered into the regression model in order to minimize the effect of colinearity. The selection process was guided by consistency (less than 5% missing values) and maximal imbalances between groups (as estimated by absolute standardized differences), as follows: cardiac disease was selected among supra-ventricular arrhythmias, left ventricle ejection fraction and cardiac disease; septic shock was selected among fluid balance between ICU admission and first SBT and septic shock; PaO$_2$/FiO$_2$ ratio was selected among acute respiratory failure as cause of intubation and PaO$_2$/FiO$_2$ ratio; duration of MV before the first SBT was selected among neuromuscular blockade, duration of MV before the first SBT, VAP, and ARDS. The multivariable model showed a good calibration as assessed by the Hosmer and Lemeshow goodness-of-fit test [χ^2 (8 df) = 6.8, $p = 0.56$] and a fair discrimination as assessed by the receiver operating characteristics curve [area under the curve of 0.76 (0.69–0.82), $p < 0.001$]

[4] Service de Réanimation Médicale, Centre Hospitalier Universitaire de Poitiers, Poitiers 86021, France. [5] AP-HP, Service de Réanimation Médicale, Hôpital Européen Georges Pompidou, 75015 Paris, France. [6] AP-HP, Réanimation Médicale et des Maladies Infectieuses, Hôpital Bichat Claude Bernard, Paris, France. [7] Département de Médecine Intensive, Groupe Hospitalier Sud Ile-de-France, Hôpital de Melun, 77011 Melun, France. [8] Service de Réanimation, Centre Hospitalier de Villeneuve-Saint-Georges, 94190 Villeneuve-Saint-Georges, France.

Acknowledgements
This study was carried out as part of our routine clinical work.

Competing interests
The authors declare that they have no competing interests.

Funding
None.

References
1. Fartoukh M, Azoulay E, Galliot R, Le Gall J-R, Baud F, Chevret S, et al. Clinically documented pleural effusions in medical ICU patients: how useful is routine thoracentesis? Chest. 2002;121:178–84.
2. Mattison LE, Coppage L, Alderman DF, Herlong JO, Sahn SA. Pleural effusions in the medical ICU: prevalence, causes, and clinical implications. Chest. 1997;111:1018–23.
3. Chiumello D, Marino A, Cressoni M, Mietto C, Berto V, Gallazzi E, et al. Pleural effusion in patients with acute lung injury: a CT scan study. Crit Care Med. 2013;41:935–44.
4. Razazi K, Thille AW, Carteaux G, Beji O, Brun-Buisson C, Brochard L, et al. Effects of pleural effusion drainage on oxygenation, respiratory mechanics, and hemodynamics in mechanically ventilated patients. Ann Am Thorac Soc. 2014;11:1018–24.
5. De Troyer A, Leduc D, Cappello M, Gevenois PA. Mechanics of the canine diaphragm in pleural effusion. J Appl Physiol Bethesda Md. 1985;2012(113):785–90.
6. Estenne M, Yernault JC, De Troyer A. Mechanism of relief of dyspnea after thoracocentesis in patients with large pleural effusions. Am J Med. 1983;74:813–9.
7. Goligher EC, Leis JA, Fowler RA, Pinto R, Adhikari NKJ, Ferguson ND. Utility and safety of draining pleural effusions in mechanically ventilated patients: a systematic review and meta-analysis. Crit Care Lond Engl. 2011;15:R46.
8. Esteban A, Alía I, Ibañez J, Benito S, Tobin MJ. Modes of mechanical ventilation and weaning. A national survey of Spanish hospitals. The Spanish lung failure collaborative group. Chest. 1994;106:1188–93.
9. Dres M, Roux D, Pham T, Beurton A, Ricard J-D, Fartoukh M, et al. Prevalence and impact on weaning of pleural effusion at the time of liberation from mechanical ventilation: a multicenter prospective observational study. Anesthesiology. 2017;126:1107–15.
10. Boles J-M, Bion J, Connors A, Herridge M, Marsh B, Melot C, et al. Weaning from mechanical ventilation. Eur Respir J. 2007;29:1033–56.
11. Girault C, Bubenheim M, Abroug F, Diehl JL, Elatrous S, Beuret P, et al. Noninvasive ventilation and weaning in patients with chronic hypercapnic respiratory failure: a randomized multicenter trial. Am J Respir Crit Care Med. 2011;184:672–9.
12. Thille AW, Boissier F, Ben-Ghezala H, Razazi K, Mekontso-Dessap A, Brun-Buisson C, et al. Easily identified at-risk patients for extubation failure may

benefit from noninvasive ventilation: a prospective before-after study. Crit Care Lond Engl. 2016;20:48.

13. Béduneau G, Pham T, Schortgen F, Piquilloud L, Zogheib E, Jonas M, et al. Epidemiology of Weaning Outcome according to a New Definition. The WIND Study. Am J Respir Crit Care Med. 2017;195:772–83.

14. Mekontso Dessap A, Roche-Campo F, Kouatchet A, Tomicic V, Beduneau G, Sonneville R, et al. Natriuretic peptide-driven fluid management during ventilator weaning: a randomized controlled trial. Am J Respir Crit Care Med. 2012;186:1256–63.

15. Yang PC, Luh KT, Chang DB, Wu HD, Yu CJ, Kuo SH. Value of sonography in determining the nature of pleural effusion: analysis of 320 cases. AJR Am J Roentgenol. 1992;159:29–33.

16. Volpicelli G, Elbarbary M, Blaivas M, Lichtenstein DA, Mathis G, Kirkpatrick AW, et al. International evidence-based recommendations for point-of-care lung ultrasound. Intensive Care Med. 2012;38:577–91.

17. Balik M, Plasil P, Waldauf P, Pazout J, Fric M, Otahal M, et al. Ultrasound estimation of volume of pleural fluid in mechanically ventilated patients. Intensive Care Med. 2006;32:318–21.

18. Lichtenstein D, Hulot JS, Rabiller A, Tostivint I, Mezière G. Feasibility and safety of ultrasound-aided thoracentesis in mechanically ventilated patients. Intensive Care Med. 1999;25:955–8.

19. Austin PC. Balance diagnostics for comparing the distribution of baseline covariates between treatment groups in propensity-score matched samples. Stat Med. 2009;28:3083–107.

20. Havelock T, Teoh R, Laws D, Gleeson F, BTS Pleural Disease Guideline Group. Pleural procedures and thoracic ultrasound: British Thoracic Society Pleural Disease Guideline 2010. Thorax. 2010;65(Suppl 2):ii61–76.

21. Walker SP, Morley AJ, Stadon L, De Fonseka D, Arnold DA, Medford AR, et al. Non-malignant pleural effusions (NMPE): a prospective study of 356 consecutive unselected patients. Chest. 2017;151(5):1099–105.

22. Mccabe WR, Jackson G. Gram-negative bacteremia: I. etiology and ecology. Arch Intern Med. 1962;110:847–55.

23. Light RW. Clinical practice. Pleural effusion. N Engl J Med. 2002;346:1971–7.

24. Umbrello M, Mistraletti G, Galimberti A, Piva IR, Cozzi O, Formenti P. Drainage of pleural effusion improves diaphragmatic function in mechanically ventilated patients. Crit Care Resusc J Australas Acad Crit Care Med. 2017;19:64–70.

25. Mayo P, Volpicelli G, Lerolle N, Schreiber A, Doelken P, Vieillard-Baron A. Ultrasonography evaluation during the weaning process: the heart, the diaphragm, the pleura and the lung. Intensive Care Med. 2016;42:1107–17.

26. Begot E, Grumann A, Duvoid T, Dalmay F, Pichon N, François B, et al. Ultrasonographic identification and semiquantitative assessment of unloculated pleural effusions in critically ill patients by residents after a focused training. Intensive Care Med. 2014;40:1475–80.

27. Giglioli C, Spini V, Landi D, Chiostri M, Romano SM, Calabretta R, et al. Congestive heart failure and decongestion ability of two different treatments: continuous renal replacement and diuretic therapy: experience of a cardiac step down unit. Acta Cardiol. 2013;68:355–64.

18

Driving pressure and long-term outcomes in moderate/severe acute respiratory distress syndrome

Carlos Toufen Junior[1]*📷, Roberta R. De Santis Santiago[1], Adriana S. Hirota[1], Alysson Roncally S. Carvalho[2,3], Susimeire Gomes[1], Marcelo Brito Passos Amato[4] and Carlos Roberto Ribeiro Carvalho[1]

Abstract

Background: Acute respiratory distress syndrome (ARDS) patients may present impaired in lung function and structure after hospital discharge that may be related to mechanical ventilation strategy. The aim of this study was to evaluate the association between functional and structural lung impairment, N-terminal-peptide type III procollagen (NT-PCP-III) and driving pressure during protective mechanical ventilation. It was a secondary analysis of data from randomized controlled trial that included patients with moderate/severe ARDS with at least one follow-up visit performed. We obtained serial measurements of plasma NT-PCP-III levels. Whole-lung computed tomography analysis and pulmonary function test were performed at 1 and 6 months of follow-up. A health-related quality of life survey after 6 months was also performed.

Results: Thirty-three patients were enrolled, and 21 patients survived after 6 months. In extubation day an association between driving pressure and NT-PCP-III was observed. At 1 and 6 months forced vital capacity (FVC) was negatively correlated to driving pressure ($p < 0.01$). At 6 months driving pressure was associated with lower FVC independently on tidal volume, plateau pressure and baseline static respiratory compliance after adjustments ($r^2 = 0.51$, $p = 0.02$). There was a significant correlation between driving pressure and lung densities and nonaerated/poorly aerated lung volume after 6 months. Driving pressure was also related to general health domain of SF-36 at 6 months.

Conclusion: Even in patients ventilated with protective tidal volume, higher driving pressure is associated with worse long-term pulmonary function and structure.

Background

Acute respiratory distress syndrome (ARDS) is a rapidly progressive illness associated with high mortality and morbidity [1–3]. Up to 5 years after discharge from the intensive care unit (ICU), ARDS survivors still present persistent disabilities, including muscle weakness, altered lung function (e.g., decreased lung volumes, or decreased lung diffusion capacity) and an impaired mental health and cognition [4].

About 25% of ARDS survivors present some reduction in the forced vital capacity (FVC) and in diffusion capacity 6 months after discharge [5]. Among ARDS survivors, abnormal findings in chest tomography correlate with restrictive lung changes and poorer health-related quality of life (HRQoL), suggesting that pulmonary dysfunction could be associated with limited activity in these patients [6].

The risk factors for a reduced long-term lung function in ARDS patients are unknown. As protective mechanical ventilation is an important intervention to reduce mortality of ARDS, probably by decreasing lung inflammation, we hypothesized that the parameters used during the ventilation strategy could be related to long-term lung fibrosis, impairing the lung function among ARDS survivors.

*Correspondence: toufenjr@usp.br
[1] Divisão de Pneumologia, Cardiopulmonary Department, Heart Institute (InCor) University of São Paulo, INCOR Av. Dr. Enéas de Carvalho Aguiar, 44 Pinheiros, São Paulo, SP CEP 05403-900, Brazil
Full list of author information is available at the end of the article

During a recent ARDS trial [7] comparing two strategies of protective mechanical ventilation, we collected lung function data for survivors, during the first 6 months after ARDS onset. We decided to explore the relationship between ventilator settings and long-term outcomes for the entire cohort. Supporting this analysis, we also assessed the acute production of N-terminal-peptide type III procollagen (NT-PCP-III), from enrollment till weaning, as well as other long-term outcomes such as quantitative computed tomography (which enabled us to estimate excess tissue reorganization), 6-min walk test (6MWT) and quality of life (QoL).

Methods

Study design

We conducted a prospective longitudinal cohort study of 22 survivors of moderate/severe ARDS, recruited from six different ICUs located in Hospital das Clínicas, São Paulo, Brazil, from November 2008 to January 2012.

Patient selection

Patients were enrolled in this study in conjunction with a clinical trial in mechanical ventilation, the "ARDSnet Protocol versus Open Lung Approach in ARDS" trial (NCT 00431158) [7]. The institutional review committee approved the study that included the follow-up, and informed consent was obtained from each patient or legal representative. Briefly, this was a randomized controlled trial in which patients were ventilated with a ARDSnet protocol, which uses low tidal volumes, relatively high respiratory rates, with oxygenation managed according to PEEP and FIO2 relationships as defined in a table, or with an open lung approach strategy, which uses a technique to recruit collapsed lung areas and then uses the lowest PEEP level that prevents recollapse of recruited lung units, being the best PEEP level determined by a decremental PEEP trial involving a series of pressure measurements taken after the recruitment maneuver. Both the ARDSnet protocol and the open lung approach require low tidal volumes and plateau pressures. In conclusion, open lung approach improved oxygenation and driving pressure, without detrimental effects on mortality, ventilator-free days or barotrauma.

The inclusion criteria for the study were as follows: Patients intubated and mechanically ventilated, with diagnosis of ARDS using American–European Consensus Criteria and enrollment in study < 48 h since diagnosis of ARDS. For 12–36 h (ideally 12–24 h), after diagnosis of ARDS, patient must be ventilated as follows: volume A/C, tidal volume of 4–8 mL/kg PBW, plateau pressure ≤ 30 cmH$_2$O, PEEP/FIO$_2$ adjustments using ARDSnet table, and ventilator rate to keep PaCO$_2 = 35$–60 mmHg. During the 12–36-h (ideally

12–24-h) period, PaO$_2$/FIO$_2$ must remain < 200 mm Hg for an ABG obtained 30 min after placement on the following specific ventilator settings: volume A/C, tidal volume = 6 mL/kg PBW, plateau pressure ≤ 30 cmH$_2$O, inspiratory time ≤ 1 s, PEEP ≥ 10 cmH$_2$O, FIO$_2 \geq 0.5$, ventilator rate to keep PaCO$_2 = 35$–60 mmHg. No lung recruitment maneuvers or adjunct therapy. Total time on mechanical ventilation < 96 h at time of randomization.

Patients were excluded if they presented one of the following criteria: age < 18 years or > 80 years, weight < 35 kg PBW, body mass index > 60, intubated 2° to acute exacerbation of a chronic pulmonary disease, acute brain injury (ICP > 18 mmHg), immunosuppression 2° to chemo- or radiation therapy, severe cardiac disease (one of the following): New York Heart Association Class 3 or 4, acute coronary syndrome or persistent ventricular tachyarrhythmias, positive laboratory pregnancy test, sickle cell disease, neuromuscular disease, high risk of mortality within 3 months from cause other than ARDS, e.g., cancer, more than 2 organ failures (not including pulmonary system), documented lung barotrauma, i.e., chest tube placement other than for fluid drainage, persistent hemodynamic instability or intractable shock, penetrating chest trauma, enrollment in another interventional study. Randomization in the pivotal study was stratified by center, age and APACHE II scores.

Measurements

Baseline data collected at enrollment included age, sex, height, severity of illness measured by the Acute Physiology and Chronic Health Evaluation (APACHE) II score, ratio between arterial oxygen tension and fraction of inspired oxygen (PaO$_2$/F$_1$O$_2$) with a positive end-expiratory pressure (PEEP) of at least 10 cmH$_2$O and FIO$_2 \geq 0.5$, and static compliance (respiratory system) 30 min before protocol enrollment. Twenty-four hours after patient enrollment, we collected respiratory variables, including tidal volume (mL/kg of predicted body weight), PEEP and plateau pressure. Airway driving pressure was defined as plateau pressure minus total PEEP. To measure the plateau pressure we used neuromuscular blocking agents and volume-controlled ventilation.

Blood samples were obtained on the day of randomization (day 0) and on days 1, 3, 7, and the day of extubation. Blood samples were centrifuged, and plasma was stored at 70 C. NT-PCP-III was assayed by a sandwich ELISA method according to the methodology specifications of the manufacturer (Elabscience, Texas, USA). The normal range of serum levels of nonsmoking individuals was determined to be 1.6–4.0 ng/L.

Pulmonary function testing (PFT) was performed at 1 and 6 months after the onset of ARDS using the Med-Graphics Cardiorespiratory Diagnostic System (Medical

Graphics Corporation, USA). All tests were done according to Brazilian guidelines [8]. Reference ranges were calculated based on statistics formulated from the Brazilian population [9–11].

High-resolution computed tomography (HRCT) scan of the lungs was also performed 1 and 6 months after the onset of ARDS in supine position during inspiration, close to total lung capacity. All CT scans were segmented by applying the region growing algorithm to select the lung parenchyma using OsiriX (OsiriX 64-bits, Pixmeo Sarl, Geneva, Switzerland). After the segmentation, the original images (DICOM files) as well as each respective ROI were exported and analyzed with a purpose-built routine (QALI-DV software) written in MATLAB (MathWorks, USA). Manual correction was applied to the segmented images containing peripheral atelectasis. Total lung volume (TLV), total air volume (TAV) and total lung mass (TLM) were extracted from the segmented whole lung in 3D [11, 12]. The percentages of hyperaerated (-1000 to -900 HU), normally aerated (-900 to -500 HU), poorly aerated (-500 to -100 HU) and nonaerated (-100 to $+100$ HU) compartments of the lung parenchyma were calculated [12, 13]. To assess the occurrence and progression of emphysema in this longitudinal study we used the percentile point [14–17] using a threshold of 15% (P15). The sensitivity of the percentile point method has been shown to be similar within a broad range of percentiles from the 10th to the 30th [14].

Six months after ARDS onset, we also performed a standardized 6MWT [18] and fulfilled the Medical Outcomes Study 36-item Short-Form General Health Survey (SF-36), which measures the HRQoL [19]. The SF-36 includes eight multiple-item scales that assess physical functioning, social functioning, physical role, emotional role, mental health, pain, vitality and general health. Scores for each aspect can range from 0 (worst) to 100 (best).

Statistical analysis

Categorical values are described as frequency and percentages, and continuous variables as the mean and SD, or median and interquartile range. The Fisher exact test was used to compare independent categorical variables. Continuous variables were compared with the Student t test or the Mann–Whitney test for dependent or independent data. The Friedman test was used for one-way repeated-measures analysis. The strength of the association between two variables was measured using correlation coefficient (r). We used Pearson correlation to parametric variable and Spearman correlation to nonparametric variable. We used linear regression to get r^2 in parametric variable. In order to determine clinical variables independently associated with lung function,

we performed a multivariable linear regression. For NT-PCP-III regression we used log10 transformations as is commonly performed for biomarkers with a right-tailed distribution. Statistical significance was set at a two-tailed p value of ≤ 0.05, and analyses were performed with R, version 3.0.2 (http://www.r-project.org).

Results

Characteristics of the population

Over the 58-month (2007–2012) recruitment period, we enrolled 33 patients. The patients in cohort were predominantly male. Mortality at 28th day was 33% (Fig. 1).

Of those enrolled, we lost the follow-up of 5 patients at month-1 and 2 between month-1 and month-6. Reasons for exclusion are outlined in Fig. 1. There was no difference in terms of severity score, age and static compliance measurement between patients followed up at month-6 and patients that were lost.

The descriptive baseline and hospital data for all randomized patients and for survivors are described in Table 1. Monitored variables during mechanical ventilation at baseline and 24 h after randomization are also shown in Table 1. Driving pressure at 24 h was related to driving pressure at 48 h ($r=0.58$, $P=0.006$) and 72 h ($r=0.56$, $P=0.009$) after randomization.

Pulmonary function tests analysis

Pulmonary function tests showed a mildly reduced FVC and a moderately reduced DL_{CO} after 6 months (Table 2). The FVC was below normal ($< 80\%$ of predicted) in eleven (65%) patients at month-1, and in five (33%) patients at month-6. Twelve patients (70%) showed a reduced DL_{CO} at month-1, whereas four (29%) patients showed a reduced DL_{CO} after 6 months of follow-up (Table 2).

Driving pressure was the only ventilation variable significantly correlated with FVC at 1- ($r=0.65$) and 6-month ($r=0.67$) follow-up (Fig. 2). Driving pressure ($r=0.51$) and APACHE II ($r=0.59$) were correlated with DL_{CO} at month-1. Of note, tidal volume and respiratory system compliance were very weakly correlated with pulmonary function tests.

After testing for the confounding effects of tidal volumes, plateau pressures and baseline static respiratory compliance ($R^2=0.51$, $F(4,10)=4.66$, $p=0.022$), the association between driving pressures and FVC at month-6 remained the only statistically significant one ($\beta=-4.62$, IC95% (-7.11 to -2.13), $P=0.002$).

When comparing the effects of the randomized treatments (OLA vs. ARDSnet) on FVC at month-6, there was a marginal difference between arms, with FVC of 4.54 ± 0.93 L versus 3.41 ± 1.04 L (OLA vs. ARDSnet, respectively, $P=0.06$), representing $96\pm20\%$ versus $86\pm15\%$ of predicted, respectively ($P=0.32$).

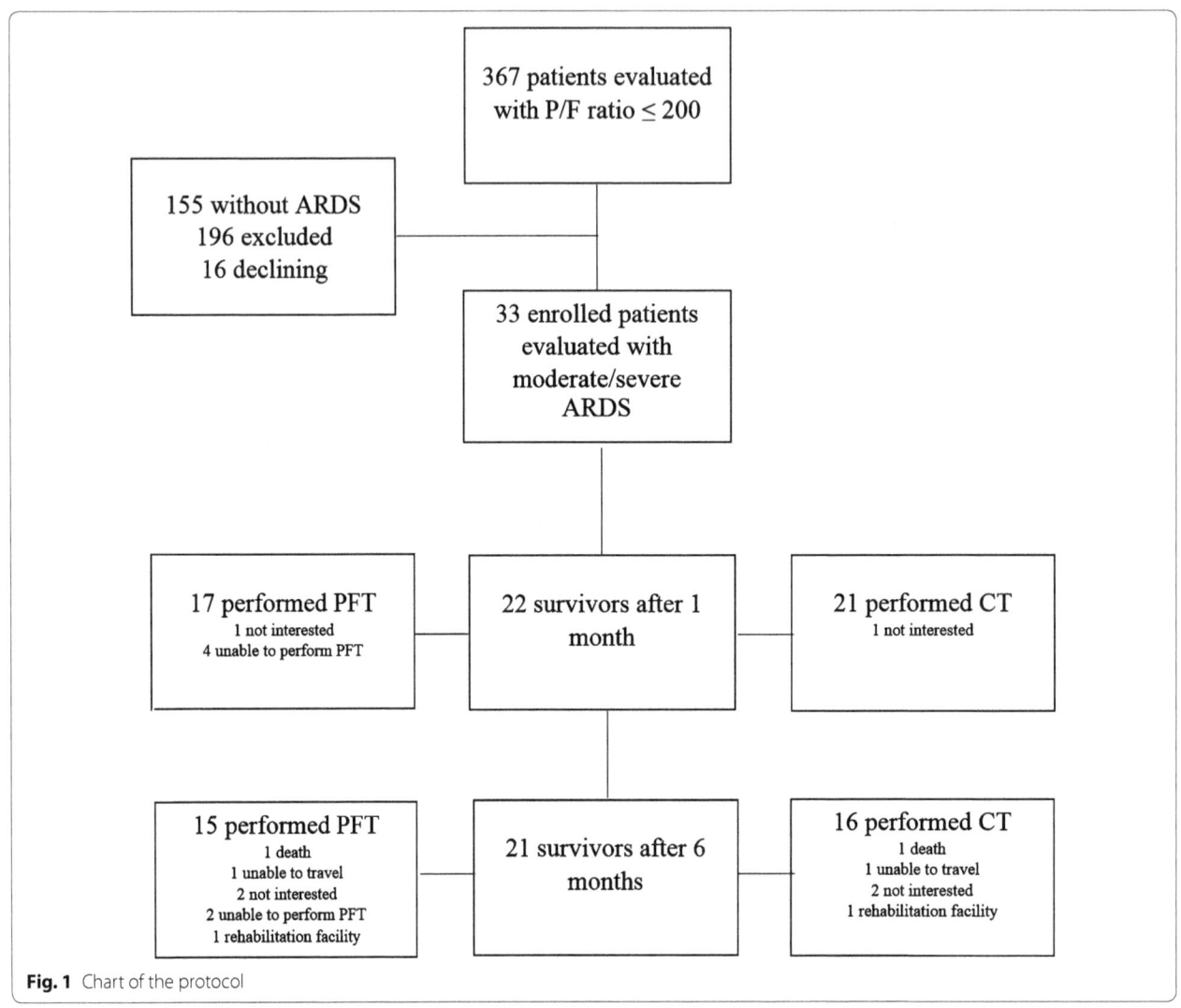

Fig. 1 Chart of the protocol

CT scan analysis

Twenty-one patients were performed a HRCT at month-1 of follow-up. The median and interquartile range of the total lung volume (TLV) was 3.54 L (2.29–4.37); the total lung weight (TLW) was 1194 g (861–1873), and the mean pulmonary density (MPD) was 451 g/L (243–610). The P_{15} (percentile 15% for lowest lung densities) was 72 g/L (42–117).

At month-6, 16 patients were performed a HRCT. The median and interquartile range of TLV increased ($P=0.01$) to 4.99 L (3.73–6.20), the TLW decreased ($P=0.01$) to 762 g (652–934 g), the MPD decreased ($P<0.001$) to 164 g/L (133–183), and P_{15} decreased ($P=0.02$) to 49 g/L (23–65). Those longitudinal reductions in MPD, TLM and percent of nonaerated/poorly

aerated lung volumes were all significant, as well as the increase in TLV.

Lung image parameters were significantly correlated with driving pressure and pulmonary function. After 6 months, individual MPD was significantly correlated with individual driving pressure ($r=0.53$, $P=0.03$), but not with respiratory system compliance ($P=0.95$). Consistently, FVC at month-6 strongly correlated with CT parameters: MPD ($r=-0.86$, $P=0.00005$), % of nonaerated/poorly aerated volume ($r=-0.70$, $P=0.003$), TLV ($r=0.65$, $P=0.008$) and air/tissue volume ratio ($r=0.70$, $P=0.003$).

Dividing patients based on median into high (HDP) or low (LDP) driving pressure groups (≥ 13 and <13 cmH$_2$O, respectively), MDP was higher in HDP group ($P=0.04$; Fig. 3).

Table 1 Demographic characteristics and mechanical ventilation variables from randomized and surviving ARDS patients

Characteristics	Randomized patients (N = 33)	Surviving patients (N = 22)	Nonsurviving patients (n = 11)	P value
Age, year	49 ± 14.9	48.5 ± 13.9	50 ± 16.7	0.80
Sex, % male	22 (66.7)	15 (68)	7 (46.7)	1.00
Smokers (%)	10 (30)	7 (28)	3 (27)	1.00
Origin of ARDS				
Primary N, %	23 (70)	17 (77)	6 (55)	0.24
Secondary N, %	10 (30)	5 (23)	5 (45)	
Baseline data				
APACHE II	19.6 ± 10.5	17.1 ± 5.3	24.5 ± 16.0	0.16
P/F ratio	129 ± 32	135 ± 34	118 ± 23	0.09
Tidal volume, mL/kg PBW	5.9 (5.7–6.0)	5.9 (5.5–6.0)	5.9 (5.9–6.4)	0.78
Driving pressure, cmH$_2$O	13.5 ± 4	13.2 ± 3.9	14.1 ± 4.3	0.58
Plateau pressure, cmH$_2$O	25.4 ± 3.8	25.3 ± 4.2	25.6 ± 3.3	1.00
PEEP, cmH$_2$O	10 (10–14)	10 (10–14)	10 (10–13)	0.69
C_{stat}, mL/cmH$_2$O/kg PBW	0.48 ± 0.15	0.47 ± 0.15	0.50 ± 0.16	0.69
Data 24 h after inclusion				
OLA arm patients, %	18 (54%)	11(50%)	7 (63%)	0.71
P/F ratio	173 ± 62	174 ± 57	170 ± 70	0.96
Tidal volume, mL/PBW	5.3 ± 1.1	5.5 ± 0.9	4.9 ± 1.4	0.20
Driving pressure, cmH$_2$O	11 (10–14)	11 (10–14)	12 (10–12.5)	0.92
Plateau pressure, cmH$_2$O	28 (26–30)	27.5 (26.2–30)	30 (24.5–31)	0.48
PEEP, cmH$_2$O	15.4 ± 5.1	15.3 ± 4.9	15.5 ± 5.5	0.93
C_{stat}, mL/cmH$_2$O/kg PBW	0.44 (0.40–0.53)	0.45 (0.41–0.54)	0.43 (0.37–0.47)	0.19
Days of ventilator use	9 (6.5–13.5)	9 (6.2–11.7)	12 (10–14.5)	0.14
ICU length of stay, days	16 (11.7–24)	18.5 (12–24.7)	15 (12.5–17)	0.26
Hosp. length of stay, days	27.5 (16.7–56.7)	34 (20.7–73.5)	21 (15–25)	0.02

Parametric data are presented as mean ± 1 standard deviation or median (first and third quartiles)

P/F ratio PaO$_2$/FIO$_2$ ratio, PBW predicted body weight and C_{stat} static compliance

Table 2 Lung function during the follow-up

	1 Month (N = 17)	6 Months (N = 15)
FVC (L)	3.34 ± 0.77	3.78 ± 1.11
FVC (% predicted)	80 ± 16	89 ± 17
FEV1/FVC ratio	0.81 ± 0.05	0.78 ± 0.06
FEV1/FVC ratio (% predicted)	99 ± 5	97 ± 8
TLC (L)	4.96 ± 1.18	5.57 ± 1.36
TLC (% of predicted)	82 ± 17	89 ± 18
RV (L)	1.71 ± 0.55	1.75 ± 0.49
RV (% predicted)	98 ± 27	97 ± 21
DLco	17.8 ± 6.1	24.0 ± 8.1
DLco (% predicted)	55 ± 17	71 ± 17

All data are presented as mean ± 1 standard deviation

FVC forced vital capacity, FEV1 forced expiratory volume in 1 s, TLC total lung capacity, RV residual volume and DLco diffusing capacity of the lung for carbon monoxide

When comparing the effects of the randomized treatments (OLA vs. ARDSnet) on MPD at month-6, there was no difference, with MPD of 175 (131–176) g/L versus 171 (138–195) g/L (OLA vs. ARDSnet, respectively, $P=0.92$). There was no difference in terms of TLV ($P=0.38$) and TLW ($P=0.35$).

NT-PCP-III

From the 28 patients, 106 blood specimens were available for analysis of NT-PCP-III levels. All plasma samples had elevated levels, considering normal values, and considering the samples collected after 24 h from inclusion, after 3 days, and after 7 days or weaning time, the level increased over time ($P=0.03$).

Individual increments in log$_{10}$NT-PCP-III levels, from baseline till extubation, correlated with individual values of driving pressures at 24 h ($\beta=0.006$, IC95% (0.001–0.011), $r^2=0.35$, $F(1,13)=8.55$, $p=0.011$; Fig. 4): the higher the driving pressure, the higher the increment in log$_{10}$NT-PCP-III difference.

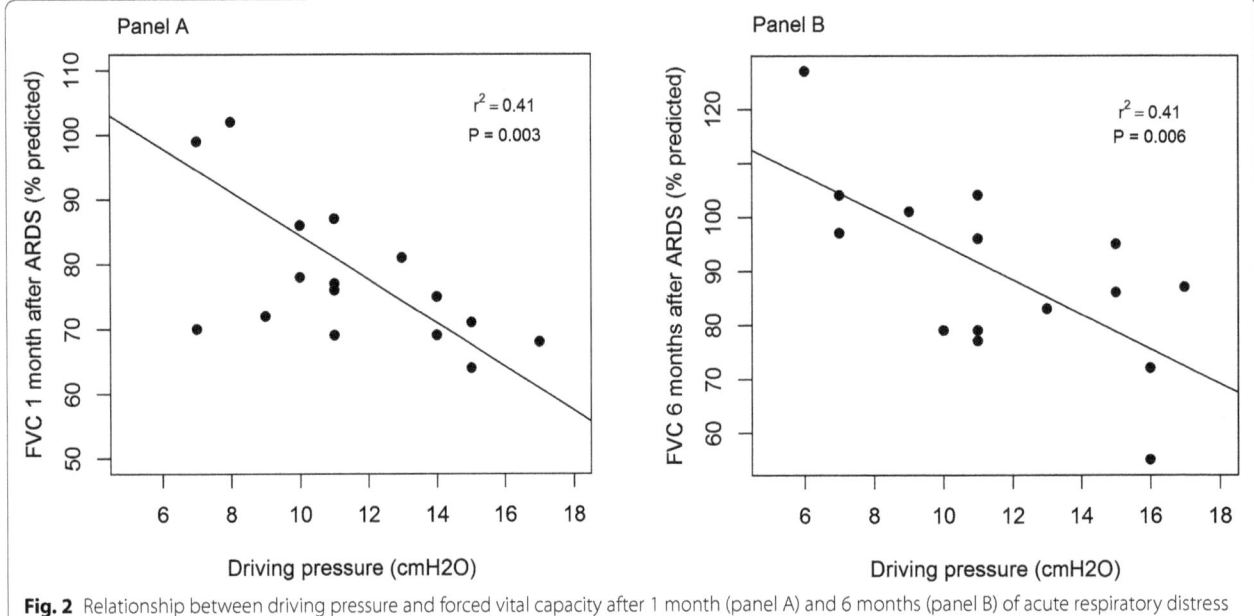

Fig. 2 Relationship between driving pressure and forced vital capacity after 1 month (panel A) and 6 months (panel B) of acute respiratory distress syndrome

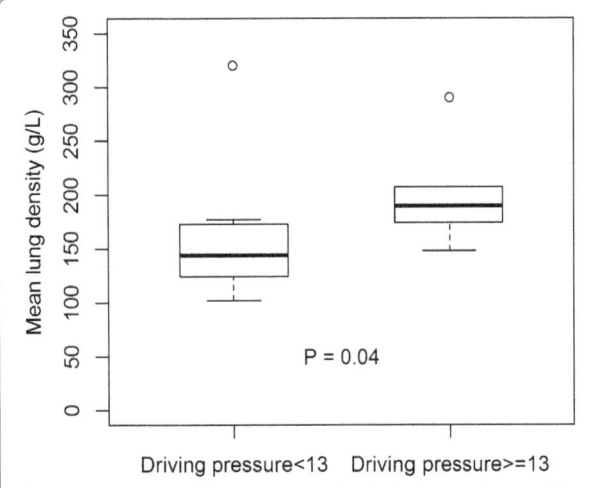

Fig. 3 Mean pulmonary parenchyma density in the whole-lung CT scan in 17 ARDS patients after 6 months of follow-up split based on driving pressure median

Mean pulmonary density (MPD) at month-6 was related to $\log_{10}$NT-PCP-III level during the first week of mechanical ventilation: at day 0 ($\beta = 0.005$, IC95% (0.001–0.010), $r^2 = 0.35$, $F(1,12) = 8.06$, $p = 0.014$), day 1 ($\beta = 0.006$, IC95% (0.002–0.010), $r^2 = 0.34$, $F(1,14) = 8.84$, $p = 0.010$), day 3 ($\beta = 0.005$, IC95% (0.0003–0.009), $r^2 = 0.25$, $F(1,12) = 5.38$, $p = 0.038$).

Dividing patients into high (HDP) or low (LDP) driving pressure groups (≥ 13 and < 13 cmH$_2$O, respectively), LDP group did not change levels over time ($P = 0.15$), while HDP group increased ($P = 0.03$; Fig. 5).

When comparing the effects of the randomized treatments (OLA vs. ARDSnet) on $\log_{10}$NT-PCP-III, there was no statistic significant difference at day 0 ($P = 0.89$), day 1 ($P = 0.55$), day 3 ($P = 0.19$) and on extubation ($P = 0.65$). There was a difference in terms of $\log_{10}$NT-PCP-III at day 7 (median $\log_{10}$NT-PCP-III 1.69 in OLA arm vs. 1.99 in ARDSnet, $P = 0.03$). There was no difference in the change between day 0 to day 1 ($p = 0.69$), to day 3 ($p = 0.23$), to day 7 ($p = 0.31$) and to extubation ($p = 0.18$).

Other tests' analysis

A standardized 6MWT was performed in 11 patients, but we could not observe any relationship between the walked distance and the ventilation variables selected. In terms of HRQoL, 10 patients completed SF-36 survey and we found a correlation between driving pressure (24 h after randomization) and the general health domain ($r = -0.69$, $p = 0.02$).

Discussion

In a population of patients surviving an episode of moderate to severe ARDS, there was a negative correlation between airway driving pressures, measured during the first 24 h of mechanical ventilation, and forced vital capacity (FVC) measured after 6 months of ARDS onset. This early measurement of driving pressure was representative of the applied strategy of protective ventilation, adjusted right after randomization and persisting at similar levels during the following days [20], and did not correlate with baseline compliance of the respiratory system.

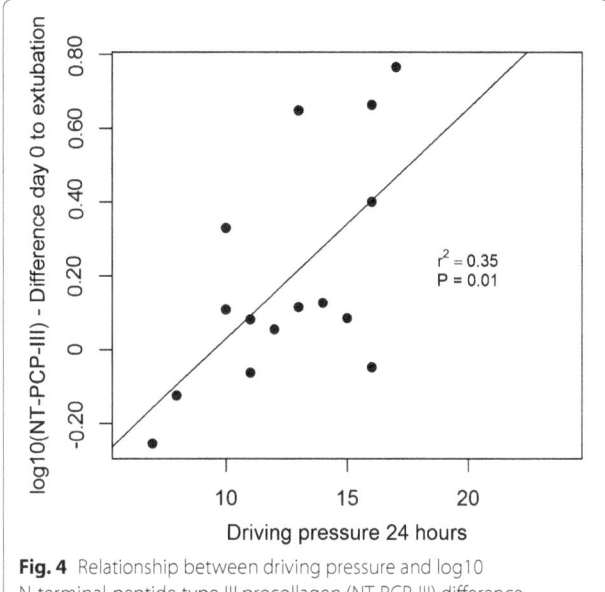

Fig. 4 Relationship between driving pressure and log10 N-terminal-peptide type III procollagen (NT-PCP-III) difference between extubation day and day 0 of acute respiratory distress syndrome

Also, we did not observe any relationship between tidal volumes (expressed in mL/PBW) and long-term pulmonary function tests.

Several studies involving ARDS survivors have shown a significant reduction in long-term lung function in a substantial proportion of patients, with a quarter of the patients presenting a FVC lower than 70% of predicted

[5, 21]. In this subgroup of patients, the reduction in FVC was correlated with higher CT scores, but not with higher weakness score (acquired ICU weakness score), suggesting that the reduction in pulmonary function was related to lung fibrosis [6]. In fact, we observed an association between driving pressure and NT-PCP-III, a marker of fibrogenesis, paralleled by increased mean densities of the parenchyma, especially in those patients ventilated with higher driving pressure (Fig. 3). In those long-term studies, the changes in HRCT and in pulmonary function tests were both related to a poorer QoL [22]. In our study, the QoL could be further related to the level of driving pressures applied during mechanical ventilation.

Some investigators had previously correlated the total duration of mechanical ventilation and the levels of plateau pressure with the long-term results of pulmonary function tests and high-resolution CT studies, suggesting a relationship between mechanical ventilation and pulmonary dysfunction [6, 23]. This is the first time, however, that driving pressure was evaluated as a risk factor for long-term outcomes in survivors, and especially so after the general adoption of protective ventilation. In recent studies, driving pressures have been correlated with ARDS mortality, independently of tidal volume, PEEP and severity of illness, suggesting a causal role in the process of ventilator lung injury [24]. Commonly—as in this study—driving pressures and tidal volumes were weakly correlated, because lung compliance and ventilation strategies vary widely among patients [20]. Thus, we showed, similarly to the study of Amato et al. [20], that

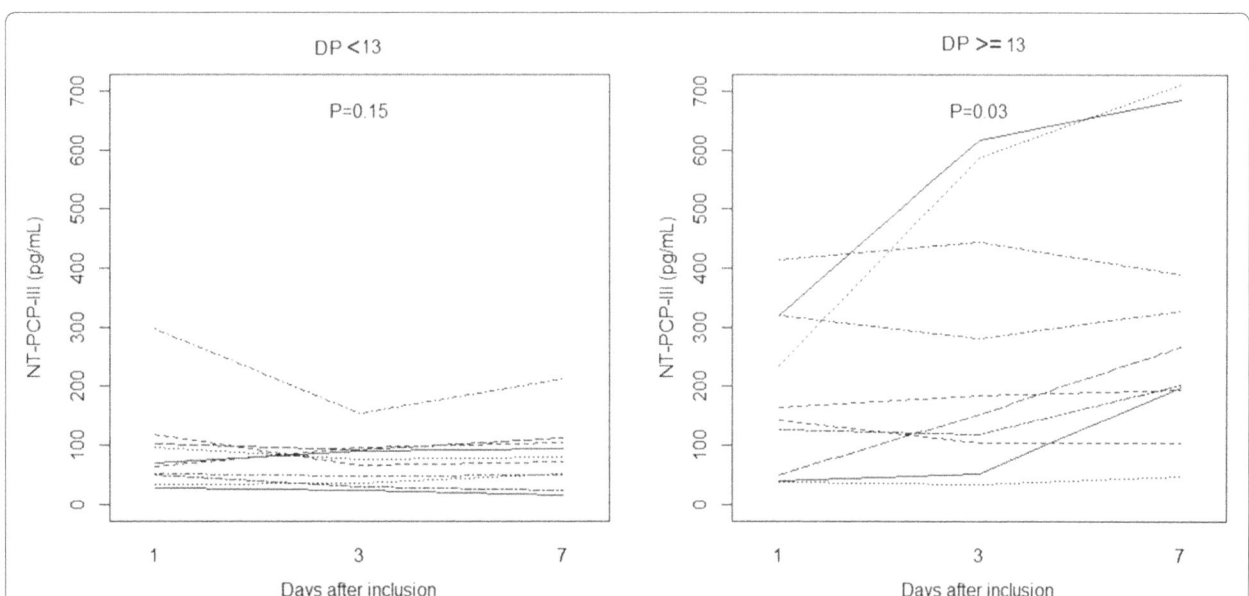

Fig. 5 Changes in serum level of N-terminal peptide for type III procollagen over time in patients ventilated with driving pressure < 13 cmH$_2$O 24 h after inclusion (N = 9) and patients ventilated with driving pressure ≥ 13 cmH$_2$O 24 h after inclusion (N = 9). (NT-PCP-III = type III procollagen, 1 = day 1 after inclusion, 3 = day 3 after inclusion, 7 = level after extubation or at day 7 after inclusion)

whereas a lower driving pressure was strongly correlated to better long-term outcomes, lower tidal volumes and higher baseline compliance (this latter reflecting lower severity of illness) were not.

A pro-fibrotic response to ARDS might be responsible for the physiologic abnormalities observed. Biomechanical interactions between cells and the extracellular matrix (ECM) proteins may be associated with the reorganization and remodeling of the ECM [25]. Collagen is the most important stress-bearing constituent of the parenchymal tissue and plays a critical role in mechanotransduction in lung repair and fibrosis development [26]. In the isolated rat lung or lung parenchymal strips, mechanical stretch resulted in enhanced NT-PCP-III gene expression, a by-product of type III collagen synthesis and a potential marker of collagen secretion [27, 28]. Interestingly, these studies suggested that the driving force (stress) applied to the tissue, but not the amplitude of resulting stretch, was responsible for collagen production.

Diffuse alveolar damage (DAD) is considered absent in approximately half of patients undergoing lung biopsy for nonresolving ARDS. The main alternatives to DAD were interstitial pneumonia and lung fibrosis, infections, cryptogenic organizing pneumonia and alveolar hemorrhage [29, 30]. In our study, the increase in NT-PCP-III, associated with higher mean lung densities and lower lung volumes, was very suggestive of an intense fibrosis. Similarly to patients with idiopathic pulmonary fibrosis, the intense remodeling concomitantly reduced the total lung weight and volume, with a progressive increase in lung densities—but not necessarily an increase in lung tissue mass [31]. The reductions in FVC in our patients were not accompanied by an increased residual volume, a finding that might otherwise suggest some weakness associated with severity of illness [32]. Thus, we believe that most of the reduction in FVC observed in our patients was related to fibrosis and remodeling of lung tissue.

In the general population, a low FVC has been associated with increased respiratory symptoms, functional limitation and mortality [33–35]. Thus, the observed relationship between driving pressure and long-term QOL might be mediated by the low FVC, secondary to lung fibrosis. Of note, some of our patients presented FVC values of less than 70% of predicted values, and studies have shown that even smaller changes in FVC can strongly influence the QoL.

Limitations

The modest number of patients enrolled in a single center (representing 10% of the total number of patients included in the multicenter trial) may have compromised the power of this study to identify statistically significant relationships. The identified relationships, however, were consistent across different long-term variables, measured independently by CT, function tests and questionnaire, suggesting the strength of the association. The independent blood samples also added consistency to our results.

Another limitation of our study was the unknown functional status of the enrolled patients, who were lost during follow-up. Additionally, though patients with an exacerbation of previous lung diseases were excluded before randomization, preexisting lung disease may have interfered in the results, as patients were not evaluated by pulmonary function tests prior to enrollment.

Finally, driving pressure was measured at 24 h of the beginning of the protocol. Ideally, we should consider some average exposition during the whole mechanical ventilation period. In this study, however, similarly to the previous study of Amato et al. [20], the values of driving pressure measured at day-one were strongly correlated to the levels measured during the next days. We may not exclude, however, that additional adjustments in mechanical ventilation after 24 h of the protocol could also be associated with late pulmonary function and structure.

Conclusion

In patients surviving after a moderate to severe ARDS there is an association between driving pressure measured 24 h after enrollment and lung function measured at 1 and 6 months after the ARDS onset, and this relationship was independent of tidal volume and independent of baseline compliance. These results suggest that, even in the context of protective tidal volume and plateau pressure, mechanical ventilation can still promote lung injury and fibrosis, highlighting the possible role of driving pressure in long-term outcomes.

Abbreviations

ARDS: acute respiratory distress syndrome; HRQoL: health-related quality of life; NT-PCP-III: N-terminal-peptide type III procollagen; 6MWT: 6-min walk test; QoL: quality of life; ICU: intensive care unit; COPD: chronic obstructive pulmonary disease; APACHE II: Acute Physiology and Chronic Health disease Classification System II; PEEP: positive end-expiratory pressure; PaO_2: arterial partial pressure of oxygen; F_iO_2: inspired O_2 fraction; ELISA: enzyme-linked immunosorbent assay; PFT: pulmonary function test; HRCT: high-resolution computed tomography; MPD: mean pulmonary density; TLV: total lung volume; TAV: total air volume; TLM: total lung mass; HU: Hounsfield unit; P15: threshold of 15%; SF-36: 36-item Short-Form General Health Survey; SD: standard deviation; P/F: PaO_2/FIO_2; C_{stat}: static compliance; PBW: predicted body weight; OLA: open lung approach; DAD: diffuse alveolar damage; HDP: high driving pressure; LDP: low driving pressure.

Authors' contributions

CTJ designed the work; acquired, analyzed, or interpreted the data for the work; and drafted the work. RRSS acquired and interpreted the data for the work and critically revised the work; ASH acquired and interpreted the data for the work and critically revised the work; ARSC analyzed and interpreted the data and critically revised the work; SG analyzed and interpreted the data and critically revised the work; MBPA designed the work, interpreted the data, and critically revised the work; CRRC designed the work, interpreted the data, and critically revised the work. All authors read and approved the final manuscript.

Author details
[1] Divisão de Pneumologia, Cardiopulmonary Department, Heart Institute (InCor) University of São Paulo, INCOR Av. Dr. Enéas de Carvalho Aguiar, 44 Pinheiros, São Paulo, SP CEP 05403-900, Brazil. [2] Laboratory of Pulmonary Engineering, Biomedical Engineering Program, Alberto Luiz Coimbra Institute of Post-Graduation and Research in Engineering, Federal University of Rio de Janeiro, Rio de Janeiro, Brazil. [3] Laboratory of Respiration Physiology, Carlos Chagas Filho Institute of Biophysics, Federal University of Rio de Janeiro, Rio de Janeiro, Brazil. [4] Respiratory Intensive Care Unit, University of São Paulo School of Medicine Hospital das Clínicas, São Paulo, Brazil.

Acknowledgements
Not applicable.

Competing interests
The authors declare that they have no competing interests.

Funding
Not applicable.

References
1. Phua J, Badia JR, Adhikari NKJ, Friedrich JO, Fowler RA, Singh JM, et al. Has mortality from acute respiratory distress syndrome decreased over time?: A systematic review. Am J Respir Crit Care Med. 2009;179(3):220–7.
2. Azevedo LC, Park M, Salluh JI, Rea-Neto A, Souza-Dantas VC, Varaschin P, et al. Clinical outcomes of patients requiring ventilatory support in Brazilian intensive care units: a multicenter, prospective, cohort study. Crit Care. 2013;17(2):R63.
3. Franca SA, Toufen C, Hovnanian ALD, Albuquerque ALP, Borges ER, Pizzo VRP, et al. The epidemiology of acute respiratory failure in hospitalized patients: a Brazilian prospective cohort study. J Crit Care. 2011;26(3):330.e1–8.
4. Herridge MS, Tansey CM, Matté A, Tomlinson G, Diaz-Granados N, Cooper A, et al. Functional disability 5 years after acute respiratory distress syndrome. N Engl J Med. 2011;364(14):1293–304.
5. Herridge MS, Cheung AM, Tansey CM, Matte-Martyn A, Diaz-Granados N, Al-Saidi F, et al. One-year outcomes in survivors of the acute respiratory distress syndrome. N Engl J Med. 2003;348(8):683–93.
6. Burnham EL, Hyzy RC, Paine R, Coley C, Kelly AM, Quint LE, et al. Chest CT features are associated with poorer quality of life in acute lung injury survivors. Crit Care Med. 2013;41(2):445–56.
7. Kacmarek RM, Villar J, Sulemanji D, Montiel R, Ferrando C, Blanco J, et al. Open lung approach for the acute respiratory distress syndrome: a pilot, randomized controlled trial. Crit Care Med. 2016;44(1):32–42.
8. Espirometria Pereira C. Diretrizes para testes de função pulmonar. J Bras Pneumol. 2002;28(Supl 3):S1–82.
9. Pereira CAdeC, Sato T, Rodrigues SC. New reference values for forced spirometry in white adults in Brazil. J Bras Pneumol. 2007;33(4):397–406.
10. Neder JA, Andreoni S, Castelo-Filho A, Nery LE. Reference values for lung function tests. I. Static volumes. Braz J Med Biol Res. 1999;32(6):703–17.
11. Neder JA, Andreoni S, Peres C, Nery LE. Reference values for lung function tests. III. Carbon monoxide diffusing capacity (transfer factor). Braz J Med Biol Res. 1999;32(6):729–37.
12. Camilo GB, Carvalho ARS, Machado DC, Mogami R, Kasuki L, Gadelha MR, et al. Correlations between forced oscillation technique parameters and pulmonary densitovolumetry values in patients with acromegaly. Braz J Med Biol Res = Rev Bras Pesqui médicas e biológicas/Soc Bras Biofísica. 2015;48(10):877–85.
13. Carvalho AR, Spieth PM, Pelosi P, Beda A, Lopes AJ, Neykova B, et al. Pressure support ventilation and biphasic positive airway pressure improve

oxygenation by redistribution of pulmonary blood flow. Anesth Analg. 2009;109(3):856–65.
14. Dirksen A, Friis M, Olesen KP, Skovgaard LT, Sørensen K. Progress of emphysema in severe alpha 1-antitrypsin deficiency as assessed by annual CT. Acta Radiol. 1997;38(5):826–32.
15. Dirksen A, Dijkman JH, Madsen F, Stoel B, Hutchison DC, Ulrik CS, et al. A randomized clinical trial of alpha(1)-antitrypsin augmentation therapy. Am J Respir Crit Care Med. 1999;160(5 Pt 1):1468–72.
16. Dowson LJ, Guest PJ, Stockley RA. Longitudinal changes in physiological, radiological, and health status measurements in alpha(1)-antitrypsin deficiency and factors associated with decline. Am J Respir Crit Care Med. 2001;164(10 Pt 1):1805–9.
17. Stolk J, Ng WH, Bakker ME, Reiber JHC, Rabe KF, Putter H, et al. Correlation between annual change in health status and computer tomography derived lung density in subjects with alpha1-antitrypsin deficiency. Thorax. 2003;58(12):1027–30.
18. ATS Committee on Proficiency Standards for Clinical Pulmonary Function Laboratories. ATS statement: guidelines for the six-minute walk test. Am J Respir Crit Care Med. 2002;166(1):111–7.
19. Ciconelli R, Ferraz M, Santos W, Meinão I. Brazilian–Portuguese version of the SF-36. A reliable and valid quality of life outcome measure. Rev Bras Reum. 1999;39(3):145–50.
20. Amato MBP, Meade MO, Slutsky AS, Brochard L, Costa ELV, Schoenfeld DA, et al. Driving pressure and survival in the acute respiratory distress syndrome. N Engl J Med. 2015;372(8):747–55.
21. Cheung AM, Tansey CM, Tomlinson G, Diaz-Granados N, Matté A, Barr A, et al. Two-year outcomes, health care use, and costs of survivors of acute respiratory distress syndrome. Am J Respir Crit Care Med. 2006;174(5):538–44.
22. Heyland DK, Groll D, Caeser M. Survivors of acute respiratory distress syndrome: relationship between pulmonary dysfunction and long-term health-related quality of life. Crit Care Med. 2005;33(7):1549–56.
23. Desai SR, Wells AU, Rubens MB, Evans TW, Hansell DM. Acute respiratory distress syndrome: CT abnormalities at long-term follow-up. Radiology. 1999;210(1):29–35.
24. Baedorf Kassis E, Loring SH, Talmor D. Mortality and pulmonary mechanics in relation to respiratory system and transpulmonary driving pressures in ARDS. Intensive Care Med. 2016;42(8):1206–13.
25. Cabrera-Benitez NE, Laffey JG, Parotto M, Spieth PM, Villar J, Zhang H, et al. Mechanical ventilation-associated lung fibrosis in acute respiratory distress syndrome: a significant contributor to poor outcome. Anesthesiology. 2014;121(1):189–98.
26. Suki B, Ito S, Stamenovic D, Lutchen KR, Ingenito EP. Biomechanics of the lung parenchyma: critical roles of collagen and mechanical forces. J Appl Physiol. 2005;98(5):1892–9.
27. Parker JC, Breen EC, West JB. High vascular and airway pressures increase interstitial protein mRNA expression in isolated rat lungs. J Appl Physiol. 1997;83(5):1697–705.
28. Garcia CSNB, Rocco PRM, Facchinetti LD, Lassance RM, Caruso P, Deheinzelin D, et al. What increases type III procollagen mRNA levels in lung tissue: stress induced by changes in force or amplitude? Respir Physiol Neurobiol. 2004;144(1):59–70.
29. Cardinal-Fernández P, Bajwa EK, Dominguez-Calvo A, Menéndez JM, Papazian L, Thompson BT. The presence of diffuse alveolar damage on open lung biopsy is associated with mortality in patients with acute respiratory distress syndrome. Chest. 2016;149(5):1155–64.
30. Gerard L, Bidoul T, Castanares-Zapatero D, Wittebole X, Lacroix V, Froidure A, et al. Open lung biopsy in nonresolving acute respiratory distress syndrome commonly identifies corticosteroid-sensitive pathologies, associated with better outcome. Crit Care Med. 2018;46(6):907–14.
31. Coxson HO, Hogg JC, Mayo JR, Behzad H, Whittall KP, Schwartz DA, et al. Quantification of idiopathic pulmonary fibrosis using computed tomography and histology. Am J Respir Crit Care Med. 1997;155(5):1649–56.
32. Hart N, Cramer D, Ward SP, Nickol AH, Moxham J, Polkey MI, et al. Effect of pattern and severity of respiratory muscle weakness on carbon monoxide gas transfer and lung volumes. Eur Respir J. 2002;20(4):996–1002.

33. Mannino DM, Ford ES, Redd SC. Obstructive and restrictive lung disease and functional limitation: data from the Third National Health and Nutrition Examination. J Intern Med. 2003;254(6):540–7.
34. Guerra S, Sherrill DL, Venker C, Ceccato CM, Halonen M, Martinez FD. Morbidity and mortality associated with the restrictive spirometric pattern: a longitudinal study. Thorax. 2010;65(6):499–504.
35. Wan ES, Hokanson JE, Murphy JR, Regan EA, Make BJ, Lynch DA, et al. Clinical and radiographic predictors of GOLD-unclassified smokers in the COPDGene study. Am J Respir Crit Care Med. 2011;184(1):57–63.

19

Physiological predictors of respiratory and cough assistance needs after extubation

Nicolas Terzi[1,2,3]*, Frédéric Lofaso[4,5,6], Romain Masson[3], Pascal Beuret[7], Hervé Normand[8,9,10], Edith Dumanowski[10], Line Falaize[11,12], Bertrand Sauneuf[3,13], Cédric Daubin[3], Jennifer Brunet[3], Djillali Annane[14], Jean-Jacques Parienti[15] and David Orlikowski[4,5,16,17]

Abstract

Background: Identifying patients at high risk of post-extubation acute respiratory failure requiring respiratory or mechanical cough assistance remains challenging. Here, our primary aim was to evaluate the accuracy of easily collected parameters obtained before or just after extubation in predicting the risk of post-extubation acute respiratory failure requiring, at best, noninvasive mechanical ventilation (NIV) and/or mechanical cough assistance and, at worst, reintubation after extubation.

Methods: We conducted a multicenter prospective, open-label, observational study from April 2012 through April 2015. Patients who passed a weaning test after at least 72 h of endotracheal mechanical ventilation (MV) were included. Just before extubation, spirometry and maximal pressures were measured by a technician. The results were not disclosed to the bedside physicians. Patients were followed until discharge or death.

Results: Among 3458 patients admitted to the ICU, 730 received endotracheal MV for longer than 72 h and were then extubated; among these, 130 were included. At inclusion, the 130 patients had mean ICU stay and endotracheal MV durations both equal to 11 ± 4.2 days. After extubation, 36 patients required curative NIV, 7 both curative NIV and mechanical cough assistance, and 8 only mechanical cough assistance; 6 patients, all of whom first received NIV, required reintubation within 48 h. The group that required NIV after extubation had a significantly higher proportion of patients with chronic respiratory disease ($P = 0.015$), longer endotracheal MV duration at inclusion, and lower Medical Research Council (MRC) score ($P = 0.02$, $P = 0.01$, and $P = 0.004$, respectively). By multivariate analysis, forced vital capacity (FVC) and peak cough expiratory flow (PCEF) were independently associated with (NIV) and/or mechanical cough assistance and/or reintubation after extubation. Areas under the ROC curves for pre-extubation PCEF and FVC were 0.71 and 0.76, respectively.

Conclusion: In conclusion, FVC measured before extubation correlates closely with FVC after extubation and may serve as an objective predictor of post-extubation respiratory failure requiring NIV and/or mechanical cough assistance and/or reintubation in heterogeneous populations of medical ICU patients.

ClinicalTrials.gov as #NCT01564745

Background

Weaning patients off endotracheal positive-pressure ventilation involves two steps: separation of the patient from the ventilator and extubation. The day of extubation is a critical time during an intensive care unit (ICU) stay, as extubation failure occurs in 10–20% of patients and is associated with up to 50% hospital mortality [1–6]. There is some evidence that extubation failure can directly worsen patient outcomes independently of underlying illness severity [5]. Several factors may contribute to extubation failure, including cough impairment and presence of thick and/or excessive mucus, in addition to hypoventilation [4]. Cough assistance and noninvasive

*Correspondence: nterzi@chu-grenoble.fr
[3] Service de réanimation médicale, Centre Hospitalier Universitaire Grenoble - Alpes, CS10217, Grenoble Cedex 09, France
Full list of author information is available at the end of the article

mechanical ventilation (NIV) can help to prevent post-extubation respiratory failure. However, as these techniques are time-consuming, criteria for selecting those patients most likely to benefit would be useful. Ideally, these criteria would be objective, easily measured parameters obtained immediately before and/or after extubation. Adequate respiratory muscle strength is essential to generate the pressures and flows needed to clear airway secretions during coughing. Accordingly, peak cough expiratory flow (PCEF) was found in many studies to predict successful decannulation and extubation [7–12]. However, the tracheal tube can alter PCEF values via two mechanisms: it elevates airway resistance [13]; and it eliminates the role of the glottis in coughing [14].

Here, our objective was to evaluate the accuracy of parameters easily collected before versus after extubation in predicting the risk of post-extubation respiratory failure requiring, at best, NIV and/or mechanical cough assistance and, at worst, reintubation. We assessed cough performance and other easily collected respiratory parameters obtained before and after extubation, with the goal of determining which parameters and measurement conditions best identified patients who would require NIV and/or mechanical cough assistance after extubation.

Methods

Study population

We conducted a multicenter, prospective, observational study in two university-affiliated hospitals (Caen and Garches) and one general hospital (Roanne) in France from April 2012 through April 2015. The appropriate ethics committee (CPP Nord-Ouest III) approved the study (#2011-A00849-32), which was registered on ClinicalTrials.gov (#NCT01564745). All patients provided written informed consent.

Patients 18 years of age or older and sufficiently cooperative without sedation were eligible if they were admitted to the ICU and received invasive mechanical ventilation (MV) for at least 72 h then passed a weaning test performed according to recommendations [4, 15, 16]. Exclusion criteria were previous long-term NIV at home and unavailability of an lung function test (LFT) technician.

Study procedures

Weaning from the ventilator was performed following a standardized protocol. Patients were screened daily for predefined weaning-readiness criteria, i.e., improvement in clinical signs, peripheral capillary oxygen saturation (SpO_2) > 92% with fraction of inspired oxygen < 50% and positive end-expiratory pressure < 5 cm H_2O, no infusion of vasopressor agents or sedatives, and adequate responses to simple commands. When these criteria were met, a spontaneous breathing test (SBT) was performed, by having the patient either breathe spontaneously from the ventilator on a T piece or receive pressure-support ventilation with an inspiratory pressure of 7 cmH₂O and zero end-expiratory pressure. The test was interrupted if any of the following signs of poor tolerance was observed: respiratory rate > 35/min, SpO_2 < 90%, heart rate > 140/min, and arterial systolic blood pressure > 180 mmHg or < 90 mmHg. Patients who successfully completed the test were considered for a trial of extubation. Decisions to perform a cuff-leak test and/or give corticosteroid therapy were based on standard practice at each study center.

Patients who passed an SBT and were considered for extubation underwent lung function testing (LFT) (see Additional file 1). After extubation, the patients breathed spontaneously with an oxygen flow titrated to maintain SpO_2 > 90%.

Physicians were blinded to LFT results. Patients were followed until ICU discharge or death.

Lung function testing (LFT)

LFT was repeated after extubation provided and there was no laryngeal edema (see Additional file 1).

Clinical data

At ICU admission, we recorded the following: comorbidities, MV duration at inclusion, number of tracheal aspirates within 24 h before extubation, Glasgow Coma Scale score, Medical Research Council (MRC) scale combined score for muscle strength [17], and Borg Scale [18] score for subjective dyspnea.

Extubation care and definitions

According to guidelines, patients were extubated by the physician if they passed an SBT [4, 15, 16]. We evaluated the accuracy of easily collected parameters obtained before or just after extubation in predicting weaning failure defined as a need for NIV and/or mechanical cough assistance and/or reintubation within 48 h after extubation.

Patients received NIV if they met at least one of the following predefined criteria: respiratory rate > 30 breaths/min; SpO_2 < 90%; ≥ 20% variation in heart rate or blood pressure; clinical signs of respiratory distress (i.e., cyanosis, sweating, involvement of accessory respiratory muscles, paradoxical abdominal motion, consciousness impairment); PaO_2 < 60 mm Hg with ≥ 6 L/min O_2; and hypercapnia with respiratory acidosis (i.e., $PaCO_2$ > 45 mm Hg and pH < 7.35). All patients received chest physiotherapy twice daily to promote secretion clearance, with deep inspiration and manual cough assistance. Mechanical cough assistance was used, alone or with NIV, when conventional chest physiotherapy failed to prevent secretion accumulation with severe hypoxemia defined as SaO_2 < 90% with ≥ 6 L/min O_2 or FiO_2 > 50%. Reintubation was considered when there was no improvement within 2 h and was performed according to guidelines [15, 16].

Statistical analysis

Quantitative variables were described as mean ± SD and qualitative variables as number (%). To compare demographics, clinical data, and LFT results between groups with and without weaning failure as defined above (NIV and/or mechanical cough assistance and/or reintubation, within 48 h after extubation), we used the Chi-square test for categorical variables and the Wilcoxon t test for quantitative co-variables. Multivariate logistic regression was performed to identify pre-extubation measurements independently associated with weaning failure. The close correlations among respiratory parameters precluded the use of a single multivariate model. Therefore, we built a separate multivariate logistic regression model to assess the ability of each LFT variable to predict weaning failure. All models were adjusted for MV duration (< 7 vs. ≥ 7 days), MRC scale score (< 48 vs. ≥ 48), and previous chronic respiratory failure. Model discrimination was assessed by the concordance index (c-index) and plotted on a receiver operating characteristic (ROC) curve. For each LFT variable, we identified the cutoff that maximized the Youden index, and we computed the sensitivity and specificity of this cutoff for predicting weaning failure. In addition, correlations between each LFT parameter before and after extubation were assessed by Pearson's correlation coefficient.

All P values were two-tailed with no adjustment for multiple comparisons. P values < 0.05 were considered significant. The statistical analyses were performed using SAS statistical software, version 9.4 (SAS Institute Inc., Cary, NC, USA).

Results

Study population

Among 3458 patients admitted to the study ICUs, 730 received MV for more than 72 h and were then extubated; among these, 130 were included in the study (Fig. 1). Table 1 reports their main characteristics at ICU admission. At study inclusion, mean values for ICU stay and MV duration were both 11.0 ± 4.2 days. Five patients were excluded from the analysis because they required immediate reintubation due to either laryngeal edema ($n = 3$) or acute coma ($n = 2$) and consequently could not undergo post-extubation testing.

After extubation, 36 patients required curative NIV, including 7 who also needed mechanical cough assistance, and 8 required only mechanical cough assistance.

Reintubation was performed within 2 days after extubation in 6 patients and on day 6 in 1 patient. All reintubated patients received NIV within 2 days following extubation, and none died in the ICU. Patients who were reintubated were significantly younger and had a lower BMI than those who received only NIV and/or mechanical cough assistance.

Comparison of lung function parameters before and after extubation

Vital capacity (VC), forced vital capacity (FVC), peak expiratory flow (PEF), and PCEF were significantly higher after than before extubation. Maximal inspiratory pressure (MIP) and maximal expiratory pressure (MEP) were significantly higher before than after extubation (all P values < 0.001). As shown in Table 2, the pre-extubation and post-extubation values correlated with each other for all variables (all P values < 0.0001); the correlation was strongest for FVC ($R = 0.89$).

Comparison of patients who did ($n = 44$) and did not (81) require NIV or mechanical cough assistance after extubation

As shown in Table 3, the group that required post-extubation NIV or mechanical cough assistance had a significantly higher proportion of patients with chronic respiratory disease, longer ICU stay and MV durations at study inclusion, and lower MRC scores compared to the other group.

By univariate analysis, pre-extubation LFT variables significantly associated with post-extubation NIV and/or mechanical cough assistance were $PaCO_2$, VC, FVC, MIP, MEP, PEF, and PCEF (Table 2). Post-extubation LFT variables significantly associated with post-extubation NIV and/or mechanical cough assistance were VC, FVC, MEP, PEF, and PCEF (Table 2).

By multivariate logistic regression adjusted for MV duration, MRC score, and the existence of chronic respiratory failure, variables independently associated with post-extubation NIV and/or mechanical cough assistance were VC, FVC, MIP, MEP, PEF, and PCEF (Table 4).

ROC curve analysis of performance of the independent predictors

As shown in Fig. 2, the areas under the ROC curves for pre-extubation PCEF, PEF, FVC, MIP, and MEP were 0.71, 0.67, 0.76, 0.61, and 0.69, respectively. The cutoffs that performed best in predicting post-extubation NIV and/or mechanical cough assistance were 85 L/min for PCEF, 62 L/min for PEF, and 1412 mL for FVC. The PCEF cutoff had 74% sensitivity and 62% specificity, the PEF cutoff 51% sensitivity and 76% specificity, and the FVC cutoff 65% sensitivity and 81% specificity.

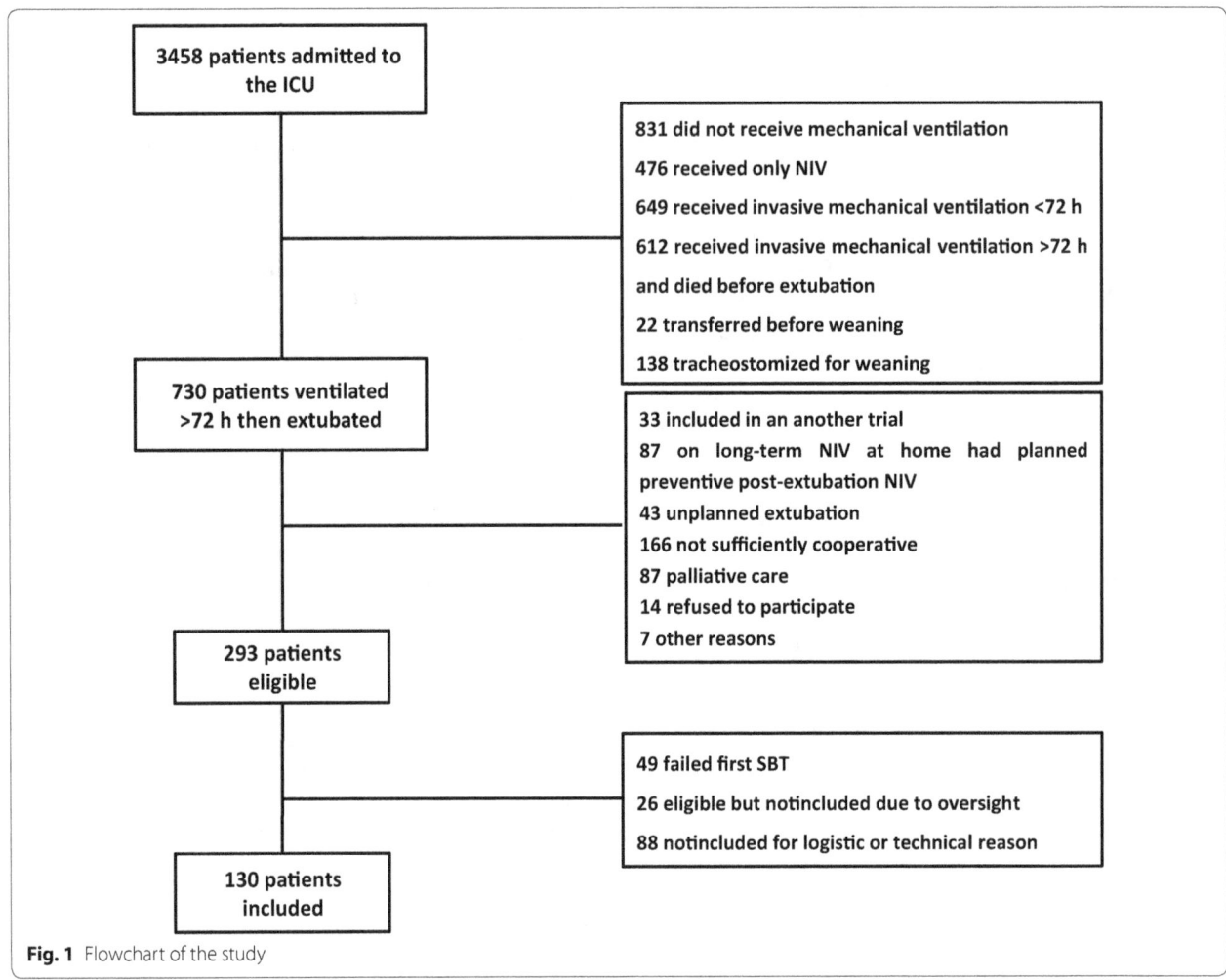

Fig. 1 Flowchart of the study

As shown in Fig. 3, the areas under the ROC curves for post-extubation PCEF, PEF, FVC, MIP, and MEP were 0.76, 0.68, 0.80, 0.62, and 0.73, respectively. The cutoffs that performed best in predicting post-extubation NIV and/or mechanical cough assistance were 113 L/min for PCEF, 151 L/min for PEF, and 1430 mL for FVC. The PCEF cutoff had 56% sensitivity and 90% specificity, the PEF cutoff 57% sensitivity and 76% specificity, and the FVC cutoff 72% sensitivity and 85% specificity.

Discussion

The main finding from this study is that the parameter with the closet correlation between pre- and post-extubation values was FVC. FVC may be an objective marker for identifying patients in whom NIV and/or mechanical cough assistance might prevent reintubation. Hypoventilation, cough impairment, and presence of thick and/or excessive mucus can contribute to extubation failure. Most of the previous studies evaluating cough efficiency before extubation focused on PCEF. However, the PCEF

cutoffs varied widely [9, 12], perhaps due to differences in study populations and MV durations. Moreover, the diversity of devices used to measure PCEF, presence of a cannula used to bypass the upper airway [19], and differences in the degree of patient coordination and cooperation during measurements may influence the results [12, 20, 21]. In our study, the optimal PCEF cutoff was 85 L/min before extubation and 113 L/min just after extubation. Our pre-extubation PCEF cutoff was higher than in earlier studies. However, our objective was to predict a need for post-extubation NIV and/or mechanical cough assistance, whereas previous studies [12, 20] sought to predict reintubation. Furthermore, the correlation between pre- and post-extubation PCEF values was weak. Several hypotheses can be suggested to explain this finding. The inability of intubated patients to close their glottis limits the pressure generated during coughing and therefore limits the PCEF values compared to those measured without the tube. Also, resistances are higher with than without the endotracheal tube. Finally, in a

Table 1 Characteristics of the patients at ICU admission

Parameters	Mean ± SD or n (%)
Total (n = 130)	
Age (years)	59.4 ± 15.6
Male	71 (54.6)
BMI	27.2 ± 6.7
Chronic disease	
Chronic obstructive pulmonary disease	16 (12.3%)
Chronic restrictive pulmonary disease	11 (8.4%)
Chronic heart disease	13 (10%)
SAPS II	45 ± 21
SOFA	7 ± 5
Main reason for ICU admission	
Acute respiratory failure	91 (70)
Heart failure	14 (10.8)
Neurologic failure	9 (6.9)
Septic shock	12 (9.2)
Postoperative	1 (0.8)
Other	3 (2.3)

BMI body mass index, *SAPS II* Simplified Acute Physiology Score II [30], *SOFA* Sequential Organ Failure Assessment

recent study in tracheostomized patients with neuromuscular disease, PCEF was higher after than before decannulation [13, 22].

Interestingly, Bach and Saporito [7] were the first to use PCEF as a criterion for extubation in patients with neuromuscular disease. However, they measured PCEF immediately after extubation and enhanced performance by combining maximal insufflation with an abdominal thrust timed to glottis opening. The results showed that PCEF > 160 L/min predicted successful extubation. More recently, they challenged their previous PCEF cutoff by demonstrating that professionals who had extensive experience with the noninvasive management of respiratory failure were able to extubate continuously ventilator-dependent patients who had severe cough impairment [8]. Finally, they demonstrated that using noninvasive techniques to improve cough performance and minute ventilation could drastically modify the outcomes of extubated patients, including those dependent on a ventilator [8]. These studies and our data suggest that identifying both the optimal PCEF value and the best PCEF measurement conditions in critically ill patients remains

Table 2 Correlations between physiological parameters before and after extubation

	VC Before extubation	FVC Before extubation	MIP Before extubation	MEP Before extubation	PEF Before extubation	PECF Before extubation
VC After extubation						
R	0.61					
P value	< 0.0001					
FVC After extubation						
R		0.89				
P value		< 0.0001				
MIP After extubation						
R			0.70			
P value			< 0.0001			
MEP After extubation						
R				0.66		
P value				< 0.0001		
PEF After extubation						
R					0.60	
P value					< 0.0001	
PCEF After extubation						
R						0.58
P value						< 0.0001

For each parameter, the table shows the correlation coefficient and P value

Italics indicate significant data

VC vital capacity, *FVC* forced vital capacity, *MIP* maximal inspiratory pressure, *MEP* maximal expiratory pressure, *PEF* peak expiratory flow, *PCEF* peak cough expiratory flow

Table 3 Univariate analyses

Parameters	No NIV or mechanical cough assistance after extubation ($n = 81$) Mean ± SD or n (%)	NIV or mechanical cough assistance after extubation			P value*
		All patients ($n = 44$) Mean ± SD or n (%)	Patients who required NIV ($n = 36$) Mean ± SD or n (%)	Patients who required Mechanical cough assistance ($n = 8$) Mean ± SD or n (%)	
Age, years	58.8 ± 14.8	59.8 ± 16.4	59.6 ± 15.7	60.8 ± 20.3	0.71
SOFA at admission	7.7 ± 5	7.2 ± 4.2	7.5 ± 4.1	5.9 ± 4.8	0.59
Coma Glasgow Scale score	15 ± 0	15 ± 0	15 ± 0	15 ± 0	1.00
Chronic respiratory failure	11 (14%)	14 (32%)	14 (39%)	0	*0.015*
Chronic heart disease	10 (12%)	3 (7%)	3 (8%)	0	0.34
Duration of MV, days	12.7 ± 8.8	17.8 ± 15.6	17.4 ± 14.4	19.8 ± 21.2	*0.02*
Diameter of the endotracheal tube, mm	7.5 ± 0.3	7.4 ± 0.3	7.3 ± 0.3	7.6 ± 0.3	0.17
MRC score	51.1 ± 12	43 ± 15.5	43.2 ± 12.2	42.2 ± 12.2	*0.004*
Tracheal aspiration before extubation (n/24 h)	7.8 ± 3	7.7 ± 2.7	7.7 ± 2.5	7.6 ± 3.6	0.89
Respiratory rate (breaths/min)	23.2 ± 11.8	24.5 ± 5.6	24.8 ± 5.9	23.4 ± 4.2	0.50
Borg Scale score (/10)	1.9 ± 2.3	2.1 ± 2.2	2 ± 2	2.3 ± 3.5	0.60
$PaCO_2$ before extubation	5.0 ± 0.6	5.6 ± 1	5.8 ± 1	4.9 ± 0.7	*0.00007*
VC (mL) before extubation	1574 ± 498	1281 ± 536	1220 ± 513	1558 ± 586	*0.003*
FVC (mL) before extubation	1571 ± 520	1146 ± 457	1121 ± 464	1257 ± 439	*0.00002*
MIP (cmH_2O) before extubation	37 ± 15	31 ± 15	32 ± 15	26 ± 12	*0.025*
MEP (cmH_2O) before extubation	53 ± 28	41 ± 24	44 ± 25	30 ± 16	*0.021*
PEF (L/min) before extubation	80 ± 32	62 ± 30	60 ± 29	71 ± 36	*0.004*
PCEF (L/min) before extubation	97 ± 36	72 ± 33	71 ± 33	75 ± 36	*0.0003*
VC (mL) after extubation	1838 ± 637	1364 ± 499	1343 ± 511	1463 ± 464	*0.00017*
FVC (mL) after extubation	1766 ± 554	1284 ± 433	1284 ± 440	1282 ± 441	*0.00003*
MIP (cmH_2O) after extubation	28 ± 13	23 ± 11	23 ± 11	22 ± 10	*0.07*
MEP (cmH_2O) after extubation	43 ± 22	29 ± 17	31 ± 17	21 ± 12	*0.002*
PEF (L/min) after extubation	142 ± 77	107 ± 63	109 ± 66	95 ± 47	*0.02*
PCEF (L/min) after extubation	166 ± 76	107 ± 66	110 ± 72	94 ± 39	*0.0001*

Italics indicate significant data

SOFA Sequential Organ Failure Assessment, *MRC* Medical Research Council sum score, *PaO₂* partial pressure of O_2 in arterial blood, *PaCO₂* partial pressure of CO_2 in arterial blood, *FiO₂* fraction of inspired O_2, *VC* vital capacity, *FVC* forced vital capacity, *MIP* maximal inspiratory pressure, *MEP* maximal expiratory pressure, *PEF* peak expiratory flow, *PCEF* peak cough expiratory flow, *NS* nonsignificant

*P values compare patients with and without NIV and/or mechanical cough assistance

challenging because many factors, including the use of assistive devices, can influence the measurement result.

We tested the usefulness of various LFT parameters for evaluating voluntary cough at the bedside. PCEF and PEF were significantly higher in the successfully extubated group, and low PCEF and PEF values independently predicted postextubation NIV and/or mechanical cough assistance.

As described previously [23–25], expiratory muscle strength as assessed by the MEP correlated with PCEF. MIP and MEP measurements require a static maneuver with maintenance of a maximal pressure for at least 1.5 s [26]. Nevertheless, contrary to FVC and PCEF, MIP and MEP cannot be measured easily in all mechanically ventilated patients without a specific device.

Table 4 Multivariate analysis of extubation predictors

Model	Odds Ratio (IC 95%)	P value
Model 1 FVC	0.998 (0.997–0.999)	*0.0005*
Model 2 VC	0.999 (0.998–1.000)	*0.0078*
Model 2 MIP	0.973 (0.947–1.000)	*0.05*
Model 3 MEP	0.983 (0.967–0.999)	*0.043*
Model 4 PEF	0.980 (0.965–0.996)	*0.012*
Model 5 PCEF	0.980 (0.967–0.993)	*0.0022*

One separate model was used for each predictor. All the models were used in multivariable analysis adjusting for the duration of mechanical ventilation (< 7-day vs. 7 days or more), chronic respiratory failure (Yes/No) and MRC (< 48 vs. 48 or more). An odds ratio (OR) > 1 signified an increased probability of necessity of mechanical ventilator assistance

Italics indicate significant data

VC vital capacity, *FVC* forced vital capacity, *MIP* maximal inspiratory pressure, *MEP* maximal expiratory pressure, *PEF* peak expiratory flow, *PCEF* peak cough expiratory flow

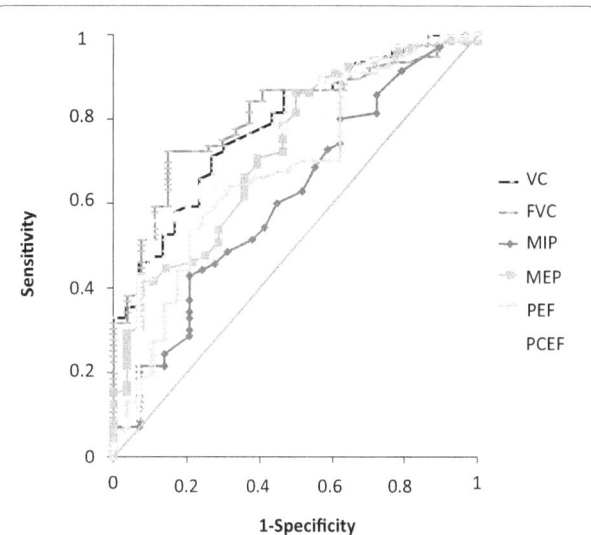

Fig. 3 Receiver operating characteristic (ROC) curves for data recorded after extubation: peak cough expiratory flow (PCEF), peak expiratory flow (PEF), forced vital capacity (FVC), slow VC, and maximal inspiratory (MIP) and expiratory (MEP) mouth pressures AUC, area under the ROC curve

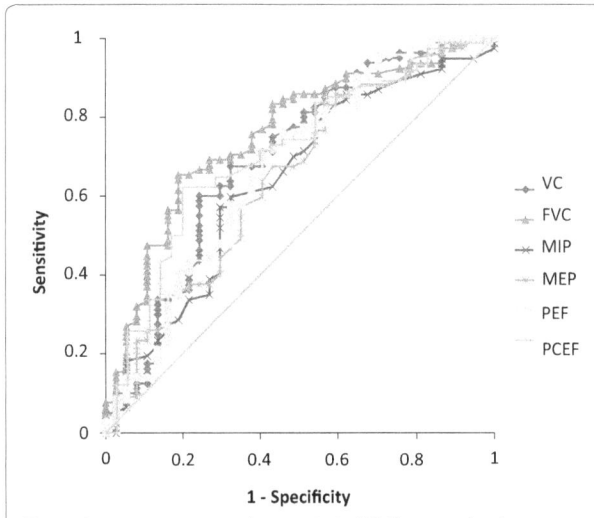

Fig. 2 Receiver operating characteristic (ROC) curves for data recorded before extubation: peak cough expiratory flow (PCEF), peak expiratory flow (PEF), forced vital capacity (FVC), slow VC, and maximal inspiratory (MIP) and expiratory (MEP) mouth pressures. AUC, area under the ROC curve

Our study provides the first evidence that FVC correlates well with PCEF and outperforms PCEF for predicting a need for NIV and/or mechanical cough assistance after extubation. In addition, FVC was the parameter least affected by the presence of a tracheal tube, so that pre-extubation FVC < 1420 mL was 64% sensitive and 81% specific, with improvements to 72 and 85%, respectively, when FVC remained < 1420 mL after extubation.

This is not surprising given that FVC diminishes only in the event of air trapping, which is generally due to peripheral airway obstruction and not to increased central airway resistance due, for instance, to a tracheal tube.

Several limitations of our study should be addressed. First, we included only those patients who were sufficiently cooperative and were extubated at a time when the technician was available for pre-extubation LFT. This requirement decreased the number of included patients but allowed the physicians to remain blinded to LFT findings, thereby minimizing bias. Thus, of the 730 patients extubated during the study period, 130 (18%) were included. Second, we did not assess involuntary cough. However, recent work indicates that, in cooperative patients, voluntary PCEF is far more accurate than involuntary PCEF in predicting reintubation, due to underestimation of cough strength by involuntary PCEF in patients with high voluntary PCEF [21]. We deliberately confined our study to cooperative patients, since we used noninvasive but volitional measurement techniques. Third, we excluded patients with MV for less than 72 h, since extubation failure is rare in this situation. Fourth, we did not measure the rapid shallow breathing index or fluid balance, two variables significantly associated with extubation failure in a previous study [27]. However, all study patients passed an SBT. Surprisingly, maximal pressures decreased after extubation, whereas the other parameters increased. This finding may be ascribable to the difference in patient-measurement device interface between pre- and post-extubation [28, 29]. In addition, upper-airway muscle activation and coordination are usually required when using a flanged mouthpiece but are not required when a tracheal tube bypasses the upper airway, which allows the patient to concentrate the effort on the inspiratory or expiratory muscles. Finally, a tracheal tube may diminish airway compliance and, therefore, the volume change during breathing, resulting in higher pressures for the same effort. Fifth, as this study used a prospective observational design, we did not change the practices in each center regarding the use of preventive NIV. The percentage of reintubated patients was surprisingly small in our study, i.e., 3 times lower than in the study by Esteban et al. among patients receiving NIV (48 vs. 16%). This difference may be ascribable to the high prevalence in our study of patients with COPD or restrictive pulmonary disease (20.7%), who may derive particularly large benefits from NIV [30]. Although ERS/ATS guidelines do not recommend using NIV to avoid reintubation in patients with overt respiratory distress and/or respiratory failure after planned extubation, this recommendation is not considered definitive and may not apply to patients with COPD [31]. Furthermore, reported benefits of curative NIV include improved oxygenation and alveolar ventilation, better alveolar recruitment in patients with atelectasis, improved left ventricular function in patients with heart failure, and decreases in intrinsic PEEP and work of breathing [32].

A legitimate issue is whether postponing extubation might have decreased the reintubation rate in our patients, who had longer MV durations before extubation compared to those in recent studies [5, 33, 34]. This difference is due to the inclusion in our study of only those patients already on MV for 72 h. However, our patients were extubated as soon as the daily conventional SBT was successful, in keeping with recent guidelines about the optimal assessment of weaning readiness [35].

Another factor that may have contributed to the low reintubation rate in our population is the considerable experience of our staff in the noninvasive treatment of patients with chronic and complete ventilator dependency [36–38]. We share this high level of experience with teams specialized in neuromuscular diseases [39]. Moreover, the addition to NIV of mechanical insufflation-exsufflation when appropriate may have further decreased the reintubation needs, as shown in a recent randomized trial [40]. Given the persistent challenges in identifying patients at high risk of post-extubation respiratory failure requiring, at best, NIV or mechanical cough assistance and, at worst, reintubation, we chose weaning failure defined as the use of NIV, cough assistance, and/or reintubation as the study endpoint.

Finally, as demonstrated by Thille et al. [41] the ability of healthcare staff to predict extubation failure is poor. The results reported here should help to identify patients likely to benefit from preventive NIV or cough assistance, using simple physiological parameters. These results need to be confirmed in a large epidemiological study including clinical and physiological variables [33].

Conclusion

In conclusion, our main finding is that FVC measurements before and after extubation are well correlated. FVC may serve as an objective predictor of post-extubation respiratory failure requiring NIV and/or mechanical cough assistance and/or reintubation in heterogeneous populations of medical ICU patients. FVC measurement may deserve consideration as an inexpensive tool to be used in combination with easily identified risk factors for assessing patients after a successful SBT, with the goal of identifying those likely to require prophylactic post-extubation NIV and/or mechanical cough assistance. However, further studies are necessary to confirm our results in different conditions and populations.

Abbreviations
FVC: Forced vital capacity; ICU: Intensive care unit; LFT: Lung function testing; MEP: Maximal expiratory pressure; MIP: Maximal inspiratory pressure; MRC sum score: Medical Research Council sum score; MV: Endotracheal mechanical ventilation; NIV: Noninvasive ventilation; PaO_2: Partial pressure of O_2 in arterial blood; $PaCO_2$: Partial pressure of CO_2 in arterial blood; PCEF: Peak cough expiratory flow; PEF: Peak expiratory flow; ROC curve: Receiver operating characteristic curve; SBT: Spontaneous breathing trial; SOFA: Sequential Organ Failure Assessment; VC: Vital capacity.

Authors' contributions
NT, FL, and DO conceived the original protocol then initiated and conducted the study. RM, ED, LF, and PB recorded the data. JJP and NT performed the statistical analysis. NT analyzed the data and drafted the manuscript. RM, PB, HN, BS, CD, JB, and DA helped to conduct the study and to draft the final manuscript. HN, NT, FL, DO, DA, and PB participated in coordinating the study. All authors read and approved the final manuscript.

Author details
[1] INSERM, Université Grenoble-Alpes, U1042, HP2, 38000 Grenoble, France. [2] CHU Grenoble Alpes, Service de réanimation médicale, 38000 Grenoble, France. [3] Service de réanimation médicale, Centre Hospitalier Universitaire Grenoble - Alpes, CS10217, Grenoble Cedex 09, France. [4] Université de Versailles Saint Quentin en Yvelines, INSERM U1179, Garches, France. [5] CIC 1429, INSERM, AP-HP, Hôpital Raymond Poincaré, 92380 Garches, France. [6] Service d'Explorations Fonctionnelles Respiratoires, AP-HP, Hôpital Raymond Poincaré, 92380 Garches, France. [7] Service de Réanimation, Centre Hospitalier de Roanne, 42300 Roanne, France. [8] INSERM, U1075, 14000 Caen, France. [9] Université de Caen, 14000 Caen, France. [10] CHRU Caen, Service d'Explorations Fonctionnelles Respiratoire, 14000 Caen, France. [11] INSERM U 1179, Université de Versailles-Saint Quentin en Yvelines, 104 Bd Raymond Poincaré, 92380 Garches, France. [12] CIC 1429, Inserm-APHP, Hôpital Raymond Poincaré, 104 Bd Raymond Poincaré, 92380 Garches, France. [13] Service de Réanimation Médicale Polyvalente, Centre Hospitalier Public du Cotentin, BP 208,

50102 Cherbourg-en-Cotentin, France. [14] General Intensive Care Unit, Raymond Poincaré Hospital (AP-HP), Laboratory of Inflammation and Infection, U1173, INSERM and University of Versailles SQY, 92380 Garches, France. [15] Unité de Biostatistique et de Recherche Clinique, Centre Hospitalier Universitaire de Caen, Avenue de la Côte de Nacre, 14033 Caen, France. [16] Pôle de ventilation à domicile, AP-HP, Hôpital Raymond Poincaré, 92380 Garches, France. [17] Service de Santé Publique, AP-HP, Hôpital Raymond Poincaré, 92380 Garches, France.

Acknowledgements
The authors are indebted to all the ICU physicians who participated in the study. We thank Damien du Cheyron, Amélie Seguin, Xavier Valette for contributing to the study as well as A Wolfe, MD, for revising the manuscript.

Competing interests
The authors declare that they have no competing interests related to this manuscript.

References

1. Epstein SK. Decision to extubate. Intensive Care Med. 2002;28(5):535–46.
2. Esteban A, Anzueto A, Frutos F, Alia I, Brochard L, Stewart TE, Benito S, Epstein SK, Apezteguia C, Nightingale P, Arroliga AC, Tobin MJ. Characteristics and outcomes in adult patients receiving mechanical ventilation: a 28-day international study. JAMA. 2002;287(3):345–55.
3. Esteban A, Frutos F, Tobin MJ, Alia I, Solsona JF, Valverdu I, Fernandez R, de la Cal MA, Benito S, Tomas R, Carriedo D, Macias S, Blanco J. A comparison of four methods of weaning patients from mechanical ventilation. Spanish Lung Failure Collaborative Group. N Engl J Med. 1995;332(6):345–50.
4. Thille AW, Cortes-Puch I, Esteban A. Weaning from the ventilator and extubation in ICU. Curr Opin Crit Care. 2013;19(1):57–64.
5. Thille AW, Harrois A, Schortgen F, Brun-Buisson C, Brochard L. Outcomes of extubation failure in medical intensive care unit patients. Crit Care Med. 2011;39(12):2612–8.
6. Vallverdu I, Calaf N, Subirana M, Net A, Benito S, Mancebo J. Clinical characteristics, respiratory functional parameters, and outcome of a two-hour T-piece trial in patients weaning from mechanical ventilation. Am J Respir Crit Care Med. 1998;158(6):1855–62.
7. Bach JR, Saporito LR. Criteria for extubation and tracheostomy tube removal for patients with ventilatory failure. A different approach to weaning. Chest. 1996;110(6):1566–71.
8. Bach JR, Goncalves MR, Hamdani I, Winck JC. Extubation of patients with neuromuscular weakness: a new management paradigm. Chest. 2010;137(5):1033–9.
9. Beuret P, Roux C, Auclair A, Nourdine K, Kaaki M, Carton MJ. Interest of an objective evaluation of cough during weaning from mechanical ventilation. Intensive Care Med. 2009;35(6):1090–3.
10. Khamiees M, Raju P, DeGirolamo A, Amoateng-Adjepong Y, Manthous CA. Predictors of extubation outcome in patients who have successfully completed a spontaneous breathing trial. Chest. 2001;120(4):1262–70.
11. Su WL, Chen YH, Chen CW, Yang SH, Su CL, Perng WC, Wu CP, Chen JH. Involuntary cough strength and extubation outcomes for patients in an ICU. Chest. 2010;137(4):777–82.
12. Smina M, Salam A, Khamiees M, Gada P, Amoateng-Adjepong Y, Manthous CA. Cough peak flows and extubation outcomes. Chest. 2003;124(1):262–8.
13. McKim DA, Hendin A, LeBlanc C, King J, Brown CR, Woolnough A. Tracheostomy decannulation and cough peak flows in patients with neuromuscular weakness. Am J Phys Med Rehabil. 2012;91(8):666–70.
14. McCool FD. Global physiology and pathophysiology of cough: ACCP evidence-based clinical practice guidelines. Chest. 2006;129(1 Suppl):48S–53S.
15. Perren A, Brochard L. Managing the apparent and hidden difficulties of weaning from mechanical ventilation. Intensive Care Med. 2013;39(11):1885–95.
16. Boles JM, Bion J, Connors A, Herridge M, Marsh B, Melot C, Pearl R, Silverman H, Stanchina M, Vieillard-Baron A, Welte T. Weaning from mechanical ventilation. Eur Respir J. 2007;29(5):1033–56.
17. Kress JP, Hall JB. ICU-acquired weakness and recovery from critical illness. N Engl J Med. 2014;370(17):1626–35.
18. Borg GA. Psychophysical bases of perceived exertion. Med Sci Sports Exerc. 1982;14(5):377–81.
19. Lofaso F, Louis B, Brochard L, Harf A, Isabey D. Use of the Blasius resistance formula to estimate the effective diameter of endotracheal tubes. Am Rev Respir Dis. 1992;146(4):974–9.
20. Salam A, Tilluckdharry L, Amoateng-Adjepong Y, Manthous CA. Neurologic status, cough, secretions and extubation outcomes. Intensive Care Med. 2004;30(7):1334–9.
21. Duan J, Liu J, Xiao M, Yang X, Wu J, Zhou L. Voluntary is better than involuntary cough peak flow for predicting re-intubation after scheduled extubation in cooperative subjects. Respir Care. 2014;59(11):1643–51.
22. Kang SW, Choi WA, Won YH, Lee JW, Lee HY, Kim DJ. Clinical Implications of Assisted Peak Cough Flow Measured with an External Glottic Control Device for Tracheostomy Decannulation in Patients with Neuromuscular Diseases and Cervical Spinal Cord Injuries: A Pilot Study. Arch Phys Med Rehabil. 2016;97(9):1509–14.
23. Mahajan RP, Singh P, Murty GE, Aitkenhead AR. Relationship between expired lung volume, peak flow rate and peak velocity time during a voluntary cough manoeuvre. Br J Anaesth. 1994;72(3):298–301.
24. Suleman M, Abaza KT, Gornall C, Kinnear WJ, Wills JS, Mahajan RP. The effect of a mechanical glottis on peak expiratory flow rate and time to peak flow during a peak expiratory flow manoeuvre: a study in normal subjects and patients with motor neurone disease. Anaesthesia. 2004;59(9):872–5.
25. Park JH, Kang SW, Lee SC, Choi WA, Kim DH. How respiratory muscle strength correlates with cough capacity in patients with respiratory muscle weakness. Yonsei Med J. 2010;51(3):392–7.
26. American Thoracic Society/European Respiratory Society. ATS/ERS statement on respiratory muscle testing. Am J Respir Crit Care. 2002;166:518–624.
27. Frutos-Vivar F, Ferguson ND, Esteban A, Epstein SK, Arabi Y, Apezteguia C, Gonzalez M, Hill NS, Nava S, D'Empaire G, Anzueto A. Risk factors for extubation failure in patients following a successful spontaneous breathing trial. Chest. 2006;130(6):1664–71.
28. Montemezzo D, Vieira DS, Tierra-Criollo CJ, Britto RR, Velloso M, Parreira VF. Influence of 4 interfaces in the assessment of maximal respiratory pressures. Respir Care. 2012;57(3):392–8.
29. Koulouris N, Mulvey DA, Laroche CM, Green M, Moxham J. Comparison of two different mouthpieces for the measurement of Pimax and Pemax in normal and weak subjects. Eur Respir J. 1988;1(9):863–7.
30. Peter JV, Moran JL, Phillips-Hughes J, Warn D. Noninvasive ventilation in acute respiratory failure—a meta-analysis update. Crit Care Med. 2002;30(3):555–62.
31. Rochwerg B, Brochard L, Elliott MW, Hess D, Hill NS, Nava S, Navalesi PMOTSC, Antonelli M, Brozek J, Conti G, Ferrer M, Guntupalli K, Jaber S, Keenan S, Mancebo J, Mehta S, Raoof SMOTTF. Official ERS/ATS clinical practice guidelines: noninvasive ventilation for acute respiratory failure. Eur Respir J. 2017;50(2):1602426.
32. Vitacca M, Ambrosino N, Clini E, Porta R, Rampulla C, Lanini B, Nava S. Physiological response to pressure support ventilation delivered before and after extubation in patients not capable of totally spontaneous autonomous breathing. Am J Respir Crit Care Med. 2001;164(4):638–41.
33. Thille AW, Boissier F, Ben-Ghezala H, Razazi K, Mekontso-Dessap A, Brun-Buisson C, Brochard L. Easily identified at-risk patients for extubation failure may benefit from noninvasive ventilation: a prospective before-after study. Crit Care (London, England). 2016;20:48.
34. Beduneau G, Pham T, Schortgen F, Piquilloud L, Zogheib E, Jonas M, Grelon F, Runge I, Nicolas T, Grange S, Barberet G, Guitard PG, Frat JP, Constan A, Chretien JM, Mancebo J, Mercat A, Richard JM, Brochard L, Group WS, The RNdd. Epidemiology of weaning outcome according to a new definition. The WIND Study. Am J Respir Crit Care Med. 2017;195(6):772–83.
35. Quintard H, l'Her E, Pottecher J, Adnet F, Constantin JM, De Jong A, Diemunsch P, Fesseau R, Freynet A, Girault C, Guitton C, Hamonic Y, Maury E, Mekontso-Dessap A, Michel F, Nolent P, Perbet S, Prat G, Roquilly A, Tazarourte K, Terzi N, Thille AW, Alves M, Gayat E, Donetti L. Intubation and extubation of the ICU patient. Anaesth Crit Care Pain Med. 2017;36(5):327–41.
36. Nardi J, Leroux K, Orlikowski D, Prigent H, Lofaso F. Home monitoring of daytime mouthpiece ventilation effectiveness in patients with neuromuscular disease. Chronic Respir Dis. 2016;13(1):67–74.

37. Lacombe M, Del Amo Castrillo L, Bore A, Chapeau D, Horvat E, Vaugier I, Lejaille M, Orlikowski D, Prigent H, Lofaso F. Comparison of three cough-augmentation techniques in neuromuscular patients: mechanical insufflation combined with manually assisted cough, insufflation-exsufflation alone and insufflation-exsufflation combined with manually assisted cough. Respir Int Rev Thorac Dis. 2014;88(3):215–22.

38. Lofaso F, Prigent H, Tiffreau V, Menoury N, Toussaint M, Monnier AF, Stremler N, Devaux C, Leroux K, Orlikowski D, Mauri C, Pin I, Sacconi S, Pereira C, Pepin JL, Fauroux B, Association Francaise Contre les Myopathies research g. Long-term mechanical ventilation equipment for neuromuscular patients: meeting the expectations of patients and prescribers. Respir Care. 2014;59(1):97–106.

39. Bach JR. Noninvasive respiratory management of patients with neuromuscular disease. Ann Rehabil Med. 2017;41(4):519–38.

40. Goncalves MR, Honrado T, Winck JC, Paiva JA. Effects of mechanical insufflation-exsufflation in preventing respiratory failure after extubation: a randomized controlled trial. Crit Care (London, England). 2012;16(2):48.

41. Thille AW, Boissier F, Ben Ghezala H, Razazi K, Mekontso-Dessap A, Brun-Buisson C. Risk factors for and prediction by caregivers of extubation failure in ICU patients: a prospective study. Crit Care Med. 2015;43(3):613–20.

20

Biomarker kinetics in the prediction of VAP diagnosis: results from the BioVAP study

Pedro Póvoa[1,2]*, Ignacio Martin-Loeches[3,4], Paula Ramirez[4,5], Lieuwe D. Bos[6], Mariano Esperatti[4,7], Joana Silvestre[1,2], Gisela Gili[3,4], Gema Goma[3,4], Eugenio Berlanga[8], Mateu Espasa[8], Elsa Gonçalves[2,9], Antoni Torres[4,7] and Antonio Artigas[3,4]

Abstract

Background: Prediction of diagnosis of ventilator-associated pneumonia (VAP) remains difficult. Our aim was to assess the value of biomarker kinetics in VAP prediction.

Methods: We performed a prospective, multicenter, observational study to evaluate predictive accuracy of biomarker kinetics, namely C-reactive protein (CRP), procalcitonin (PCT), mid-region fragment of pro-adrenomedullin (MR-proADM), for VAP management in 211 patients receiving mechanical ventilation for >72 h. For the present analysis, we assessed all ($N = 138$) mechanically ventilated patients without an infection at admission. The kinetics of each variable, from day 1 to day 6 of mechanical ventilation, was assessed with each variable's slopes (rate of biomarker change per day), highest level and maximum amplitude of variation (Δ^{max}).

Results: A total of 35 patients (25.4 %) developed a VAP and were compared with 70 non-infected controls (50.7 %). We excluded 33 patients (23.9 %) who developed a non-VAP nosocomial infection. Among the studied biomarkers, CRP and CRP ratio showed the best performance in VAP prediction. The slope of CRP change over time (adjusted odds ratio [aOR] 1.624, confidence interval [CI]$_{95\%}$ [1.206, 2.189], $p = 0.001$), the highest CRP ratio concentration (aOR 1.202, CI$_{95\%}$ [1.061, 1.363], $p = 0.004$) and Δ^{max} CRP (aOR 1.139, CI$_{95\%}$ [1.039, 1.248], $p = 0.006$), during the first 6 days of mechanical ventilation, were all significantly associated with VAP development. Both PCT and MR-proADM showed a poor predictive performance as well as temperature and white cell count.

Conclusions: Our results suggest that in patients under mechanical ventilation, daily CRP monitoring was useful in VAP prediction.

Keywords: Biomarkers, C-reactive protein, Procalcitonin, Mid-region fragment of pro-adrenomedullin, Ventilator-associated pneumonia, Clinical Pulmonary Infection Score, Diagnosis, Prediction

Background

Ventilator-associated pneumonia (VAP) is usually caused by bacteria and is the most common serious intensive care unit (ICU)-acquired infection in patients undergoing invasive mechanical ventilation [1]. The widespread implementation of several preventive measures is, at least in part, associated with the observed decrease in VAP incidence [2].

One of the most challenging problems in VAP is its correct identification, resulting from the lack of a "gold standard" method of diagnosis [1]. The commonly used criteria are too sensitive but poorly specific [3]; as a result, up to 50 % of patients diagnosed with VAP do not have the condition and up to 30 % of cases of VAP are not correctly identified [4].

The accuracy of several biomarkers in the diagnosis and management of infection, namely VAP, have been evaluated repeatedly [5–9] with soluble triggering receptor

*Correspondence: pedrorpovoa@gmail.com
[1] Polyvalent Intensive Care Unit, Centro Hospitalar de Lisboa Ocidental, São Francisco Xavier Hospital, Estrada do Forte do Alto do Duque, 1449-005 Lisbon, Portugal
Full list of author information is available at the end of the article

expressed on myeloid cells (sTREM-1), C-reactive protein (CRP) and procalcitonin (PCT) being the most frequently studied.

The majority of the published studies assessed the usefulness of a single biomarker measurement in VAP diagnosis [3, 10]. Few have studied the value of serial measurements in the assessment of VAP, either before the diagnosis or after initiation of antibiotic therapy. In addition, these studies on biomarkers present discordant results [11–14], not achieving sufficient specificity or sensitivity to be routinely employed in clinical practice.

Our hypothesis was that the course of plasma concentrations of biomarkers after endotracheal intubation and invasive mechanical ventilation could be useful in VAP prediction. With that purpose, we assessed the predictive performance of kinetics of several biomarkers, namely CRP, PCT and MR-proADM, in all non-infected patients during the first 6 days of mechanical ventilation. Besides we also assessed the diagnostic performance of a single biomarker measurement at the day of VAP diagnosis.

Methods

Study design

The BioVAP study (biomarkers in the diagnosis and management of VAP) is a prospective, multicenter, observational study, designed to evaluate the additional information biomarkers can bring in the clinical decision-making process of VAP at the bedside (NCT02078999). The ICU recruitment was by direct invitation with no financial incentive. Local hospital ethics committees approved the study design, and written informed consent was obtained from all patients or their legally authorized surrogates in accordance with local requirements.

Study subjects

During the study period (September 2008 till September 2010), all patients admitted to the participating ICU were screened for inclusion if they were mechanically ventilated for >72 h. A total of 211 included adult (>18 years) patients were divided into three groups: (1) non-infected, (2) pulmonary infection and (3) non-pulmonary infection (for details, see Fig. 1; Additional file 1). For each patient, only the first ICU admission and the first VAP episode were included in the study.

Data collection and management

Data collection included demographic data and comorbid diseases (for data management, see Additional file 1). Clinical and laboratory data, namely the reason of mechanical ventilation at ICU admission, were recorded. The Simplified Acute Physiology Score (SAPS) II [15] was calculated from the worst values within the first 24 h after ICU admission. Microbiological and clinical infectious

data were reported as well as the antibiotics prescribed, their changes and the duration of therapy. Organ dysfunctions were evaluated at ICU admission and during the duration of mechanical ventilation according to the Sequential Organ Failure Assessment (SOFA) score [16].

Day 1 (D1) was considered the day of initiation of invasive mechanical ventilation. Patients were monitored till D21, the day of successful weaning and extubation, the day of a non-VAP infection or the day of clinical diagnosis of VAP whatever arrived first (for definitions see Additional file 1).

The following clinical variables were collected daily: mechanical ventilation parameters at 08:00, American College of Chest Physicians/Society of Critical Care Medicine (ACCP/SCCM) consensus conference on sepsis criteria, simplified Clinical Pulmonary Infection Score (CPIS) [17, 18], SOFA score, daily registry of the renal support therapy, surgery (type and reason), steroids (drug, dose and reason), any ICU-acquired infection other than VAP, antibiotic therapy if applied.

Blood samples were obtained from an arterial line at ICU admission and subsequently daily every morning for the routine assessment of CRP, PCT, MR-proADM and arterial blood gases. In all patients, a quantitative tracheal aspirate (QTA) was performed at ICU admission and subsequently twice a week (Mondays–Thursdays or Tuesdays–Fridays).

Patients were followed up till death or ICU discharge as well as hospital discharge. At 90th day, a telephonic interview was performed for outcome assessment.

For the present analysis, we compared biomarker kinetics of VAP patients and non-infected controls during the first 6 days of mechanical ventilation as well as at the day of VAP diagnosis. All VAP have microbiological documentation (for definitions, see Additional file 1).

Statistical analysis

Continuous variables were expressed as mean and standard deviation (SD) or median and interquartile range (IQR) if the distribution was clearly asymmetric. Comparisons between groups were performed with two-tailed unpaired Student's t test or Mann–Whitney U tests for continuous variables according to data distribution. Fisher's exact test and Chi-square test were used to carry out comparisons between categorical variables as appropriate.

In addition to CRP evaluation, we also assessed the relative changes in CRP concentration and the CRP ratio. The relative changes were calculated in relation to D1 CRP concentration.

Time-dependent analysis of different variables from D1 to D6 of mechanical ventilation was performed with general linear models univariate repeated measures analysis using a split-plot design approach.

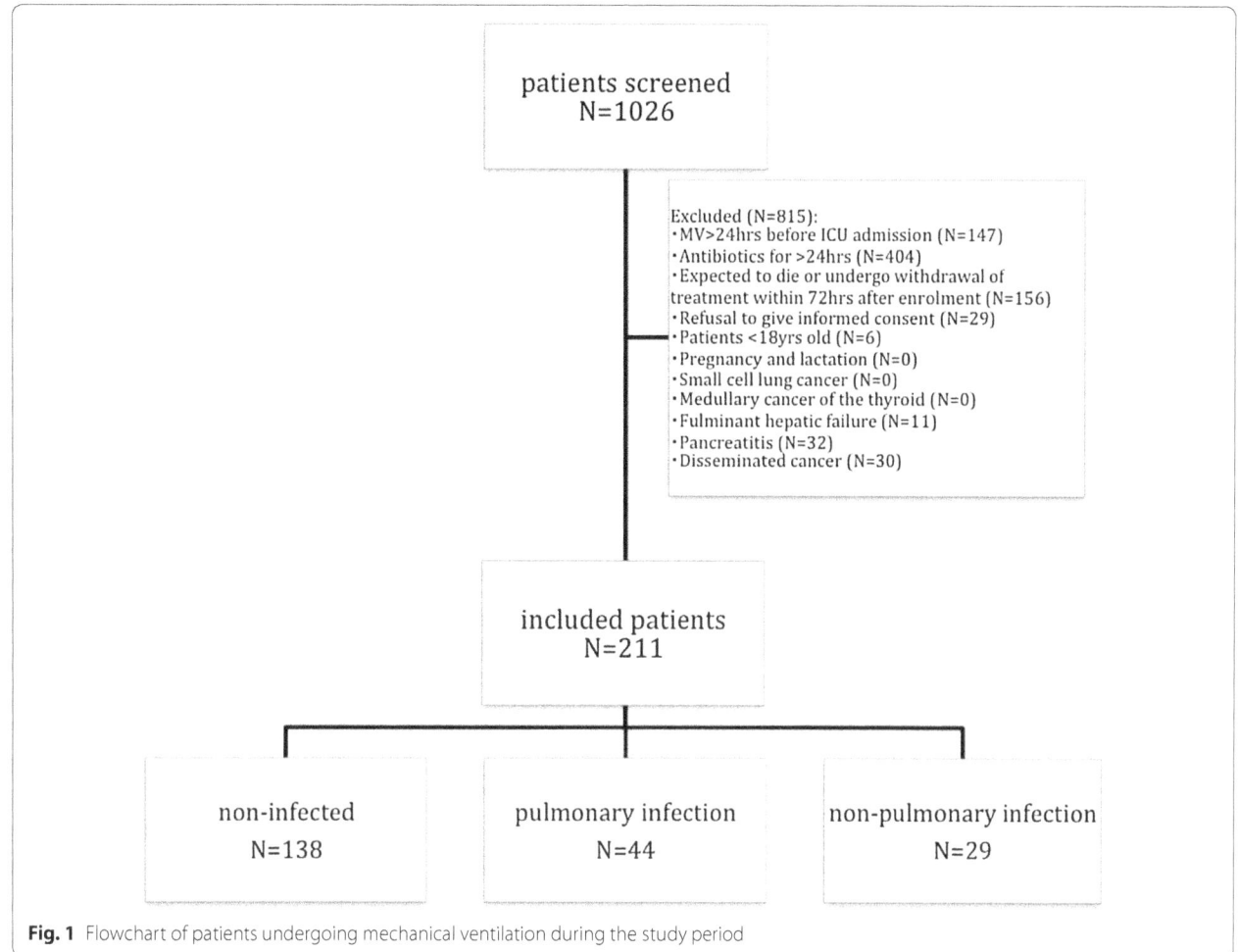

Fig. 1 Flowchart of patients undergoing mechanical ventilation during the study period

For the statistical analysis of the patient's infectious status, VAP versus non-infected controls, as function of a longitudinal covariate, obtained from the six measurements of the variables of interest between D1 and D6 (CRP, PCT, MR-proADM, white cell count (WCC), temperature and CPIS), we used a two-step approach as previously described elsewhere [19] (for additional details, see Additional file 1), in order to evaluate the slope of each variable over time (see Additional file 2: Figure S1).

Receiver operating characteristics curves (ROC) were plotted for the day of VAP diagnosis of the studied variables. The accuracy of these variables was assessed calculating its area under the curve (AUC), assessment of the best cutoff value, sensitivity and specificity calculation as well as the likelihood ratios.

Data were analyzed using PASW version 20.0 for MAC (SPSS, Chicago, IL, USA) and R (R Development Core Team: A Language and Environment for Statistical Computing. Vienna, Austria: 2005). Adjusted odds ratios (OR) with 95 % confidence interval (CI) were computed. All

statistics were two-tailed, and significance level was set at 0.05.

Results
During the study period, a total of 211 patients were included in the BioVAP study (Fig. 1). For the present analysis, we assessed all non-infected mechanically ventilated patients ($N = 138$). A total of 35 patients (25.4 %) developed VAP, 70 (50.7 %) had no infection and did not receive antibiotics (controls), and 33 (23.9 %) developed another non-VAP nosocomial infection. The last group was excluded.

The baseline patients' characteristics are presented in Table 1. At the day of initiation of mechanical ventilation, patients that develop a VAP and non-infected controls presented similar characteristics, with the two exceptions; at admission, in VAP group, CRP was significantly lower and SOFA score was significantly higher when compared with controls. From the 35 VAP episodes (35/211—25.4 %), with 41 bacterial isolates (see

Table 1 Baseline characteristics of all patients mechanically ventilated for non-infectious reasons

	Total (N = 138)	VAP (N = 35)	No infection (N = 70)	p
Male, N (%)	93 (67.4 %)	26 (74.3 %)	41 (58.6 %)	0.116
Age (years)	59.8 ± 18.4	57.9 ± 16.2	60.6 ± 20.5	0.501
SAPS II	49.1 ± 18.4	52.6 ± 18.3	49.8 ± 19.0	0.479
SOFA	7.2 ± 3.0	8.1 ± 2.9	6.8 ± 2.9	0.045
CPIS	2.6 ± 1.9	2.7 ± 2.0	2.7 ± 1.9	0.971
Cause of admission, N (%)				0.581
Medical	96 (69.6 %)	25 (71.4 %)	50 (71.4 %)	
Trauma	2 (1.4 %)	8 (22.9 %)	11 (15.7 %)	
Elective surgery	27 (19.6 %)	0	1 (1.4 %)	
Emergency surgery	13 (9.4 %)	2 (5.7 %)	8 (11.4 %)	
Comorbidities, N (%)				
COPD	19 (13.8 %)	7 (20.0 %)	6 (8.6 %)	0.119
Steroids	1 (0.7 %)		1 (1.4 %)	
Diabetes	19 (13.8 %)	3 (8.6 %)	12 (17.1 %)	0.375
Immunosuppression	3 (2.2 %)		1 (1.4 %)	
CHF	23 (16.7 %)	3 (8.6 %)	14 (20.0 %)	0.167
CLD	1 (0.7 %)	1 (2.9 %)		
CRF	9 (6.5 %)	3 (8.6 %)	6 (8.6 %)	1.0
HIV	3 (2.2 %)	1 (2.9 %)	2 (2.9 %)	1.0
Admission diagnosis, N (%)				0.501
CVA	16	6	10	
AECB	6	2	4	
Decompensated CHF	17	5	12	
TBI	19	10	9	
Others	28	14	14	
Reason of MV, N (%)				0.1
Respiratory failure	40 (29.0 %)	8 (22.9 %)	23 (32.9 %)	
Shock	17 (12.3 %)	8 (22.9 %)	5 (7.1 %)	
Coma	76 (55.1 %)	17 (48.6 %)	40 (51.7 %)	
Other	5 (3.6 %)	2 (5.7 %)	2 (2.9 %)	
Tidal volume (mL)	458 [146]	488 [97]	442 [160]	0.21
Plateau pressure (cmH$_2$O)	19 [7]	21 [9]	19 [6]	0.213
PEEP	5 [2]	5 [3]	5 [2]	0.686
PaO$_2$/FiO$_2$	245 [172]	245 [122]	224 [213]	0.828
CPR (mg/dL)	6.00 [8.62]	4.33 [6.20]	8.40 [9.39]	0.003
PCT (μg/L)	0.40 [1.76]	0.94 [2.37]	0.34 [1.48]	0.167
MR-proADM (nmol/L)	1.85 [2.64]	1.70 [2.87]	1.91 [2.82]	0.470
WCC (×10^3/mm^3)	12.46 ± 4.55	12.58 ± 4.92	11.85 ± 4.54	0.456
Temperature (°C)	36.7 ± 1.3	36.9 ± 1.3	36.4 ± 1.3	0.126
Nosocomial infection[a]	68 (49.3 %)			
VAP	35 (25.4 %)			
VAT	14 (10.1 %)			
CVC bacteremia	2 (1.4 %)			
UTI	6 (4.3 %)			
Surgical infection	5 (3.6 %)			
Other	6 (4.3 %)			
Duration of MV (days)	7.5 [9.8]	14.0 [8.0]	5.0 [5.5]	<0.001
LOS ICU (days)	12.0 [12.0]	18.0 [12.0]	10.0 [8.5]	<0.001
LOS hospital (days)	25.0 [30.3]	27.0 [31.5]	24.0 [30.5]	0.55

Table 1 continued

	Total (*N* = 138)	VAP (*N* = 35)	No infection (*N* = 70)	*p*
Mortality D28, *N* (%)	16 (18.6)	15 (40.5)	1 (2)	<0.001
Mortality D90, *N* (%)	20 (23.3)	15 (40.5)	5 (10.2)	0.004

AECB acute exacerbation of chronic bronchitis, *CHF* chronic heart failure, *CVA* cerebrovascular accident, *CLD* chronic liver disease, *COPD* chronic obstructive pulmonary disease, *simplified CPIS* Clinical Pulmonary Infection Score, *CRF* chronic renal failure, *CRP* C-reactive protein, *CVC* central venous catheter, *HIV* human immunodeficiency virus, *ICU* intensive care unit, *LOS* length of stay, *MV* mechanical ventilation, *MR-proADM* mid-region fragment of pro-adrenomedullin, *PaO₂/FiO₂* ratio of partial pressure of arterial O_2 to the fraction of inspired O_2, *PCT* procalcitonin, *PEEP* positive end-expiratory pressure, *SAPS* Simplified Acute Physiology Score, *SOFA* Sequential Organ Failure Assessment, *TBI* traumatic brain injury, *UTI* urinary tract infection, *VAP* ventilator-associated pneumonia, *VAT* ventilator-associated tracheobronchitis, *WCC* white cell count

Additional file 1), 18 were early VAP and 77.1 % were diagnosed during the first week of mechanical ventilation. The duration of mechanical ventilation till the diagnosis of VAP was (median) 5.0 days (IQR 4.0).

Kinetics of biomarkers and inflammatory variables

Figure 2 presents the variables' values during the study period from D1 to D6. The time-dependent analysis of CRP and CRP ratio was significantly different between non-infected controls and patients that went on to develop a VAP ($p < 0.001$ and $p < 0.001$, respectively). In VAP patients, we found no differences in CRP kinetics between early and late VAP ($p = 0.304$). When we compared CRP and CRP ratio at the different time points, their values were significantly higher from D5 of mechanical ventilation onwards in VAP patients. The time-dependent analysis of PCT (log transform), MR-proADM, WCC and temperature values was not significantly different between groups ($p = 0.685$, $p = 0.753$, $p = 0.681$ and $p = 0.835$, respectively).

To study the value in VAP prediction of the kinetics of each variable, we evaluated the absolute changes from D1 to D6 of mechanical ventilation assessed with the previously calculated slopes, as well the highest value and the Δ^{max}.

The slope describes the rate of change per day of a particular variable in each patient from the beginning of mechanical ventilation, that is D1, till D6. Additional file 2: Figure S1 presents some examples of predictions of individual CRP slopes that describe the CRP rate of change per day in an individual patient. Among all the studied slopes (Additional file 1), only CRP and CRP ratio were significantly different between groups ($p = 0.001$, $p < 0.001$, respectively). The slopes of CRP and CRP ratio showed a reasonable diagnostic performance with a ROC–AUC >0.7. Besides, CRP and CRP ratio were significantly associated with VAP prediction (Table 2). After adjustment for confounders, the slope of CRP was significantly associated with VAP development (aOR 1.624, CI₉₅% [1.206, 2.189], $p = 0.001$). The ability of the model to predict VAP assessed by the area under the ROC curve

was 0.71 (CI₉₅% [0.60; 0.82]). As an example, a patient with an average increase in CRP concentration of 1 mg/dL/day from D1 till D6 of mechanical ventilation has 62 % greater chance of having VAP when compared with a patient with no CRP increase. The same is shown in Fig. 3, with the CRP-slope calibration plot showing that the higher the slope, the higher the VAP probability.

We evaluated the highest value reached by a variable from the beginning of mechanical ventilation, that is D1, till D6 in VAP patients and non-infected controls. Of the studied variables (Additional file 1), only highest CRP ratio, MR-proADM and temperature were significantly different between groups ($p < 0.001$, $p = 0.014$, $p = 0.027$, respectively). However, only the highest value of CRP ratio showed a reasonable diagnostic performance with a ROC–AUC above 0.7. Moreover, the highest value of CRP ratio and MR-proADM were significantly associated with VAP prediction (Table 2). After adjustment for confounders, highest CRP ratio was significantly associated with VAP development (aOR 1.202, CI₉₅% [1.061, 1.363], $p = 0.004$). The ability of the model to predict VAP assessed by the area under the ROC curve was 0.75 (CI₉₅% [0.64; 0.87]) for the highest CRP ratio. As an example, for each 10 % increase in the highest CRP ratio concentration from D1 to D6 was associated with a 20 % greater chance of having VAP when compared with a patient with no CRP ratio change. The same is shown in Fig. 3, with the calibration plot showing that the higher the highest CRP ratio, the higher the VAP probability.

The maximum delta (Δ^{max}) evaluates the difference between the lowest and the highest value of each variable from the beginning of mechanical ventilation, that is D1, till D6 in VAP patients and non-infected controls. Of the studied variables (Additional file 1), only CRP, CRP ratio and MR-proADM were significantly different between groups ($p < 0.001$, $p < 0.001$, $p = 0.01$, respectively). The Δ^{max} of CRP showed a good diagnostic performance with a ROC–AUC >0.75 but was outperformed by Δ^{max} of CRP ratio with an ROC–AUC of 0.82. Besides, Δ^{max} of CRP and CRP ratio was significantly associated with VAP prediction (Table 2). After adjustment for confounders,

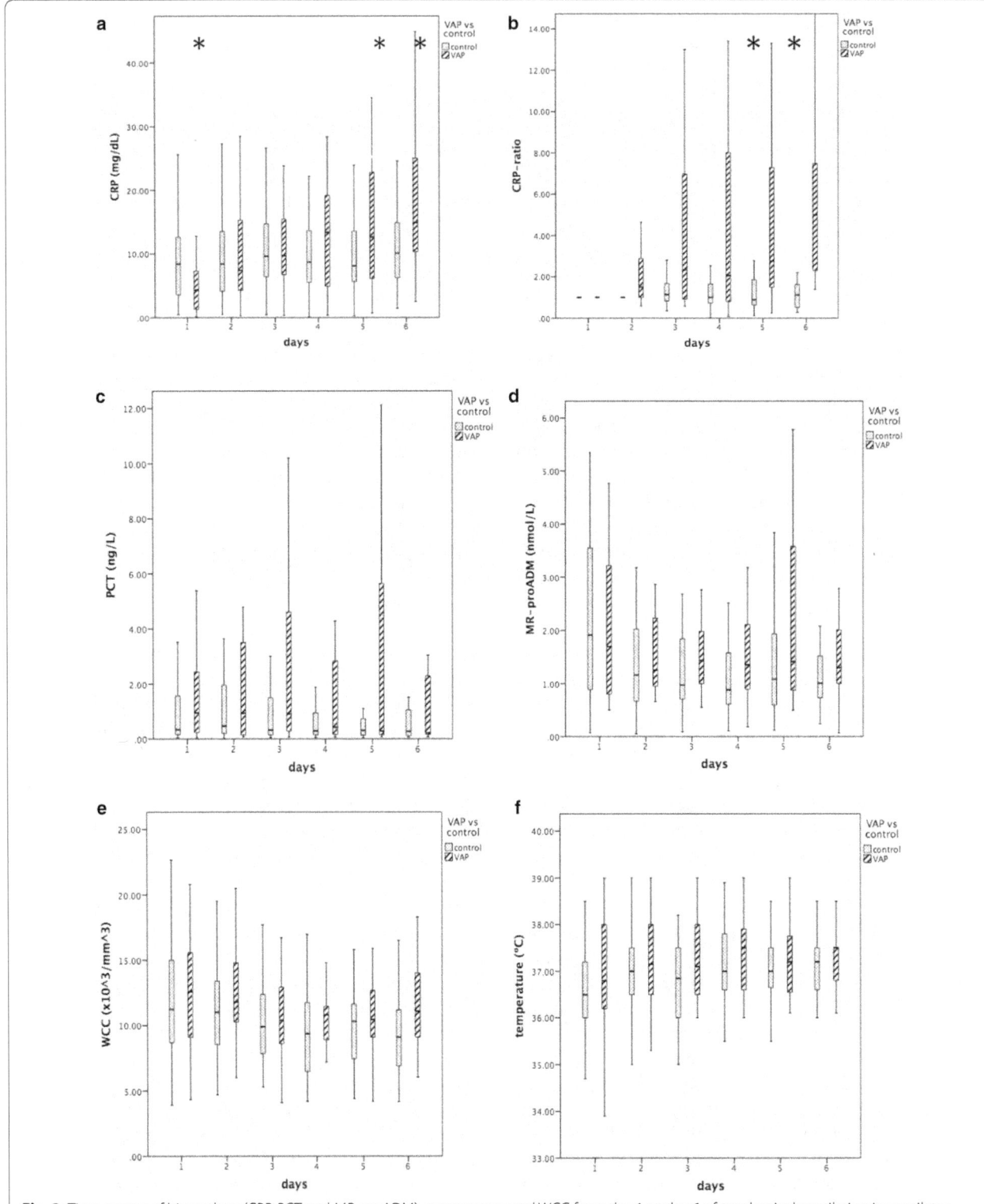

Fig. 2 Time course of biomarkers (CRP, PCT and MR-proADM), temperature and WCC from day 1 to day 6 of mechanical ventilation in ventilator-associated pneumonia (VAP) patients and non-infected controls (**a** CRP, **b** CRP ratio, **c** PCT, **d** MR-proADM, **e** WCC, **f** temperature). Time-dependent analysis of CRP, CRP ratio and CPIS was significantly different between VAP patients and controls ($p < 0.001$, $p < 0.001$ and $p = 0.019$, respectively). Some variables, namely CRP and CRP ratio, became significantly higher by day 5 in patients that will develop a VAP in comparison with controls (*$p < 0.05$). *CRP* C-reactive protein, *MR-proADM* mid-region fragment of pro-adrenomedullin, *PCT* procalcitonin, *VAP* ventilator-associated pneumonia, *WCC* white cell count

Table 2 Evaluation of studied variables in ventilator-associated pneumonia prediction

	OR	95 % CI	p	aOR	95 % CI	p
Slope						
CRP (mg/dL)	1.641	1.229–2.192	<0.001	1.624	1.206–2.189	0.001
CRP ratio	1.516	1.021–2.250	0.039	1.480	1.060–2.067	0.021
PCT (µg/L)	0.803	0.544–1.183	0.267	0.844	0.559–1.274	0.419
ADM (nmol/L)	0.740	0.147–3.742	0.716	0.730	0.137–3.902	0.713
WCC ($\times 10^3$/mm^3)	1.182	0.807–1.729	0.391	1.225	0.809–1.855	0.338
Temperature (°C)	0.288	0.033–2.540	0.262	0.270	0.028–2.590	0.256
Highest						
CRP (mg/dL)	1.044	1.000–1.090	0.052	1.037	0.992–1.085	0.11
CRP ratio	1.201	1.065–1.355	0.003	1.202	1.061–1.363	0.004
PCT (µg/L)	1.032	0.987–1.079	0.168	1.020	0.974–1.068	0.392
ADM (nmol/L)	1.335	1.022–1.744	0.034	1.369	1.035–1.809	0.028
WCC ($\times 10^3$/mm^3)	1.032	0.987–1.079	0.168	1.020	0.974–1.068	0.392
Temperature (°C)	2.043	1.170–3.536	0.012	2.053	1.126–3.744	0.019
$\Delta^{\max}$						
CRP (mg/dL)	1.151	1.057–1.252	0.001	1.139	1.039–1.248	0.006
CRP ratio	1.213	1.030–1.428	0.021	1.186	1.018–1.381	0.029
PCT (µg/L)	1.036	0.984–1.089	0.178	1.023	0.971–1.078	0.399
ADM (nmol/L)	1.395	0.964–2.020	0.078	1.372	0.943–1.996	0.099
WCC ($\times 10^3$/mm^3)	1.044	0.963–1.131	0.294	1.046	0.959–1.140	0.312
Temperature (°C)	1.020	0.665–1.565	0.928	0.933	0.583–1.494	0.772

Variables included in the adjusted model: age, sex, SAPS II, cause of admission

Simplified CPIS Clinical Pulmonary Infection Score, *CRP* C-reactive protein, *MR-proADM* mid-region fragment of pro-adrenomedullin, *OR* odds ratio, *PCT* procalcitonin, *ROC* receiver operating characteristics, *VAP* ventilator-associated pneumonia, *WCC* white cell count

$\Delta^{\max}$ of CRP was significantly associated with VAP development (aOR 1.139, CI$_{95\%}$ [1.039, 1.248], $p = 0.006$, respectively). The ability of the adjusted model to predict VAP assessed by the area under the ROC curve was 0.82 (CI$_{95\%}$ [0.73; 0.91]) for $\Delta^{\max}$ CRP. As an example, for each 1 mg/dL increment in $\Delta^{\max}$ CRP concentration from D1 to D6 of mechanical ventilation was associated with a 14 % greater chance of having VAP when compared with a patient with no CRP concentration change.

Figure 3 also shows the calibration plots of PCT (slope, highest and $\Delta^{\max}$). The inverted U-shape of the three curves clearly shows that the kinetics of PCT assessed by the slope, the highest value as well as the $\Delta^{\max}$ was not useful in VAP prediction that is far from the ideal linear correlation that is indicative of a good diagnostic marker.

Discussion

The present analysis of the BioVAP study showed that, among the studied biomarkers, only the kinetics of serial CRP measurements during the first 6 days of mechanical ventilation was useful in VAP prediction. We showed that the rate of change per day of CRP and CRP ratio, but also the highest value of CRP ratio and the maximum change in CRP and CRP ratio during the study period were all

associated with VAP prediction. In addition, at the day of VAP diagnosis we showed that a single measurement of CRP was useful in particular to exclude VAP diagnosis, whereas CPIS was better to include VAP.

In our analysis, VAP and controls presented similar baseline characteristics, with the exception of CRP, which was higher in the control group, and SOFA score, which was higher in patients that developed VAP. Our study was not designed to assess mortality or prognosis of mechanically ventilated patients but to evaluate the predictive performance for VAP of the kinetics of different biomarkers, that is to say, to identify patients with a high probability VAP, before its clinical diagnosis. To do so, we assessed the kinetics of several biomarkers during the first 6 days of mechanical ventilation to evaluate their performance in VAP prediction, not as risk factors [20].

In VAP, some studies have previously looked at PCT and/or CRP concentration changes before diagnosis. Luyt et al. [13] found that PCT, either absolute values or concentration changes in the 5 days before diagnosis, had a poor diagnostic performance for late VAP. Charles et al. [21] showed that, within the period spanning 3 days before the day of diagnosis, PCT changed only in the last 24 h but with a very good diagnostic performance. Finally,

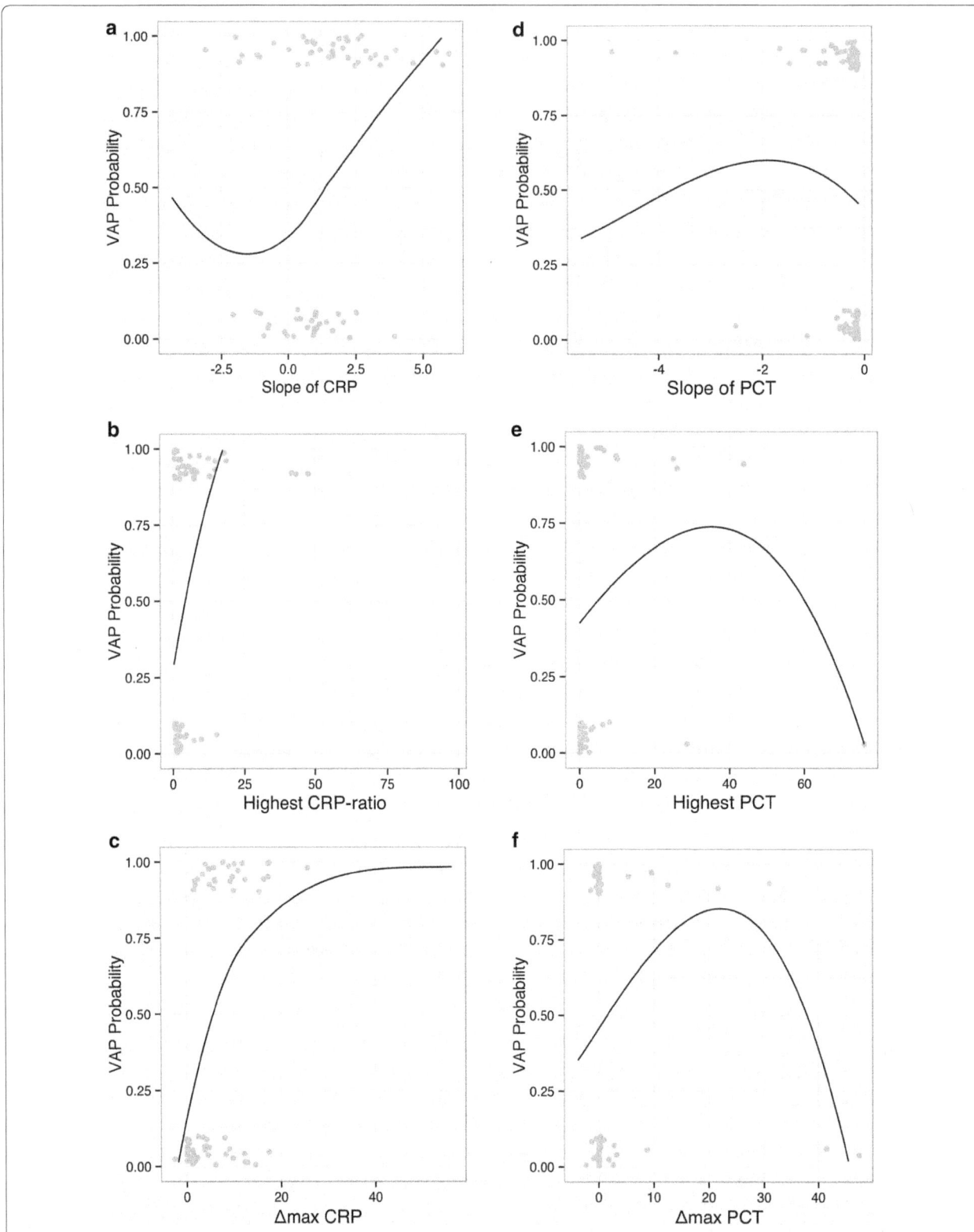

Fig. 3 Curve of disease risk probability of ventilator-associated pneumonia (VAP), for the possible range of kinetics of CRP concentration changes over time, assessed by the slope, highest value and Δ^{max} from day 1 to day 6 of mechanical ventilation (**a**–**c** CRP, **d**–**f** PCT, respectively). Ideally, the *line* should show a linear relationship between the marker and the probability of VAP. For PCT, the same calibration plots are presented (slope, highest and Δ^{max}). *CRP* C-reactive protein, *VAP* ventilator-associated pneumonia

in the diagnosis of aspiration syndromes, PCT presented a poor diagnostic performance in three studies [22–24], whereas CRP showed to be clinically helpful in the one study in which it was evaluated [22]. None of these studies performed an analysis of biomarker kinetics.

In our study, it was also clear that, from D1 to D6 of mechanical ventilation, both CRP and CRP ratio increase steadily in VAP group and became significantly higher from D5 onwards. Of the studied biomarkers, the slope of CRP was the individual variable most useful in VAP prediction. In addition, the calibration plot nicely separates those patients with low slopes and low probability of VAP from those with higher slopes and higher probability. This is particularly relevant, since monitoring the course of a single biomarker is much easier to interpret than the calculation of a score.

Besides, we also evaluated a single biomarker measurement on the day of VAP diagnosis. In doing so, we found that CRP was the best biomarker. With a similar methodology, we have previously showed that CRP presented a good performance in VAP diagnosis, and interestingly found an almost equal cutoff of 9.6 mg/dL [25].

As far as we are aware, the present study is the first using strict inclusion criteria comparing the diagnostic performance of CRP and PCT in VAP prediction. Previous studies comparing the diagnostic performance for infection of a single value of CRP and PCT in different clinical scenarios showed that, at the day of diagnosis, the AUC of CRP was always higher than of PCT [22, 26–31]. Similarly, in our study in VAP patients, CRP performed better than PCT, presenting a good negative likelihood ratio, meaning that CRP is a good biomarker to exclude that diagnosis in the presence of dubious clinical manifestations. On the opposite, the poor diagnostic performance of PCT has been attributed to the relatively low virulence of the usual microorganisms found in VAP [8, 32] as well as being considered a compartmentalized infection [32, 33].

The MR-proADM is a novel biomarker and has not yet been well evaluated in the diagnosis of infection [34], and never before in VAP. In our study, MR-proADM showed a poor diagnostic performance for VAP.

At the day of VAP diagnosis, CPIS showed to be superior to any of the studied biomarkers. It had an excellent diagnostic performance, namely a high positive likelihood ratio. Regarding CPIS, there is still controversy concerning its widespread clinical use as a surrogate of VAP diagnosis since it lacks well-done studies of validation as well as marked inter-observer variability [35]. Besides, the routine use of CPIS is time-consuming and not possible to be mentally calculated; however, in the upside, it is an inexpensive tool.

Our study has several strengths. First, this is a multicenter prospective observational study that limits the potential bias of reflecting only the practice from one center, as well as from retrospective data collection. Second, we followed a group of patients ventilated for non-infectious reasons during the first 6 days of mechanical ventilation. This way we could assess the kinetics of biomarkers in VAP prediction.

Besides, we recognize that the present study has limitations. First, the nonrandomized and observational nature of the study design bears the potential of unmeasured confounders that may have caused differences in therapeutic and supportive approach. Second, despite the use of quantitative cultures in VAP diagnosis, it is important to consider the potential false-positive and false-negative rates of quantitative cultures that could have influenced the results. Third, our findings can only be applied to non-infected patients admitted in the ICU for invasive MV and on MV for >72 h. Fourth, since measurement CRP was available daily in all centers and PCT in three centers, this could have introduced potential unmeasured bias in patient classification. Finally, it is possible that other types of patients as well as infections, not VAP, may have different biomarker time courses. Thus, the presence of non-pulmonary infections besides VAP may influence the diagnostic accuracy we report in this manuscript. Besides, our results are not applicable to patients that have a previous infection since we compared cases initially non-infected to non-infected controls.

Conclusions

In summary, we found that the combination of two cheap and widely available tools, CRP and CPIS, could be very helpful in the approach of patients undergoing mechanical ventilation with risk of VAP but always in combination with the available clinical data. On the one hand, we showed that the kinetics of CRP in the days before VAP diagnosis, namely the slope of CRP, could be useful in VAP prediction. A patient with an average increase in CRP of 1 mg/dL/day has 62 % greater chance of having a VAP when compared with a patient with no CRP increase during the first 6 days of mechanical ventilation. In addition, on the day of VAP, we could use CRP and CPIS, since CRP could be useful to exclude VAP diagnosis and CPIS to admit the diagnosis. As a result, this innovative approach needs to be further validated in different settings and with a larger sample size.

Abbreviations
AUC: area under the curve; CI: confidence interval; CPIS: Clinical Pulmonary Infection Score; CRP: C-reactive protein; ICU: intensive care unit; OR: odds ratio; MR-proADM: mid-region fragment of pro-adrenomedullin; MV: mechanical ventilation; PCT: procalcitonin; QTA: quantitative tracheal aspirate; ROC: receiver operating characteristic; SAPS: Simplified Acute Physiology Score; SOFA: Sequential Organ Failure Assessment; VAP: ventilator-associated pneumonia; WCC: white cell count.

Authors' contributions
PP conceived the study, participated in its design and coordination, participated in data analysis and drafted the manuscript. IML contributed to the
study conception and design, carried out and supervised data analysis and
helped to draft the manuscript. PR contributed to the study conception and
design and participated in data collection. LB participated in data analysis
and drafted the manuscript. ME participated in data analysis. JS contributed
to the study conception and design and participated in data collection. GG
and GG coordinated data collection. EB participated in data analysis. ME and
EG participated in data analysis and collection. AT contributed to the study
conception and design. AA conceived the study, participated in its design and
coordination, participated in data analysis and helped to draft the manuscript.
All authors read and approved the final manuscript.

Author details
[1] Polyvalent Intensive Care Unit, Centro Hospitalar de Lisboa Ocidental, São
Francisco Xavier Hospital, Estrada do Forte do Alto do Duque, 1449-005 Lis-
bon, Portugal. [2] NOVA Medical School, CEDOC, New University of Lisbon,
Lisbon, Portugal. [3] Critical Care Center, Sabadell Hospital, Corporación Sanitaria
Universitaria Parc Taulí, Universitat Autonoma de Barcelona, Sabadell, Spain.
[4] CIBER de Enfermedades Respiratorias (CIBERES), Madrid, Spain. [5] Intensive
Care Unit, University Hospital La Fe, Valencia, Spain. [6] Department of Intensive
Care, Academic Medical Center, University of Amsterdam, Amsterdam, The
Netherlands. [7] Respiratory Disease Department, Hospital Clínic i Provincial
de Barcelona, IDIBAPS, Barcelona, Spain. [8] Laboratory Department, UDIAT,
Corporación Sanitaria Universitaria Parc Taulí, Sabadell, Spain. [9] Microbiology
Department, Centro Hospitalar de Lisboa Ocidental, Egas Moniz Hospital,
Lisbon, Portugal.

Acknowledgements
We thank Dr. David Suarez as an independent biostatistician for statistical
comments and discussion of results. This study was partially supported by an
unrestricted grant from Thermo Fisher Scientific providing free of charge the
kits for PCT and MR-proADM measurement without any role in the analysis of
the data.
Institutions where the work was performed: see "Appendix."

Competing interests
PP received unrestricted research grants from Thermo Fisher Scientific. IM-L,
LB, ME, JS, GG, GG, EB, ME, EG and EG have no competing interests. PR was
invited speaker by Brahms Iberica. AT has given lectures for Brahms and had
research grants from Brahms. AA was invited as speaker in a symposium
organized by Thermo Fisher Scientific and received unrestricted research
grants from Thermo Fisher Scientific.

Appendix
Study coordinators Antonio Artigas Raventós (Area de
Críticos, Corporació Sanitaria Universitaria Parc Taulí,
Hospital de Sabadell, CIBERES, Sabadell, Spain), Pedro
Póvoa (Unidade de Cuidados Intensivos Polivalente, Hos-
pital São Francisco Xavier, Centro Hospitalar de Lisboa
Ocidental, NOVA Medical School, New University of
Lisbon, Lisbon, Portugal).

Participating intensive care units Corporación Sanitaria
Universitaria Parc Taulí, Hospital de Sabadell, Sabadell,
Spain (Ignacio Martin-Loeches, Eugenio Berlanga, Mateu

Espasa, Gisela Gili, Gemma Goma), Unidade de Cuida-
dos Intensivos Polivalente, Hospital São Francisco Xavier,
Centro Hospitalar de Lisboa Ocidental, Lisbon, Portugal
(Joana Silvestre, Elsa Gonçalves), Hospital Universitario y
Politécnico La Fe, Valencia, Spain (Paula Ramirez), Hos-
pital Clinic Provincial, Barcelona, Spain (Antoni Torres,
Mariano Esperati).

References
1. American Thoracic Society, Infectious Diseases Society of America. Guide-lines for the management of adults with hospital-acquired, ventilator-associated, and healthcare-associated pneumonia. Am J Respir Crit Care Med. 2005;171(4):388–416.
2. Alvarez Lerma F, Sanchez Garcia M, Lorente L, Gordo F, Anon JM, Alvarez J, et al. Guidelines for the prevention of ventilator-associated pneumonia and their implementation. The Spanish "Zero-VAP" bundle. Med Intensiv. 2014;38(4):226–36.
3. Rea-Neto A, Youssef NC, Tuche F, Brunkhorst F, Ranieri VM, Reinhart K, et al. Diagnosis of ventilator-associated pneumonia: a systematic review of the literature. Crit Care. 2008;12(2):R56.
4. Lisboa T, Rello J. Diagnosis of ventilator-associated pneumonia: is there a gold standard and a simple approach? Curr Opin Infect Dis. 2008;21(2):174–8.
5. Determann RM, Millo JL, Gibot S, Korevaar JC, Vroom MB, van der Poll T, et al. Serial changes in soluble triggering receptor expressed on myeloid cells in the lung during development of ventilator-associated pneumonia. Intensive Care Med. 2005;31(11):1495–500.
6. Sierra R. C-reactive protein and procalcitonin as markers of infection, inflammatory response, and sepsis. Clin Pulm Med. 2007;14:127–39.
7. Povoa P. Serum markers in community-acquired pneumonia and ventilator-associated pneumonia. Curr Opin Infect Dis. 2008;21(2):157–62.
8. Schuetz P, Albrich W, Christ-Crain M, Chastre J, Mueller B. Procalci-tonin for guidance of antibiotic therapy. Expert Rev Anti Infect Ther. 2010;8(5):575–87.
9. Prkno A, Wacker C, Brunkhorst FM, Schlattmann P. Procalcitonin-guided therapy in intensive care unit patients with severe sepsis and septic shock—a systematic review and meta-analysis. Crit Care. 2013;17(6):R291.
10. Pierrakos C, Vincent JL. Sepsis biomarkers: a review. Crit Care. 2010;14(1):R15.
11. Povoa P, Coelho L, Almeida E, Fernandes A, Mealha R, Moreira P, et al. C-reactive protein as a marker of ventilator-associated pneumonia resolu-tion: a pilot study. Eur Respir J. 2005;25(5):804–12.
12. Povoa P, Coelho L, Almeida E, Fernandes A, Mealha R, Moreira P, et al. Early identification of intensive care unit-acquired infections with daily monitoring of C-reactive protein: a prospective observational study. Crit Care. 2006;10(2):R63.
13. Luyt CE, Combes A, Reynaud C, Hekimian G, Nieszkowska A, Tonnellier M, et al. Usefulness of procalcitonin for the diagnosis of ventilator-associated pneumonia. Intensive Care Med. 2008;34(8):1434–40.
14. Jung B, Embriaco N, Roux F, Forel JM, Demory D, Allardet-Servent J, et al. Microbiogical data, but not procalcitonin improve the accuracy of the clinical pulmonary infection score. Intensive Care Med. 2010;36(5):790–8.
15. Le Gall JR, Lemeshow S, Saulnier F. A new Simplified Acute Physiology Score (SAPS II) based on a European/North American multicenter study. JAMA. 1993;270(24):2957–63.
16. Vincent JL, de Mendonca A, Cantraine F, Moreno R, Takala J, Suter PM, et al. Use of the SOFA score to assess the incidence of organ dysfunction/failure in intensive care units: results of a multicenter, prospective study. Working group on "sepsis-related problems" of the European Society of Intensive Care Medicine. Crit Care Med. 1998;26(11):1793–800.
17. Pugin J, Auckenthaler R, Mili N, Janssens JP, Lew PD, Suter PM. Diagnosis of ventilator-associated pneumonia by bacteriologic analysis of broncho-scopic and nonbronchoscopic "blind" bronchoalveolar lavage fluid. Am Rev Respir Dis. 1991;143(5 Pt 1):1121–9.
18. Luna CM, Blanzaco D, Niederman MS, Matarucco W, Baredes NC, Desmery P, et al. Resolution of ventilator-associated pneumonia: prospective evaluation of the clinical pulmonary infection score as an early clinical predictor of outcome. Crit Care Med. 2003;31(3):676–82.

19. Povoa P, Teixeira-Pinto AM, Carneiro AH, Portuguese Community-Acquired Sepsis Study Group (SACiUCI). C-reactive protein, an early marker of community-acquired sepsis resolution: a multi-center prospective observational study. Crit Care. 2011;15(4):R169.

20. Polley MY, Freidlin B, Korn EL, Conley BA, Abrams JS, McShane LM. Statistical and practical considerations for clinical evaluation of predictive biomarkers. J Natl Cancer Inst. 2013;105(22):1677–83.

21. Charles PE, Kus E, Aho S, Prin S, Doise JM, Olsson NO, et al. Serum procalcitonin for the early recognition of nosocomial infection in the critically ill patients: a preliminary report. BMC Infect Dis. 2009;9:49.

22. Schuetz P, Affolter B, Hunziker S, Winterhalder C, Fischer M, Balestra GM, et al. Serum procalcitonin, C-reactive protein and white blood cell levels following hypothermia after cardiac arrest: a retrospective cohort study. Eur J Clin Invest. 2010;40(4):376–81.

23. Mongardon N, Lemiale V, Perbet S, Dumas F, Legriel S, Guerin S, et al. Value of procalcitonin for diagnosis of early onset pneumonia in hypothermia-treated cardiac arrest patients. Intensive Care Med. 2010;36(1):92–9.

24. El-Solh AA, Vora H, Knight PR III, Porhomayon J. Diagnostic use of serum procalcitonin levels in pulmonary aspiration syndromes. Crit Care Med. 2011;39(6):1251–6.

25. Povoa P, Coelho L, Almeida E, Fernandes A, Mealha R, Moreira P, et al. C-reactive protein as a marker of infection in critically ill patients. Clin Microbiol Infect. 2005;11(2):101–8.

26. Ugarte H, Silva E, Mercan D, De Mendonca A, Vincent JL. Procalcitonin used as a marker of infection in the intensive care unit. Crit Care Med. 1999;27(3):498–504.

27. Chan YL, Tseng CP, Tsay PK, Chang SS, Chiu TF, Chen JC. Procalcitonin as a marker of bacterial infection in the emergency department: an observational study. Crit Care. 2004;8(1):R12–20.

28. Gaini S, Koldkjaer OG, Pedersen C, Pedersen SS. Procalcitonin, lipopolysaccharide-binding protein, interleukin-6 and C-reactive protein in community-acquired infections and sepsis: a prospective study. Crit Care. 2006;10(2):R53.

29. Kofoed K, Andersen O, Kronborg G, Tvede M, Petersen J, Eugen-Olsen J, et al. Use of plasma C-reactive protein, procalcitonin, neutrophils, macrophage migration inhibitory factor, soluble urokinase-type plasminogen activator receptor, and soluble triggering receptor expressed on myeloid cells-1 in combination to diagnose infections: a prospective study. Crit Care. 2007;11(2):R38.

30. Ingram PR, Inglis T, Moxon D, Speers D. Procalcitonin and C-reactive protein in severe 2009 H1N1 influenza infection. Intensive Care Med. 2010;36(3):528–32.

31. Robriquet L, Sejourne C, Kipnis E, D'herbomez M, Fourrier F. A composite score combining procalcitonin, C-reactive protein and temperature has a high positive predictive value for the diagnosis of intensive care-acquired infections. BMC Infect Dis. 2013;13(1):159.

32. Christ-Crain M, Opal SM. Clinical review: the role of biomarkers in the diagnosis and management of community-acquired pneumonia. Crit Care. 2010;14(1):203.

33. Christ-Crain M, Muller B. Biomarkers in respiratory tract infections: diagnostic guides to antibiotic prescription, prognostic markers and mediators. Eur Respir J. 2007;30:556–73.

34. Angeletti S, Battistoni F, Fioravanti M, Bernardini S, Dicuonzo G. Procalcitonin and mid-regional pro-adrenomedullin test combination in sepsis diagnosis. Clin Chem Lab Med. 2013;51(5):1059–67.

35. Zilberberg MD, Shorr AF. Ventilator-associated pneumonia: the clinical pulmonary infection score as a surrogate for diagnostics and outcome. Clin Infect Dis. 2010;51(Suppl. 1):S131–5.

21

Impact of ventilator-associated pneumonia on mortality and epidemiological features of patients with secondary peritonitis

María Heredia-Rodríguez[1,2*], María Teresa Peláez[1*], Inmaculada Fierro[3], Esther Gómez-Sánchez[1,2], Estefanía Gómez-Pesquera[1,2], Mario Lorenzo[1,2], F. Javier Álvarez-González[3], Juan Bustamante-Munguira[4], José María Eiros[2,5], Jesús F. Bermejo-Martin[2,6], José I. Gómez-Herreras[1,2] and Eduardo Tamayo[1,2]

Abstract

Background: Despite the significant impact of nosocomial infections on the morbidity and mortality of patients staying in the intensive care unit (ICU), no study over the past 20 years has focused specifically on VAP following secondary peritonitis. The objective of the present study was to determine in-hospital mortality and epidemiological features attributed to ventilator-associated pneumonia (VAP) following secondary peritonitis.

Methods: Prospective observational study involved 418 consecutive patients admitted in the ICU. Univariate and multivariate analyses were performed to identify risk factors associated with mortality and development of VAP.

Results: The incidence of VAP following secondary peritonitis was 9.6 %. Risk factors associated with the development of VAP were hospital-acquired peritonitis, requiring >48 h of mechanical ventilation, and SOFA score. The onset of VAP was late in majority of patients. VAP was developed about 16.8 days after the initiation of the peritonitis. Etiological microorganisms responsible for the peritonitis were different than for VAP. The 90-day in-hospital mortality rate was 47.5 % of VAP patients. Independent factors associated with 30- to 90-day in-hospital mortality were VAP and SOFA.

Conclusions: In light of the impact on morbidity and mortality in the ICU, more attention should be given to the concurrent features among VAP and secondary peritonitis.

Background

Intra-abdominal infections (IAIs) are one of the most important causes of mortality in the intensive care unit (ICU) [1]. Secondary peritonitis constitutes 80–90 % of cases of IAIs and is originated from the microbiological infection of the gastrointestinal tract by the perforation of hollow organs, ischemia, malignancy, and perioperative complications (anastomotic leakage, intraoperative contamination) [2, 3]. Secondary peritonitis can be classified in community-acquired and hospital-acquired, this latter associated with microorganisms presenting antibiotic resistance [2]. Mortality rate due to secondary peritonitis ranges approximately between 10 and 20 % [4–6]. During the management, the clinical outcome of the patient may be critically compromised by the development of nosocomial infections [7]. Ventilator-associated pneumonia (VAP) is a type of hospital-acquired pneumonia that is developed after at least 48 h of the patient's intubation [8]. VAP is the most frequent of the nosocomial infections occurring in the ICU, affecting to 9–27 % of all intubated patients [9]. The VAP is associated with an increased length of hospital stay, of about 4–13 days, and hospital costs [10–13]. In our knowledge, there are only in the literature three studies analyzing specifically clinical and epidemiological aspects of the development of VAP following secondary peritonitis. The first

*Correspondence: maria_her_05@hotmail.com;
mteresapelaez@gmail.com
[1] Anaesthesiology and Surgical Critical Care Department, Hospital Clínico Universitario de Valladolid, Avenida Ramón y Cajal, 3, 47005 Valladolid, Spain
Full list of author information is available at the end of the article

one was a retrospective study of 1982, which reported clinical outcomes of 143 patients with intra-abdominal abscesses, and revealing an incidence of VAP of 28.7 % of the patients, and a mortality rate attributed to VAP of 65.9 % [14]. The second one was a prospective study published in 1991 comparing clinical outcomes between nosocomial pneumonia and recurrent IAI [15]. The incidence of VAP was 19.7 % of cases, and the mortality rates were 53 % for the group of patients with pneumonia and no recurrent IAI, and 75 % of those with both conditions. Finally, the third study, of 2006, included retrospectively medical records from 618,495 patients undergoing intra-abdominal surgery [16]. From them, 13,292 patients developed subsequently pneumonia, and the mortality rate was of 10.7 %.

Although there are extensive studies analyzing secondary IAIs or VAP in the ICU, in our knowledge, studies focusing specifically on VAP following secondary peritonitis are scarce and date mainly from two decades ago. Furthermore, there are some issues that remain being characterized, such as the lapse time between the starting of the peritonitis and VAP onset, and whether or not the etiologic agents responsible for IAIs are the same that for VAP, which is critical for the selection of the empirical antibiotic therapy. Early VAP onset has been associated with better prognosis, while the late one has the highest mortality rates and is often associated with multidrug-resistant microorganisms [8]. Our working hypothesis is that pneumonia increases the mortality in patients developing peritonitis. Therefore, the objective of the study was to determine in-hospital mortality and epidemiological features attributed to VAP following secondary peritonitis.

Methods

This prospective observational study involved consecutive patients admitted in the ICU of the clinical university hospital of Valladolid between May 2008 and May 2015 for the management of a secondary peritonitis. All patients, or family members, signed the written consent form to participate in the study. The collection of respiratory and blood samples, for microbiological examinations, was required for the inclusion in the study. Patients presenting primary peritonitis or those who refused to sign the consent form were excluded from the study. One of the investigators made daily rounds in the ICU to identify eligible patients and determine the onset of VAP. Because of the observational nature of the study, investigators did not interact with ICU treating physicians for the diagnosis or management of VAP. To test our working hypothesis, the primary endpoint was to evaluate whether or not VAP patients had a higher mortality rate than non-VAP patients. Secondary endpoints included

the identification of variables potentially associated with in-hospital mortality and with the development of VAP. Procedures were performed in accordance with guidelines established by the hospital's ethics committee and the Declaration of Helsinki.

Surgical procedures and microbiological management

The surgery was performed by an experienced and trained team following the guidelines for the treatment of complicated IAIs [17]. A laparoscopy or laparotomy was performed taking into account the diagnosis and the preference of the surgeon. Peritoneal fluid was sampled to detect microbiological and mycological activity. The empirical antimicrobial therapy was started as soon as possible and consisted in the administration of amoxicillin/clavulanic acid or meropenem plus linezolid if community-acquired or hospital-acquired peritonitis, respectively. Treatment against yeast infection was only considered in the case of organ failure. Ranitidine (50 mg intravenously every 12 h) was administered for gastric protection within the first 24 h of admission in the ICU. Mouthwashes with chlorhexidine were carried out twice a day [18]. The adequacy of source control was confirmed by specialists in the ICU. The empirical antibiotic treatment for VAP was based on identifying the most common pathogens associated with VAP in the ICU, following international guidelines, including the initial empirical treatment of methicillin-resistant S. aureus with linezolid or teicoplanin and of *P. aeruginosa* with at least one of the following antibiotics: imipenem, cefepime, or piperacillin–tazobactam, in association with amikacin or ciprofloxacin [19].

Diagnosis of VAP

According to the definition of the Centers for Disease Control and Prevention, VAP was diagnosed upon the presence of new and/or progressive pulmonary infiltrates on a chest radiograph plus 2 or more of the following criteria: fever (≥ 38.5 °C) or hypothermia (< 36 °C), leukocytosis ($\geq 12 \times 10^9$/L), positive pleural fluid culture, purulent tracheobronchial secretions, or a reduction in PaO_2/FIO_2 of at least 15 % in the previous 48 h, a cavitating infiltrate, and/or evidence of bronchiolitis, neutrophilic alveolitis, and consolidation [20, 21]. The diagnosis also included those patients with a Pugin score greater than 6 [22]. The confirmation of the diagnosis included the isolation of at least one pathogenic microorganism in significant bacterial counts, i.e., $\geq 10^3$ colony-forming units (CFU)/mL for protected specimen brush, $\geq 10^4$ CFU/mL in case of bronchoalveolar lavage, and $\geq 10^5$ CFU/mL for endotracheal aspiration. These cutoffs were not modified in patients receiving antimicrobial therapy at the time of VAP diagnosis. Coagulase-negative

Staphylococcus, *Corynebacterium* spp., *Candida* spp., *Viridans* group *streptococci*, and *Neisseria* spp. were no considered pathogenic microorganisms. Special attention was given to species isolated from both peritoneal fluid and lungs.

Outcome variables and statistical analysis

In-hospital mortality (at 30 days, 30–90 days, and 90 days) was differentiated from caused by the severity of the peritonitis or intraoperative and postoperative events. Patients were evaluated for VAP during mechanical ventilation and within 48 h after extubation. Hospital-acquired infection was defined when occurred ≥48 h after admission. Early or late VAP onset was established depending on whether VAP was developed before or later the 4th day since the initiation of the peritonitis and the mechanical ventilation. Regarding the results of the antibiogram, the treatment was classified as adequate or inadequate. Multidrug resistance was considered when species showed resistance to at least three groups of antibiotics. Categorical variables were expressed as absolute and relative (%) frequencies, whereas continuous ones as the median and the standard deviation (SD) or the median and the interquartile range (IQR). Differences between groups were compared by using the t test, with continuous variables, and by Chi-square test or Fisher's exact test, with categorical ones. A univariate analysis, classifying patients in survivors and nonsurvivors, was also carried out to identify potential demographic and clinical factors associated with in-hospital mortality. Kaplan–Meier analysis was performed to compare overall survival regarding the development of VAP. Stepwise logistic regression analyses were performed to identify factors associated with in-hospital mortality and with the development of VAP (odds ratio, OR, and 95 % confidence interval, 95 % CI). Independent variables introduced in the models were carefully selected to avoid confounding effects. The statistical significance was established for $p \leq 0.05$. All statistical procedures were performed with SPSS 19.0 software.

Results

Clinical and microbiological characteristics of patients

From a total of 418 patients presenting secondary peritonitis, 40 subsequently did develop VAP (9.6 %) and 378 did not (90.4 %; Table 1). The mean lapse time between the starting of the secondary peritonitis and the development of VAP was 16.8 ± 15.1 days (community-acquired 14.6 ± 14.5 days and hospital-acquired 21.8 ± 15.7 days). The VAP onset was early in 12 patients (30.0 %) and late in 28 (70.0 %; $p < 0.001$). The mean age of patients was 71.1 ± 11.0 years for those with VAP and 70.0 ± 13.3 years for those without VAP. Septic shock

was higher in VAP patients (82.5 %) than non-VAP (61.4 %), whereas severe sepsis was opposite, 17.5 versus 38.6 % of patients, respectively. The infection was mainly hospital-acquired (70.0 %) in VAP patients, whereas community-acquired (52.1 %) in non-VAP. The main cause of peritonitis was bowel perforation in both groups (47.5 vs 43.6 %, respectively). Colon/rectum (50.0 vs 40.7 %) and small bowel (17.5 vs 19.0 %) were the most frequent locations of the peritonitis. The acute physiology and chronic health evaluation II (APACHE II) score and the Sepsis-Related Organ Failure Assessment (SOFA) score were significantly higher ($p = 0.007$ and $p < 0.001$) in VAP patients (15.95 ± 4.29 and 8.10 ± 2.50) than in non-VAP (13.65 ± 5.16 and 6.22 ± 2.46, respectively). A significantly ($p < 0.001$) higher number of VAP patients (62.5 %) received low-dose steroid therapy than non-VAP patients (25.7 %). VAP patients required significantly ($p < 0.001$) more days of mechanical ventilation (8.91 ± 14.49 days) than non-VAP (2.61 ± 6.19 days). More than 48 h of mechanical ventilation was required in a higher number of VAP patients (47.5 %) than in non-VAP (20.4 %; $p < 0.001$). The stay in the ICU and the hospital were significantly longer ($p < 0.001$) in VAP patients (median 9.0 days; IQR 7.0–30.0 days; and median 45.0 days; IQR 29.0–61.0 days, respectively) than in non-VAP (median 3.0 days; IQR 1.0–7.0 days; and median 20.0 days; IQR 11.0–34.0 days, respectively; Table 1). The most frequent species isolated from lungs of VAP patients were *Acinetobacter spp.* (45.0 % of patients), *Klebsiella spp.* (17.5 %), and *P. aeruginosa* (17.5 %) and from their peritoneal fluid were *Enterococcus spp.* (37.5 %), *E. coli* (35.0 %), *Klebsiella spp.* (25.0 %), and anaerobes (25.0 %; Table 2). All microorganisms given in Table 2 are associated with VAP. In lungs from non-VAP patients, the main species isolated were *anaerobes* (0.3 % of patients) and from their peritoneal fluid were *E. coli* (28.6 %), anaerobes (27.5 %), and *Enterococcus spp.* (24.1 %). Only three patients presented the same species in the peritoneal fluid and in lungs (two patients with *Klebsiella spp.* and one with *P. aeruginosa*; $p < 0.001$). VAP had a polymicrobial origin in four patients. None of the patients showed more than one VAP episode. Multidrug-resistant species were isolated from 25 VAP patients (62.5 %; $p = 0.02$). Regarding the antibiogram, the antibiotic treatment was therefore adequate in 22 VAP patients (55.0 %; $p = 0.37$).

Relationship between secondary peritonitis, pneumonia, and mortality

Mortality at 30 days was not different between groups and however at 90 days was significantly higher ($p = 0.008$) in VAP patients (45.0 %) than in non-VAP (5.8 %). Kaplan–Meier survival analysis revealed that the percentage of survival was different between VAP and

Table 1 Demographic and clinical characteristics 24 h after the admission in the ICU in patients presenting secondary peritonitis regarding the subsequent development of ventilator-associated pneumonia

	VAP patients ($n = 40$)	Non-VAP patients ($n = 378$)	P value
Age (mean years ± SD)	71.1 ± 11.0	70.0 ± 13.3	0.61
Sex male [n (%)]	31 (77.5)	217 (57.4)	0.014
Comorbidities [n (%)]			
Diabetes mellitus	33 (82.5)	283 (74.3)	0.02
Hypertension	21 (52.5)	194 (51.3)	0.81
Malignant neoplasm	16 (40.0)	168 (44.4)	0.63
Obesity	5 (12.5)	52 (13.8)	0.83
Chronic renal failure	5 (12.5)	34 (9.0)	0.46
Immunosuppression	1 (2.5)	13 (3.4)	
Liver disease	2 (5.0)	11 (2.9)	0.46
Acute renal failure, dialysis	2 (5.0)	7 (1.9)	
Postoperative status [n (%)]			0.001
Septic shock	33 (82.5)	232 (61.4)	
Severe sepsis	7 (17.5)	146 (38.6)	
Type of infection [n (%)]			0.007
Community-acquired	12 (30.0)	181 (47.9)	
Hospital-acquired	28 (70.0)	197 (52.1)	
Etiology of peritonitis [n (%)]			0.72
Bowel perforation	19 (47.5)	165 (43.6)	
Anastomotic leakage	6 (15.0)	74 (19.6)	
Biliary pathology	6 (15.0)	44 (11.6)	
Ischemia	3 (7.5)	34 (9.0)	
Abdominal Abscess	2 (5.0)	36 (9.5)	
Pancreatitis	4 (10.0)	18 (4.8)	
Bladder perforation	0 (0.0)	3 (0.8)	
Uterine perforation	0 (0.0)	3 (0.8)	
Vesical perforation	0 (0.0)	4 (1.1)	
Location of the peritonitis[†] [n (%)]			0.75
Colon/rectum	20 (50.0)	154 (40.7)	
Small bowel	7 (17.5)	72 (19.0)	
Biliary pathology	5 (12.5)	60 (15.9)	
Stomach and duodenum	1 (2.5)	31 (8.2)	
Pancreas	4 (10.0)	23 (6.1)	
Appendix	2 (5.0)	16 (4.2)	
Bladder	0 (0.0)	10 (2.6)	
Various	1 (2.5)	8 (2.1)	
Uterus/fallopian tubes	0 (0.0)	4 (1.1)	
Clinical score			
APACHE II (mean ± SD)	15.95 ± 4.29	13.65 ± 5.16	0.007
SOFA (mean ± SD)	8.10 ± 2.50	6.22 ± 2.46	<0.001
Postoperative management			
Low-dose steroid therapy [n (%)]	25 (62.5)	97 (25.7)	<0.001
Blood transfusions, units	3.50 ± 7.44	2.37 ± 4.89	0.192
Politransfusion (>10 units) [n (%)]	6 (15.0)	45 (11.9)	0.57
Mechanical ventilation			
Total duration (days ± SD)	8.91 ± 14.49	2.61 ± 6.19	<0.001
Patients requiring >48 h [n (%)]	19 (47.5)	77 (20.4)	<0.001
Time for VAP onset (mean days ± SD)	16.8 ± 15.1	–	

Table 1 continued

	VAP patients (*n* = 40)	Non-VAP patients (*n* = 378)	*P* value
Clinical outcome			
Stay at ICU, median days (IQR)	9.0 (7.0–30.0)	3.0 (1.0–7.0)	<0.001
Total stay at the hospital, median days (IQR)	45.0 (29.0–61.0)	20.0 (11.0–34.0)	<0.001
Mortality after 30 days [*n* (%)]	7 (17.5)	76 (20.1)	0.69
Mortality after 90 days [*n* (%)]	18 (47.5)	96 (25.4)	0.008

VAP ventilator-associated pneumonia, *SD* standard deviation, *APACHE II* Acute Physiology and Chronic Health Evaluation II, *SOFA* Sepsis-Related Organ Failure Assessment, *ICU* intensive care unit, *IQR* interquartile range

[†] In some patients, the infection extended into more than one location

Table 2 Microorganisms isolated from lungs and peritoneal fluid associated with VAP in patients with secondary peritonitis

	Lungs		Peritoneal fluid	
	VAP patients (*n* = 40)	Non-VAP patients (*n* = 378)	VAP patients (*n* = 40)	Non-VAP patients (*n* = 378)
Gram-positive cocci				
Methicillin susceptible *Staphylococcus aureus*	6 (15.0)	0 (0.0)	1 (2.5)	8 (2.1)
Methicillin-resistant *Staphylococcus aureus*	2 (5.0)	0 (0.0)	0 (0.0)	2 (0.5)
Staphylococcus epidermidis	0 (0.0)	0 (0.0)	7 (17.5)	26 (6.9)
Other *Staphylococcus* spp.	2 (5.0)	0 (0.0)	0 (0.0)	16 (4.2)
Streptococcus spp.	0 (0.0)	0 (0.0)	4 (10.0)	33 (8.7)
Enterococcus spp.	1 (2.5)	0 (0.0)	15 (37.5)	91 (24.1)
Other	0 (0.0)	0 (0.0)	4 (10.0)	10 (2.6)
Gram-negative bacilli				
Klebsiella spp.	7 (17.5)	0 (0.0)	10 (25.0)	27 (7.1)
Enterobacter spp.	1 (2.5)	0 (0.0)	6 (15.0)	25 (6.6)
Escherichia coli	4 (10.0)	0 (0.0)	14 (35.0)	108 (28.6)
Pseudomonas aeruginosa	7 (17.5)	0 (0.0)	6 (15.0)	3 (0.8)
Acinetobacter spp.	18 (45.0)	1 (0.3)	2 (5.0)	5 (1.3)
Other *Enterobacteriaceae*	2 (5.0)	0 (0.0)	0 (0.0)	8 (2.1)
Anaerobes	1 (2.5)	1 (0.3)	10 (25.0)	104 (27.5)

Percentages may sum more than 100 % because more than one pathogen could have been found in an individual patient

non-VAP patients (log rank = 5.289; *p* = 0.021; Fig. 1), indicating higher values for non-VAP patients. Both survival curves diverged after the day 40th of admission in the ICU.

Factors associated with in-hospital mortality and development of VAP

By classifying patients in survivors (*n* = 304, 72.7 %) and nonsurvivors (*n* = 114, 27.3 %), the univariate analysis demonstrated that in-hospital mortality was significantly associated with 19 demographic or clinical variables (Table 3). The logistic regression model indicated that independent factors associated with 30-day in-hospital mortality were age (OR 1.038; CI 95 % 0.003–1.013;

p = 0.003), SOFA (OR 1.329, CI 95 % 0.0001–1.171; *p* < 0.001), and severe sepsis/septic shock (OR 3.105; CI 95 % 0.013–1.271; *p* = 0.013). Stepwise logistic regression model to identify independent factors associated with in-hospital mortality at 30, 30–90, and 90 days in patients with secondary peritonitis is given in Table 4. Independent factors associated with 30- to 90-day in-hospital mortality were SOFA (OR 1.373, CI 95 % 0.0001–1.151; *p* < 0.001), and VAP (OR 3.777, CI 95 % 0.006–1.475; *p* = 0.006). Factors associated with 90-day in-hospital mortality were age (OR 1.036; CI 95 % 0.002–1.013; *p* = 0.002), SOFA (OR, 1.247, CI 95 % 0.006–1.065; *p* = 0.006), creatinine (OR 1.351; CI 95 % 0.042–1.011; *p* = 0.042), and severe sepsis/septic shock (OR 2.967;

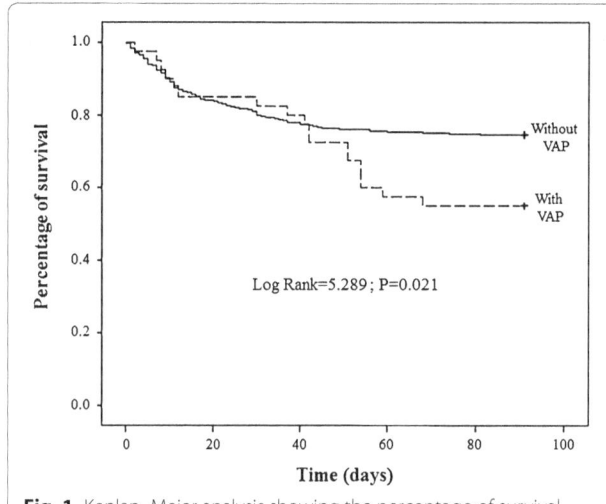

Fig. 1 Kaplan–Meier analysis showing the percentage of survival between patients with and without ventilator-associated pneumonia

CI 95 % 0.004–1.402; $p = 0.004$). Finally, independent factors associated with the development of VAP were hospital-acquired peritonitis (OR 2.873; CI 95 % 1.299–6.369; $p = 0.009$), SOFA (OR 1.325; CI 95 % 1.126–1.559;

$p = 0.001$), and requiring >48 h of mechanical ventilation (OR 2.359; CI 95 % 1.074–5.181; $p = 0.032$).

Discussion

Despite the significant impact of nosocomial infections on morbidity and mortality of patients staying in the ICU, no study over the last 20 years has determined the clinical, epidemiological, and microbiological features of VAP following secondary peritonitis. Therefore, the goal of the present study was to complete and update such lacking information. The most relevant results from our study included: (1) an updated incidence value of VAP of 9.6 %; (2) risk factors associated with the development of VAP including hospital-acquired peritonitis, requiring >48 h of mechanical ventilation, and SOFA score; (3) mainly late onset of VAP, and caused by multidrug-resistant microorganisms intrinsically different for each condition; (4) the 90-day in-hospital mortality rate of 47.5 % of VAP patients; and (5) independent factors associated with 30- to 90-day in-hospital mortality including VAP and SOFA score.

Overall incidence of VAP reported in our study was 9.6 % of patients who underwent surgery due to

Table 3 Significant demographic and clinical variables potentially associated with in-hospital mortality

	Nonsurvivors (n = 114)	Survivors (n = 304)	P value
Age (mean years ± SD)	74.69 ± 10.43	68.38 ± 13.58	0.006
Comorbidities [n (%)]			
Chronic renal failure	21 (18.4)	18 (5.9)	<0.001
Acute renal failure, dialysis	3 (2.6)	6 (2.0)	<0.001
Immunosuppression	11 (9.6)	4 (1.3)	<0.001
Postoperative status			0.001
Severe sepsis	12 (10.5)	139 (45.7)	
Septic shock	100 (87.7)	163 (53.6)	
Biochemical parameters at ICU (mean ± SD)			
Sodium (mEq/L)	137.64 ± 6.8	136.05 ± 4.81	<0.001
Creatinine (mg/dL)	2.18 ± 1.71	1.21 ± 0.77	<0.001
Lactate (mmol/L)	34.90 ± 26.16	24.13 ± 19.28	0.005
Procalcitonin (ng/mL)	24.48 ± 36.42	16.27 ± 30.28	0.043
HCO_3^- (mEq/L)	20.42 ± 7.28	21.73 ± 5.52	0.030
Postoperative management			
Low-dose steroid therapy	25 (21.9)	97 (31.9)	<0.001
Blood transfusions, units	4.43 ± 6.90	1.74 ± 4.16	<0.001
Politransfusion (>10 units) [n (%)]	26 (22.8)	25 (8.2)	<0.001
Mechanical ventilation			
Total duration (days ± SD)	7.38 ± 11.70	1.69 ± 4.48	<0.001
Patients requiring >48 h [n (%)]	50 (43.9)	46 (15.1)	<0.001
Clinical outcome			
Stay at ICU, median days (IQR)	8.0 (3.8–14.3)	3.0 (1.0–6.0)	<0.001
Total stay at the hospital, median days (IQR)	21.0 (9.3–43.8)	21.0 (12.3–35.0)	0.004
VAP	18 (15.8)	22 (7.2)	0.008

SD standard deviation, *ICU* intensive care unit, HCO_3^- bicarbonate, *VAP* ventilator-associated pneumonia, *IQR* interquartile range

Table 4 Logistic regression models to identify factors associated with in-hospital mortality and with the development of VAP

	OR	95 % CI	P value
In-hospital mortality			
30-day in-hospital mortality			
Age (years)	1.038	1.013–1.064	0.003
SOFA score	1.329	1.171–1.510	<0.001
Severe sepsis/septic shock	3.105	1.271–7.588	0.013
30- to 90-day in-hospital mortality			
SOFA score	1.373	1.151–1.637	<0.001
VAP	3.777	1.475–9.671	0.006
90-day in-hospital mortality			
Age (years)	1.036	1.013–1.060	0.002
SOFA score	1.247	1.065–1.461	0.006
Creatinine (mg/dL)	1.351	1.011–1.805	0.042
Severe sepsis/septic shock	2.967	1.402–6.278	0.004
Development of VAP			
Hospital-acquired peritonitis	2.873	1.299–6.369	0.009
SOFA score	1.325	1.126–1.559	0.001
Requiring >48 h of mechanical ventilation	2.359	1.074–5.181	0.032

OR odds ratio, *CI* confidence interval, *SOFA* Sepsis-Related Organ Failure Assessment, *VAP* ventilator-associated pneumonia

peritonitis, a value significantly lower than previous studies, ranging between 20 and 30 % [14, 15]. A possible explanation may derive from the fact that, in our study, VAP included both hospital- and community-acquired cases; however, previous studies only included hospital-acquired cases, which are associated with higher incidence rates. Moreover, the reduction in the impact of VAP over the years may be a result of the implementation of effective preventive strategies in the ICU, such as the Spanish national VAP prevention bundle called "zero VAP," based on good general practices for control of the infection and pathogenic-tailored strategies [23, 24]. The International Nosocomial Infection Control Consortium reported a decrease in incidence from 15 to 8 % in a surveillance study conducted from 2004 to 2009 [25, 26].

There are many factors potentially associated with the development of VAP, including preexisting medical conditions in the patient (such as immunosuppression or chronic obstructive lung disease), body position, level of consciousness, nasotracheal intubation, duration of the mechanical ventilation, ventilator circuit-related factors, enteral nutrition, or personnel-related factors (such as inadequate hand hygiene or change in gloves between patients) [12, 27, 28]. In our study, hospital-acquired peritonitis, requiring >48 h of mechanical ventilation, and SOFA score were independent factors for VAP development. The duration of ventilation has been positively

correlated with the development of VAP, although this potential risk seems not to be constant over the time [12]. Specifically, the risk of VAP has been estimated in 3 % per day during the first week of mechanical ventilation, 2 % in the second week, and 1 % in the subsequent weeks [27]. A high SOFA score at admission in the ICU has been associated with mortality in VAP patients [29]; for this reason, a high score in multiple organ dysfunction, concomitant with a probably immunosuppression status and/or other underlying medical conditions, may be a cause for the development of such opportunistic infection. Similarly, hospital-acquired peritonitis is associated with microorganisms presenting antibiotic resistance, poor outcomes, and longer stays in the hospital, compared with community-acquired peritonitis, which may explain its correlation with the development of VAP [2].

The onset of VAP was late in the majority of patients. More than 90 % of cases of VAP occur within the first 10 days of the intubation [30]. VAP was also developed about 16.8 days after the initiation of the peritonitis. A high percentage of the microorganisms responsible of VAP were multidrug resistant (62.5 %). Regarding the antibiogram, almost half of patients (55.0 %) received an adequate treatment. The low number of patients receiving adequate antibiotic treatment may be a consequence of: (1) the late onset of pneumonia (16.8 ± 15.1 days) since the initiation of the peritonitis. At this time, patients had received other antibiotic treatments for the peritonitis. (2) the peritonitis was the primary target of the antibiotic treatment; VAP was not so. It has been demonstrated that patients who receive inadequate empiric antibiotic treatment have longer hospital stays, higher rates of abscesses, and mortality [31]. For this reason, attention should be given to the antibiogram of each respective center, selecting adequate antibiotics taken into account potential multidrug-resistant microorganisms [1]. The high rate of multidrug resistance found in our study may be correlated with the higher proportion of patients presenting late-onset VAP. In general, etiological microorganisms responsible for the peritonitis were different than for VAP, which is consistent with previous studies [6].

According to published studies, mortality rates attributable to VAP range between 53 and 75 % [14, 15]. Since clinical outcomes depend on the length of the stay in the ICU, one goal of our study was to investigate differences in in-hospital mortality at different endpoints (30, 30–90, and 90 days). VAP patients showed a significant higher mortality rate and longer hospital stay than non-VAP. The 90-day mortality was 47.5 % of VAP patients, a value slightly lower than previous studies. Similar to the incidence, there is a decreasing tendency in the mortality rate as a result of the implementation of preventive strategies [22, 25]. In our study, the mortality rate was actually quite high, even in the non-VAP cohort, for secondary peritonitis. The recent multicenter STOP-IT trial has reported a mortality rate of 1.2 % for patients with complicated intra-abdominal infection [32]. Although this study cohort did have a much higher rate of septic shock and severe sepsis than that our study, most recent severe sepsis and septic shock studies have reported mortality rates of approximately 25 %. Risk factors associated with in-hospital mortality included VAP and SOFA score, although the univariate analysis revealed both VAP and stay at ICU as significant risk factors associated with mortality. VAP was only significant for 30- to 90-day in-hospital mortality. According to the literature, the development of VAP is associated with the percentage of nonsurvivors and survivors in a rate 2:1. It is interesting to note that Kaplan–Meier curves showed a significant divergence in survival likelihood since approximately the day 40th after admission in the ICU. Among the extensive studies evaluating the risk factors associated with worse outcomes and mortality for secondary peritonitis [31, 33–35], none of them have included VAP in their analyses. One possible reason to omit it might derive from the fact that VAP is intrinsically associated with the stay in the ICU, whatever the underlying condition of the patient. Nevertheless, results of our study highlight the importance of including VAP as a factor involved in the 30- to 90-day in-hospital mortality of patient with secondary peritonitis. Our present study had some limitations. One of them was that the study was performed in a single center. A multicenter study might have strengthen results obtained in the study and have reduced factors intrinsically associated with the center, such as the empiric antibiotic treatment or the spectrum of nosocomial pathogenic microorganisms. Another limitation of the study was the low number of patients developing VAP (40). Although similar to the sample size of the literature, a large cohort of patients might also have strengthen our results and diminish interindividual differences.

Conclusion

In light of the impact on morbidity and mortality in the ICU, more attention should be given to the concurrent features among VAP and secondary peritonitis. Additional prospective studies, involving large cohort of patients, are required to corroborate these results.

Author details
[1] Anaesthesiology and Surgical Critical Care Department, Hospital Clínico Universitario de Valladolid, Avenida Ramón y Cajal, 3, 47005 Valladolid, Spain. [2] Group of Biomedical Research in Critical Care Medicine (BioCritic), Hospital Clínico Universitario de Valladolid, Valladolid, Spain. [3] Department of Pharmacology and Therapeutics, Faculty of Medicine, University of Valladolid, Valladolid, Spain. [4] Department of Cardiovascular Surgery, Hospital Universitario de La Princesa, Madrid, Spain. [5] Department of Microbiology, Faculty of Medicine, University of Valladolid, Valladolid, Spain. [6] Investigación Médica en Infección e Inmunidad (IMI), Hospital Clínico Universitario de Valladolid-IECSCYL, Valladolid, Spain.

Acknowledgements
Authors would like to express thankfulness to the nurses from our ICU. Authors would also like to thank to Patricia Ortega and Pablo Vivanco (PhD, Meisys) for helping in the elaboration of the manuscript.

Competing interests
The authors declare that they have no competing interests.

References
1. Lopez N, Kobayashi L, Coimbra R. A comprehensive review of abdominal infections. World J Emerg Surg. 2011;6:7.
2. Eckmann C, Dryden M, Montravers P, Kozlov R, Sganga G. Antimicrobial treatment of "complicated" intra-abdominal infections and the new IDSA guidelines? A commentary and an alternative European approach according to clinical definitions. Eur J Med Res. 2011;16(3):115–26.
3. Laroche M, Harding G. Primary and secondary peritonitis: an update. Eur J Clin Microbiol Infect Dis. 1998;17(8):542–50.
4. McClean KL, Sheehan GJ, Harding GK. Intraabdominal infection: a review. Clin Infect Dis. 1994;19(1):100–16.
5. Gauzit R, Péan Y, Barth X, Mistretta F, Lalaude O, Top Study Team. Epidemiology, management, and prognosis of secondary non-postoperative peritonitis: a French prospective observational multicenter study. Surg Infect (Larchmt). 2009;10(2):119–27.
6. Jang JY, Lee SH, Shim H, Choi JY, Yong D, Lee JG. Epidemiology and microbiology of secondary peritonitis caused by viscus perforation: a single-center retrospective study. Surg Infect (Larchmt). 2015;16(4):436–42.
7. Koenig SM, Truwit JD. Ventilator-associated pneumonia: diagnosis, treatment, and prevention. Clin Microbiol Rev. 2006;19(4):637–57.
8. American Thoracic Society. Infectious Diseases Society of America. Guidelines for the management of adults with hospital-acquired, ventilator-associated, and healthcare-associated pneumonia. Am J Respir Crit Care Med. 2005;171(4):388.
9. Tamayo E, Álvarez FJ, Martínez-Rafael B, Bustamante J, Bermejo-Martin JF, Fierro I, et al. Ventilator-associated pneumonia is an important risk factor for mortality after major cardiac surgery. J Crit Care. 2012;27(1):18–25.
10. Kappstein I, Schulgen G, Beyer U, Geiger K, Schumacher M, Daschner FD. Prolongation of hospital stay and extra costs due to ventilator-associated pneumonia in an intensive care unit. Eur J Clin Microbiol Infect Dis. 1992;11(6):504–8.
11. Heyland DK, Cook DJ, Griffith L, Keenan SP, Brun-Buisson C. The attributable morbidity and mortality of ventilator-associated pneumonia in the critically ill patient. Am J Respir Crit Care Med. 1999;159(4):1249–56.
12. Bonten MJ, Kollef MH, Hall JB. Risk factors for ventilator-associated pneumonia: from epidemiology to patient management. Clin Infect Dis. 2004;38(8):1141–9.
13. Safdar N, Dezfulian C, Collard HR, Saint S. Clinical and economic consequences of ventilator associated pneumonia: a systematic review. Crit Care Med. 2005;33(10):2184–93.
14. Richardson JD, DeCamp MM, Garrison RN, Fry DE. Pulmonary infection complicating intra-abdominal sepsis: clinical and experimental observations. Ann Surg. 1982;195(6):732–8.
15. Mustard RA, Bohnen JM, Rosati C, Schouten BD. Pneumonia complicating abdominal sepsis: an independent risk factor for mortality. Arch Surg. 1991;126(2):170–5.
16. Thompson DA, Makary MA, Dorman T, Pronovost PJ. Clinical and economic outcomes of hospital acquired pneumonia in intra-abdominal surgery patients. Ann Surg. 2006;243(4):547–52.
17. Solomkin JS, Mazuski JE, Bradley JS, et al. Diagnosis and management of complicated intra-abdominal infection in adults and children: guidelines by the Surgical Infection Society and the Infectious Diseases Society of America. Clin Infect Dis. 2010;50:133–64.
18. Marshall JC, Maier RV, Jimenez M, Dellinger EP. Source control in the management of severe sepsis and septic shock: an evidence-based review. Crit Care Med. 2004;32(11):513–26.
19. Ibrahim EH, Ward S, Sherman G, Schaiff R, Fraser VJ, Kollef MH. Experience with a clinical guideline for the treatment of ventilator-associated pneumonia. Crit Care Med. 2001;29(6):1109–15.
20. Garner JS, Jarvis WR Emori TG, et al. CDC definitions for nosocomial infections. Am J Infect Control. 1988;16(4):128–40.

21. Medford AR, Husain SA, Turki HM, Millar AB. Diagnosis of ventilator-associated pneumonia. J Crit Care. 2009;24(473):e1–6.

22. Luna CM, Blanzaco D, Niederman MS, Matarucco W, Baredes NC, Desmery P, et al. Resolution of ventilator-associated pneumonia: prospective evaluation of the clinical pulmonary infection score as an early clinical predictor of outcome. Crit Care Med. 2003;31(3):676–82.

23. Mietto C, Pinciroli R, Patel N, Berra L. Ventilator associated pneumonia: evolving definitions and preventive strategies. Respir Care. 2013;58(6):990–1007.

24. Lerma FA, García MS, Lorente L, Gordo F, Añón JM, Álvarez J, et al. Guidelines for the prevention of ventilator-associated pneumonia and their implementation. The Spanish "Zero-VAP" bundle. Med Intensiva. 2014;38(4):226–36.

25. Rosenthal VD, Bijie H, Maki DG, Mehta Y, Apisarnthanarak A, Medeiros EA, et al. International Nosocomial Infection Control Consortium (INICC) report, data summary of 36 countries, for 2004–2009. Am J Infect Control. 2012;40(5):396–407.

26. Lorente L, Blot S, Rello J. Evidence on measures for the prevention of ventilator-associated pneumonia. Eur Respir J. 2007;30(6):1193–207.

27. Augustyn B. Ventilator-associated pneumonia: risk factors and prevention. Crit Care Nurse. 2007;27(4):32–9.

28. Cook DJ, Walter SD, Cook RJ, Griffith LE, Guyatt GH, Leasa D, et al. Incidence of and risk factors for ventilator-associated pneumonia in critically ill patients. Ann Intern Med. 1998;129(6):433–40.

29. Boeck L, Eggimann P, Smyrnios N, Pargger H, Thakkar N, Siegemund M, et al. The Sequential Organ Failure Assessment score and copeptin for predicting survival in ventilator-associated pneumonia. J Crit Care. 2012;27(5):523.e1–29.

30. Koulenti D, Lisboa T, Brun-Buisson C, Krueger W, Macor A, Sole-Violan J, et al. Spectrum of practice in the diagnosis of nosocomial pneumonia in patients requiring mechanical ventilation in European intensive care units. Crit Care Med. 2009;37(8):2360–8.

31. Montravers P, Gauzit R, Muller C, Marmuse JP, Fichelle A, Desmonts JM. Emergence of antibiotic-resistant bacteria in cases of peritonitis after intraabdominal surgery affects the efficacy of empirical antimicrobial therapy. Clin Infect Dis. 1996;23(3):486–94.

32. Sawyer RG, Claridge JA, Nathens AB, Rotstein OD, Duane TM, Evans HL, et al. Trial of short-course antimicrobial therapy for intraabdominal infection. N Engl J Med. 2015;372(21):1996–2005.

33. Mulier S, Penninckx F, Verwaest C, Filez L, Aerts R, Fieuws S, Lauwers P. Factors affecting mortality in generalized postoperative peritonitis: multivariate analysis in 96 patients. World J Surg. 2003;27(4):379–84.

34. Riché FC, Dray X, Laisné MJ, Matéo J, Raskine L, Sanson-Le Pors MJ, et al. Factors associated with septic shock and mortality in generalized peritonitis: comparison between community-acquired and postoperative peritonitis. Crit Care. 2009;13(3):99.

35. Inui T, Haridas M, Claridge JA, Malangoni MA. Mortality for intra-abdominal infection is associated with intrinsic risk factors rather than the source of infection. Surgery. 2009;146(4):654–62.

22

Prolonged prone positioning under VV-ECMO is safe and improves oxygenation and respiratory compliance

Antoine Kimmoun[1,2,3], Sylvain Roche[1], Céline Bridey[1], Fabrice Vanhuyse[2,3,5], Renaud Fay[6], Nicolas Girerd[6], Damien Mandry[3,4] and Bruno Levy[1,2,3]*

Abstract

Background: Data are sparse regarding the effects of prolonged prone positioning (PP) during VV-ECMO. Previous studies, using short sessions (<12 h), failed to find any effects on respiratory system compliance. In the present analysis, the effects of prolonged PP sessions (24 h) were retrospectively studied with regard to safety data, oxygenation and respiratory system compliance.

Methods: Retrospective review of 17 consecutive patients who required both VV-ECMO and prone positioning. PP under VV-ECMO was considered when the patient presented at least one unsuccessful ECMO weaning attempt after day 7 or refractory hypoxemia combined or not with persistent high plateau pressure. PP sessions had a duration of 24 h with fixed ECMO and respiratory settings. PP was not performed in patients under vasopressor treatment and in cases of recent open chest cardiac surgery.

Results: Despite optimized protective mechanical ventilation and other adjuvant treatment (i.e. PP, inhaled nitric oxide, recruitment maneuvers), 44 patients received VV-ECMO during the study period for refractory acute respiratory distress syndrome. Global survival rate was 66 %. Among the latter, 17 patients underwent PP during VV-ECMO for a total of 27 sessions. After 24 h in prone position, PaO_2/FiO_2 ratio significantly increased from 111 (84–128) to 173 (120–203) mmHg ($p < 0.0001$) while respiratory system compliance increased from 18 (12–36) to 32 (15–36) ml/cmH$_2$O ($p < 0.0001$). Twenty-four hours after the return to supine position, tidal volume was increased from 3.0 (2.2–4.0) to 3.7 (2.8–5.0) ml/kg ($p < 0.005$). PaO_2/FiO_2 ratio increased by over 20 % in 14/14 sessions for late sessions ($\geq$7 days) and in 7/13 sessions for early sessions (<7 days) ($p = 0.01$). Quantitative CT scan revealed a high percentage of non-aerated or poorly-aerated lung parenchyma [52 % (41–62)] in all patients. No correlation was found between CT scan data and respiratory parameter changes. Hemodynamics did not vary and side effects were rare (one membrane thrombosis and one drop in ECMO blood flow).

Conclusion: When used in combination with VV-ECMO, 24 h of prone positioning improves both oxygenation and respiratory system compliance. Moreover, our study confirms the absence of serious adverse events.

Keywords: ARDS, ECMO, Prone positioning

Background

One year after the publication of the PROSEVA study, the association of prone positioning (PP) and lung-protective

*Correspondence: b.levy@chu-nancy.fr
[1] CHU Nancy, Service de Réanimation Médicale Brabois, Pole Cardiovasculaire et Réanimation Médicale, Hôpital Brabois, 54511 Vandoeuvre les Nancy, France
Full list of author information is available at the end of the article

ventilation has become routine management for patients with acute respiratory distress syndrome (ARDS) [1]. However, refractory ARDS is still observed in all recent observational and randomized trials [1–3]. In these cases, veno-venous extra-corporeal membrane oxygenation (VV-ECMO) is indicated while awaiting lung function recovery [4]. Indeed, in the CESAR trial, a protocol including VV-ECMO was associated with a decreased mortality rate when compared to a conventional lung protective strategy [2].

The management of persistent severe hypoxemia under VV-ECMO requires a multi-step clinical approach including the optimization of VV-ECMO blood flow, red blood cell transfusion, moderate hypothermia, optimization of native lung function, short-action beta-blockers and finally PP [5]. PP can be effective in patients with VV-ECMO given that the use of ultra-protective ventilation [i.e. 3–4 mL/kg Vt] may increase the proportion of poorly-aerated areas in dependent lung regions [6]. As a result, PP during VV-ECMO may recruit the dorsal regions of the lungs, facilitate lung drainage and therefore improve oxygenation. The value of PP during VV-ECMO has furthermore been previously described in a few studies, the largest being a study by Guervilly et al. in which 12 h of PP significantly improved the PaO_2/FiO_2 ratio in 15 ARDS patients on VV-ECMO after a median of 9 days [7]. Altogether, data from this and other previously published studies suggest that PP during VV-ECMO is safe when performed by a referent team and ultimately improves oxygenation. Of note, these studies failed to find any improvement in respiratory system compliance [6–11].

Since PP during VV-ECMO also carries potentially harmful effects, it is thus imperative to better delineate its effects and putative indications.

Previous studies, using short sessions (>12 h), failed to find any effects on respiratory system compliance. In light of the above, the present study was aimed at retrospectively analyzing the effects of prolonged PP sessions (24 h) on safety data, oxygenation and respiratory system compliance.

Methods

The ECMO database of our 14-bed ICU was retrospectively reviewed to identify patients who received PP during VV-ECMO between January 2012 (first treatment in our ICU) and January 2014. The study protocol was evaluated by the local Ethics Committee (Comité de Réflexion Ethique Nanceien Hospitalo-Universitaire) which waived written informed consent due to both the retrospective study design and because PP and VV-ECMO are an integral part of care provided to patients with ARDS. All patients or their relatives were informed that some data could be used for clinical research. We included patients with severe ARDS as defined by the BERLIN consensus [12].

ARDS management

All patients were treated in accordance with the latest recommended guidelines. In particular, treatment in ICU included the systematic use of protective ventilation,

transient use of paralyzing agents, diuresis to dry weight, prone positioning, recruitment maneuvers, transient use of inhaled nitric oxide and high positive end expiratory pressure (PEEP) levels [2].

Indication of ECMO

VV-ECMO was considered in patients with an optimal protective ventilator setting (Vt at 6 mL/kg of predicted body weight, PEEP adjusted to maintain a plateau pressure (pPlat) between 27 and 30 cmH_2O) after the failure of at least one prone positioning session with one of the following criteria adapted from the ongoing EOLIA trial: (1) $PaO_2/FiO_2 < 50$ mmHg for more than 3 h under $FiO_2 > 80$ %; (2) $PaO_2/FiO_2 < 85$ mmHg for more than 6 h; (3) pPlat > 35 cmH_2O despite adjustment of Vt and PEEP; (4) pH < 7.25 for more than 6 h despite an increase in respiratory rate to 35/min. VV-ECMO was either initiated in our intensive care unit (ICU) or in another hospital. In the latter instance, all patients were transferred to our ICU immediately after instituting VV-ECMO by our mobile ECMO team.

ECMO management

All VV-ECMOs were performed using percutaneous cannulation under echocardiography. A femoro-jugular circuit was implanted whenever possible, with femoro–femoral jugular circuit as an alternative. A servo-controlled centrifugal pump (Rotaflow console, Maquet, Hirrlingen, Germany) and poly-methyl pentene oxygenators (Quadrox Bioline oxygenator system Maquet, Hirrlingen, Germany) were used. The circuit and the oxygenator were fully coated with heparin. VV-ECMO flow was adapted daily according to cardiac output measured by echocardiography in order to maintain an ECMO blood flow/cardiac output ratio of at least 0.7 [13]. Sweep gas flow was titrated in order to maintain $PaCO_2$ between 40 and 45 mmHg. Oxygen fraction delivered on the membrane (FDO_2) was adjusted on post-oxygenator blood gas. Heparin was continuously infused to obtain an anti-Xa activity at 0.1–0.2.

Respiratory management under VV-ECMO

All patients were ventilated in volume control mode. Ultraprotective ventilation was applied during the first 48 h with the following settings: Vt at 1.5–3 ml/kg of predicted body weight, respiratory rate between 8 and 12/min, PEEP between 10 and 18 adapted for a pPlat at 25 cmH_2O. FiO_2 was adapted for a SpO_2 between 88 and 95 %. All patients were sedated and paralyzed by besilate cisatracurium (Hospira France, France) during the first 24 h. After 24 h, besilate cisatracurium was discontinued when possible.

Weaning procedure

After the first 48 h, Vt was increased daily when possible, respecting a pPlat at 25 cmH$_2$O. When Vt was >5 ml/kg of predicted body weight and respiratory rate >15/min, ECMO and sweep gas flow were progressively decreased respecting the following criteria: (1) PaO$_2$/FIO$_2$ > 150 mmHg, (2) FiO$_2$ on ventilator <60 %, (3) PaCO$_2$ < 50 mmHg, (4) pPlat < 25 cmH$_2$O. ECMO was halted if the above criteria were respected in a non paralyzed patient after a successful 12–24 h session with a sweep gas flow at 0 L/min.

Indication for prone positioning under VV-ECMO

Prone positioning placement was only performed in one of the two following conditions: (1) Failure of attempts to wean VV-ECMO after at least 7 days under VV-ECMO combined with the need of therapeutic sedation, (2) Refractory hypoxemia with PaO$_2$/FiO$_2$ ratio <85 mmHg under FiO$_2$ 100 % both on the ventilator and the membrane despite optimal VV-ECMO and ventilator settings combined or not with persistent high plateau pressure (>25 cmH$_2$O) despite ultra-protective ventilation. Further sessions were also performed according to the same indications.

Contraindication for placement in prone position under VV-ECMO

Given the potential risks of PP during VV-ECMO, PP was not performed in patients under vasopressor treatment and in cases of recent open chest cardiac surgery. PP was proposed only in patients who were still under sedation and in whom it was not possible to use partial ventilatory support.

Protocol for prone positioning under VV-ECMO (Additional files 1, 2)

The protocol was adapted from PROSEVA guidelines for prone positioning placement and has been published elsewhere [1, 6]. The detailed protocol is described in the supplementary material.

Study parameters

The use of PP in our ICU with or without ECMO is described in an institutional procedure. For all sessions, parameters were recorded at three time intervals: prior to prone positioning placement, after 24 h in prone position and 24 h after the return to supine position. As specified in the procedure, in order to formally objectify respiratory improvement, respiratory and VV-ECMO parameters were maintained constant throughout the entire prone positioning session. An increase in FiO$_2$ and/or VV-ECMO blood flow was only considered when SpO$_2$ was below 85 %. VV-ECMO and ventilator settings were adjusted according to lung recovery after the prone positioning session. Data analysis also included the recording, at the above three pre-specified times, of complete blood gas (PaO$_2$, PaCO$_2$, pH, HCO$_3^-$, SaO$_2$), respiratory parameters (respiratory rate, Vt, PEEP, FiO$_2$, pPlat, respiratory system compliance) and VV-ECMO parameters (blood flow, sweep gas flow, oxygen delivery by VV-ECMO device: FDO$_2$). Respiratory system compliance (RS compliance) was computed by dividing tidal volume by pPlat (measured during an end-inspiratory pause (1 s) minus total PEEP. Total PEEP was measured by using an expiratory pause (5 s). Driving pressure was calculated as plateau pressure minus PEEP [14]. The pre-ECMO survival probability was also calculated according to the RESP score [15].

Chest CT analysis

In patients who underwent a computed tomography (CT) scan within the 3 days prior to placement in prone position, a measurement of the amount of non-aerated lung tissue was performed according to an adapted previously-published method by Malbouisson et al. [16]. The detailed protocol is presented in the Additional file 3 (see Figure S1) [17].

Adverse effects

Three categories were systematically reported in the procedure: (1) adverse effects related to the cannulas and VV-ECMO device during the prone position session (drop in flow necessitating fluid resuscitation, oxygenator thrombosis, cannula removal, bleeding from cannulation sites), (2) adverse effects related to the tracheal tube and the ventilator device (accidental tracheal extubation, tube displacement) and (3) adverse effects related to the other catheters (accidental wrenching of central venous or arterial lines and nasogastric tube).

Statistical analysis

All analyses were performed using SAS software R9.3 (SAS Institute, Cary, NC, USA). The two-tailed significance level was set at $p < 0.05$. Results are respectively presented as median (1st–3rd quartiles) and frequency (percentage) for continuous and discrete variables. The paired Wilcoxon test and Fisher's exact test were carried out for intra-group (before-after PP) and inter-group (respiratory response) comparisons, respectively. Since 11 intra-group comparisons were performed on the same subjects at the end of each session and 24 h thereafter, significance levels were adjusted for multiple testing at each respective time points. Results were analyzed for the first session ($n = 17$) as well as for all sessions ($n = 27$), considering that the increase in gas exchange of a given PP session does not predict survival [18]. Moreover, the sampling and the number of sessions did not allow for any intra-individual adjustment.

Results

Population description (Table 1)

Despite optimized protective mechanical ventilation and other adjuvant treatment (i.e. PP, inhaled nitric oxide, recruitment maneuvers), 44 patients received VV-ECMO during the study period for refractory acute respiratory distress syndrome. Global survival rate was 66 %. Among the latter, 17 patients underwent PP during VV-ECMO. Pre-ECMO survival probability according to the RESP score was 76 % (33–90). All of the patients had a severe ARDS according to the Berlin definition [19]. Before being placed on VV-ECMO, 13/17 (76 %) patients were prone positioned. Prior to ECMO implantation, 4/14 patients previously responded to PP in terms of oxygenation but developed major respiratory acidosis and high plateau pressure. Femoro–jugular VV-ECMO was used in 16/17 patients and femoro-femoral VV-ECMO in one patient. ARDS was related to an infectious process in all

cases. Four patients presented an influenza infection at admission.

Prone positioning was considered after a median delay of 6 days of VV-ECMO (4–12). Sixteen of 27 prone position sessions were performed after this median period. Indications for PP included unsuccessful VV-ECMO weaning attempts after at least 7 days under VV-ECMO in 11/17 patients and refractory hypoxemia with PaO_2/FiO_2 ratio <85 mmHg despite optimal VV-ECMO and ventilator settings in 6/17 patients. For three patients (6 sessions), refractory hypoxemia was associated with elevated plateau pressure despite ultra-protective ventilation. Four patients had 3 sessions and two patients had 2 sessions. The median delay between each session was 2 days (1–4).

Effects of prone position session on respiratory state

Pre-PP parameters are described in Table 2. Twenty-seven sessions were performed. All sessions had an identical duration of 24 h. In 23/27 sessions, nurses described a major increase in sputum drainage. After 24 h in PP under the same respiratory and ECMO settings, PaO_2/FiO_2 increased from 111 (84–128) to 173 (120–203) mmHg ($p < 0.0001$) (Fig. 1). PaO_2/FiO_2 increased by more than 20 % in 22/27 sessions. According to this threshold value, when PP was performed after day 7, PaO_2/FiO_2 ratio increased by more than 20 % in 14/14 sessions. Conversely, only 7/12 sessions had a higher than 20 % increase in PaO_2/FiO_2 ratio before day 7 ($p = 0.01$). RS compliance significantly increased after 24 h in PP from 18 (12–36) to 32 (15–36) ml/cmH$_2$O ($p < 0.005$) (Fig. 2). Additional file 4: Figure S2 and Additional file 5: Figure S3 (see supplemental digital content) provide individual data for plateau pressure and RS compliance, respectively. Twenty-four

Table 1 Baseline characteristics

	Median (quartiles) or n (%), n = 17
Age (years)	45 (36–55)
Male gender	12/17 (71 %)
Body mass index (kg/m²)	27 (23–34)
SAPS II score	44 (38–59)
SOFA score (at ICU admission)	12 (8–15)
SOFA score (before first PP session)	7 (5–11)
Pre-existing conditions	
Congestive heart failure	2/17 (12 %)
Neoplasia	0/17
Chronic respiratory disorders	1/17 (6 %)
Neuropsychiatric disorders	4/17 (24 %)
None	10/17 (59 %)
Causes of ARDS	
Gram-negative pneumonia	7/17 (41 %)
Gram-positive pneumonia	8/17 (47 %)
Influenza virus	4/17 (24 %)
Abdominal septic shock	2/17 (12 %)
Sarcoidosis	1/17 (6 %)
Prone positioning before ECMO	13/17 (76 %)
Pre-ECMO survival probability (%) (RESP score)	76 (33–90)
Duration of hospitalization before ICU (days)	1 (1–2)
Duration under ECMO (days)	18 (13–26)
Duration of ICU stay (days)	54 (36–66)
Survival at discharge	16/17 (94 %)

SAPS II simplified acute physiology score II, *SOFA* sequential organ failure assessment, *ARDS* acute respiratory distress syndrome, *ECMO* extracorporeal membrane oxygenation, *ICU* intensive care unit

Table 2 Baseline characteristics

PaO$_2$/FiO$_2$ (mmHg)	111 (84–128)
PaCO$_2$ (mmHg)	42 (39–43)
Tidal volume (ml/kg)	3.0 (2.2–4.0)
Arterial pH	7.42 (7.39–7.44)
PEEP (cmH$_2$O)	12 (6–13)
Plateau pressure (cmH$_2$O)	24 (22–25)
RS compliance (ml/cmH$_2$O)	18 (12–36)
Respiratory frequency (cycles/min)	17 (10–25)
ECMO settings	
FiO$_2$ (%)	70 (70–90)
ECMO blood flow (l/min)	4.7 (3.7–5.5)
Sweep gas (l/min)	5.0 (3.0–5.0)

PaO$_2$, PaO$_2$ arterial oxygen pressure, *PaCO$_2$* partial pressure of carbon dioxide in arterial blood, *FiO$_2$* fraction of expired oxygen, *PEEP* positive end expiratory pressure, *RS compliance* respiratory system compliance, *ECMO* extracorporeal membrane oxygenation

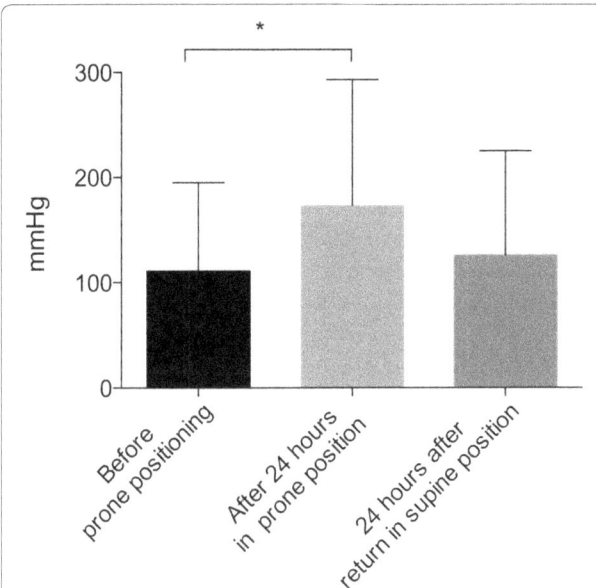

Fig. 1 Effect of prone positioning on PaO_2/FiO_2 ratio before and after 24 h of prone position as well as 24 h after the return to supine position; $*p < 0.05$

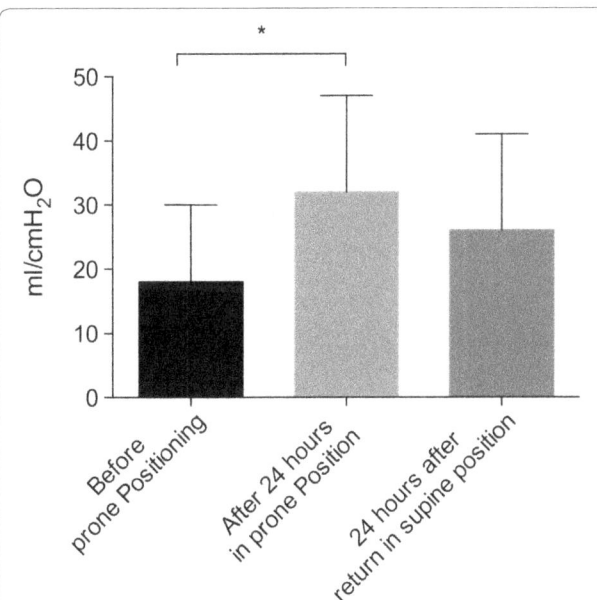

Fig. 2 Effect of prone positioning on respiratory system compliance before and after 24 h of prone position as well as 24 h after the return to supine position; $*p < 0.05$

Correlation between lung condensation and PaO_2/FiO_2 response

Fifteen CT scans were performed prior to placement in prone position. All patients exhibited a high percentage of non-aerated or poorly-aerated lung parenchyma prior to PP: 52 % (41–62). Thus, no correlation was found between the increase in PaO_2/FiO_2 ratio and the amount of non-aerated lung tissue measured on chest scans ($r = 0.064, p = 0.82$).

Adverse events attributable to PP

In one patient, an oxygenator thrombosis occurred while one other patient required fluid resuscitation in order to correct a drop in VV-ECMO flow.

No adverse event was related to either the tracheal tube, the ventilator device or other catheters.

Discussion

The main findings of the present study are that (1) in a majority of patients, PP markedly improved oxygenation during VV-ECMO and was not associated with side effects confirming the Guervilly et al. study, (2) the improvement in oxygenation appeared to be more efficient when applied after 7 days of VV-ECMO, (3) contrary to the Guervilly et al. study, PP was associated with an improvement in lung compliance therefore allowing the use of increased Vt and (4) there was no correlation between the volume of condensation and PP efficiency.

Prone positioning during VV-ECMO improves oxygenation

All currently published studies are consistent with regard to the effect of PP on oxygenation during VV-ECMO. Clearly, PP improves oxygenation in a majority of patients. Moreover, previous studies mainly studied the effects of PP when performed late after VV-ECMO initiation (8 days in the Guervilly et al. study). It appears that for some patients PP was effective under ECMO and ineffective prior to ECMO. It is likely that time is an important factor in allowing lung healing and symptomatic treatments such as antibiotics to be effective. The decrease in lung aggression secondary to ultraprotective ventilation should also be considered.

Prone positioning during VV-ECMO improves respiratory system compliance and allows increased tidal volume

Importantly, PP was associated with a marked decrease in plateau pressure in patients in whom it was not possible to maintain this pressure under 25 cmH_2O. In randomized controlled trials comparing supine and prone positions, the results on respiratory compliance have been inconsistent. Indeed, Mancebo et al. noted higher compliance of the respiratory system in the prone

hours after the return to supine position, tidal volume was significantly increased from 3 (2.2–4) before PP to 3.7 (2.8–5) ml/kg of predicted body weight ($p < 0.05$). Arterial PCO_2 did not change during and after PP.

position, whereas Guerin et al. and Taccone et al. did not [20, 21]. Previous studies using PP during VV-ECMO also failed to demonstrate any significant changes in static compliance. Guervilly et al. suggested that the improvement in oxygenation without concomitant increase in respiratory static compliance and without decrease in $PaCO_2$ at constant levels of minute ventilation and sweep gas flow do not suggest lung recruitment by PP with relatively small Vt and high levels of PEEP but rather an improvement in VA/Q mismatch. Unfortunately, no CT scan data were provided in their study. Herein, all of our patients had major posterior condensation (>50 % of lung volume) and thus it is likely that PP in this situation allows lung recruitment. Arguing in favor of this hypothesis is the fact that PP further allows the use of increased Vt. Importantly, in 23/27 sessions, nurses described a major increase in sputum drainage that may have contributed to recruitment. Another hypothesis to explain this discrepancy is that prolonged PP sessions were used in our study (24 h as opposed to 12 h), which may have contributed to the observed improvement in compliance. Finally, the discrepancy could be due to different patient populations, i.e. patients still under sedation in whom it was not possible to use partial mode of ventilatory support or to a different phase of the disease comparatively to previous reports.

The driving pressure (plateau pressure minus PEEP) is associated with ARDS prognosis, [14] but also with treatment efficiency when associated with decreases in ΔP. Interestingly, the driving pressure observed in our study was relatively low and the use of PP was associated with a further decrease in driving pressure.

Study limitations
Although the present constitutes the largest study relative to the use of PP during VV-ECMO, the number of studied patients remains relatively small. Nevertheless, severe ARDS treated with ECMO and needing prone positioning is a rare occurrence and thus it is unlikely that a multicenter randomized study will be performed. Accordingly, only 36 cases have been previously reported in the literature in which session durations differed considerably. Therefore, we firmly believe that this study adds valuable information, first in confirming previous but scarce data but also in extending these data with new findings, notably on compliance.

The small sample size may also have had a bearing on our findings regarding the comparison between early and late sessions. In addition, specific predefined criteria were chosen as to whether or not to use PP in our VV-ECMO patients. Therefore, our results and conclusions are only valuable when considering the present clinical algorithm. Finally, because of the retrospective nature of the present study, it was not possible to study the mechanism involved in PP effects during VV-ECMO.

Conclusions
When used in combination with VV-ECMO, 24 h of prone positioning improves both oxygenation and respiratory system compliance. Moreover, our study confirms the absence of serious adverse events. Currently, it remains unknown when and for which indication prone positioning should be systematically applied during VV-ECMO. Therefore, further studies are needed to better delineate prone positioning indications during VV-ECMO.

Additional files

Additional file 1: Movie S1 Protocol for prone positioning under VV-ECMO (Supplemental Digital Content movie).

Additional file 2: Protocol for prone positioning under VV-ECMO (Supplemental Digital Content movie).

Additional file 3: Figure S1. CT scan analysis. In a first step in the analysis of CT images (A), lung contours were manually delineated from chest wall, mediastinum and pleural effusion. This resulted in the crude lung volume (B). (Actual, True) lung volume (C) was obtained by excluding large vessels (densities above 150 HU on enhanced scans) and bronchi lumen and hyperinflated lungs (densities below 900 HU). Lastly, a normally-aerated lung was defined as having a density below 100 HU (D).

Additional file 4: Figure S2. Evolution of plateau pressure before and 24 h after prone positioning. Individual data.

Additional file 5: Figure S3. Evolution of respiratory system compliance before and 24 h after prone positioning. Individual data.

Authors' contributions
AK supervised development of the work, performed data interpretation and wrote the manuscript; SR recorded data and performed data interpretation; CB wrote the prone-positioning procedure; FV helped in data interpretation and manuscript evaluation; DM performed CT scan analysis and wrote CT scan methodology; NG and RF performed the statistical analysis; BL supervised development of the work, helped in data interpretation and manuscript evaluation and wrote the manuscript. All authors read and approved the final manuscript.

Author details
[1] CHU Nancy, Service de Réanimation Médicale Brabois, Pole Cardiovasculaire et Réanimation Médicale, Hôpital Brabois, 54511 Vandoeuvre les Nancy, France. [2] INSERM U 1116, Groupe Choc, Equipe 2, Faculté de Médecine, 54511 Vandoeuvre les Nancy, 54000 Nancy, France. [3] Université de Lorraine, 54000 Nancy, France. [4] CHU Nancy, Département de Radiologie, Hôpital Brabois, 54511 Vandoeuvre les Nancy, France. [5] CHU Nancy, Département de Chirugie Cardiaque Brabois, Pole Cardiovasculaire et Réanimation Médicale, Hôpital Brabois, 54511 Vandoeuvre les Nancy, France. [6] INSERM, Centre d'Investigations Cliniques-9501 and CHU de Nancy, 54511 Vandoeuvre les Nancy, France.

Acknowledgements
We thank Pierre Pothier for the English manuscript proofreading service.

Competing interests
The authors declare that they have no competing interests.

References

1. Guerin C, Reignier J, Richard JC, Beuret P, Gacouin A, Boulain T, Mercier E, Badet M, Mercat A, Baudin O, Clavel M, Chatellier D, Jaber S, Rosselli S, Mancebo J, Sirodot M, Hilbert G, Bengler C, Richecoeur J, Gainnier M, Bayle F, Bourdin G, Leray V, Girard R, Baboi L, Ayzac L, Group PS. Prone positioning in severe acute respiratory distress syndrome. N Engl J Med. 2013;368:2159–68.

2. Peek GJ, Mugford M, Tiruvoipati R, Wilson A, Allen E, Thalanany MM, Hibbert CL, Truesdale A, Clemens F, Cooper N, Firmin RK, Elbourne D. CESAR trial collaboration. Efficacy and economic assessment of conventional ventilatory support versus extracorporeal membrane oxygenation for severe adult respiratory failure (CESAR): a multicentre randomised controlled trial. Lancet. 2009;374:1351–63.

3. Schmidt M, Zogheib E, Roze H, Repesse X, Lebreton G, Luyt CE, Trouillet JL, Brechot N, Nieszkowska A, Dupont H, Ouattara A, Leprince P, Chastre J, Combes A. The PRESERVE mortality risk score and analysis of long-term outcomes after extracorporeal membrane oxygenation for severe acute respiratory distress syndrome. Intensive Care Med. 2013;39:1704–13.

4. Parhar K, Vuylsteke A. What's new in ECMO: scoring the bad indications. Intensive Care Med. 2014;40:1734–7.

5. Levy B, Taccone FS, Guarracino F. Recent developments in the management of persistent hypoxemia under veno-venous ECMO. Intensive Care Med. 2015;41(3):508–10.

6. Kimmoun A, Guerci P, Bridey C, Ducrocq N, Vanhuyse F, Levy B. Prone positioning use to hasten veno-venous ECMO weaning in ARDS. Intensive Care Med. 2013;39:1877–9.

7. Guervilly C, Hraiech S, Gariboldi V, Xeridat F, Dizier S, Toesca R, Forel JM, Adda M, Grisoli D, Collart F, Roch A, Papazian L. Prone positioning during veno-venous extracorporeal membrane oxygenation for severe acute respiratory distress syndrome in adults. Minerva Anestesiol. 2014;80:307–13.

8. Kipping V, Weber-Carstens S, Lojewski C, Feldmann P, Rydlewski A, Boemke W, Spies C, Kastrup M, Kaisers UX, Wernecke KD, Deja M. Prone position during ECMO is safe and improves oxygenation. Int J Artif Organs. 2013;36:821–32.

9. Kredel M, Bischof L, Wurmb TE, Roewer N, Muellenbach RM. Combination of positioning therapy and venovenous extracorporeal membrane oxygenation in ARDS patients. Perfusion. 2014;29:171–7.

10. Masuda Y, Tatsumi H, Imaizumi H, Gotoh K, Yoshida S, Chihara S, Takahashi K, Yamakage M. Effect of prone positioning on cannula function and impaired oxygenation during extracorporeal circulation. J Artif Organs. 2014;17:106–9.

11. Otterspoor LC, Smit FH, van Laar TJ, Kesecioglu J, van Dijk D. Prolonged use of extracorporeal membrane oxygenation combined with prone positioning in patients with acute respiratory distress syndrome and invasive Aspergillosis. Perfusion. 2012;27:335–7.

12. Force ADT, Ranieri VM, Rubenfeld GD, Thompson BT, Ferguson ND, Caldwell E, Fan E, Camporota L, Slutsky AS. Acute respiratory distress syndrome: the Berlin Definition. JAMA. 2012;307:2526–33.

13. Schmidt M, Tachon G, Devilliers C, Muller G, Hekimian G, Brechot N, Merceron S, Luyt CE, Trouillet JL, Chastre J, Leprince P, Combes A. Blood oxygenation and decarboxylation determinants during venovenous ECMO for respiratory failure in adults. Intensive Care Med. 2013;39:838–46.

14. Amato MB, Meade MO, Slutsky AS, Brochard L, Costa EL, Schoenfeld DA, Stewart TE, Briel M, Talmor D, Mercat A, Richard JC, Carvalho CR, Brower RG. Driving pressure and survival in the acute respiratory distress syndrome. N Engl J Med. 2015;372:747–55.

15. Schmidt M, Bailey M, Sheldrake J, Hodgson C, Aubron C, Rycus PT, Scheinkestel C, Cooper DJ, Brodie D, Pellegrino V, Combes A, Pilcher D. Predicting survival after extracorporeal membrane oxygenation for severe acute respiratory failure. The Respiratory Extracorporeal Membrane Oxygenation Survival Prediction (RESP) score. Am J Respir Crit Care Med. 2014;189:1374–82.

16. Malbouisson LM, Muller JC, Constantin JM, Lu Q, Puybasset L, Rouby JJ. Group CTSAS. Computed tomography assessment of positive end-expiratory pressure-induced alveolar recruitment in patients with acute respiratory distress syndrome. Am J Respir Crit Care Med. 2001;163:1444–50.

17. Protti A, Chiumello D, Cressoni M, Carlesso E, Mietto C, Berto V, Lazzerini M, Quintel M, Gattinoni L. Relationship between gas exchange response to prone position and lung recruitability during acute respiratory failure. Intensive Care Med. 2009;35:1011–7.

18. Albert RK, Keniston A, Baboi L, Ayzac L, Guerin C. Prone position-induced improvement in gas exchange does not predict improved survival in the acute respiratory distress syndrome. Am J Respir Crit Care Med. 2014;189:494–6.

19. Ferguson ND, Fan E, Camporota L, Antonelli M, Anzueto A, Beale R, Brochard L, Brower R, Esteban A, Gattinoni L, Rhodes A, Slutsky AS, Vincent JL, Rubenfeld GD, Thompson BT, Ranieri VM. The Berlin definition of ARDS: an expanded rationale, justification, and supplementary material. Intensive Care Med. 2012;38:1573–82.

20. Mancebo J, Fernandez R, Blanch L, Rialp G, Gordo F, Ferrer M, Rodriguez F, Garro P, Ricart P, Vallverdu I, Gich I, Castano J, Saura P, Dominguez G, Bonet A, Albert RK. A multicenter trial of prolonged prone ventilation in severe acute respiratory distress syndrome. Am J Respir Crit Care Med. 2006;173:1233–9.

21. Taccone P, Pesenti A, Latini R, Polli F, Vagginelli F, Mietto C, Caspani L, Raimondi F, Bordone G, Iapichino G, Mancebo J, Guerin C, Ayzac L, Blanch L, Fumagalli R, Tognoni G, Gattinoni L, Prone-Supine IISG. Prone positioning in patients with moderate and severe acute respiratory distress syndrome: a randomized controlled trial. JAMA. 2009;302:1977–84.

23

Protective effect of early low-dose hydrocortisone on ventilator-associated pneumonia in the cancer patients

David Lagier[1*], Laura Platon[1], Jérome Lambert[2], Laurent Chow-Chine[1], Antoine Sannini[1], Magali Bisbal[1], Jean-Paul Brun[1], Karim Asehnoune[3], Marc Leone[4], Marion Faucher[1] and Djamel Mokart[1]

Abstract

Background: Ventilator-associated pneumonia (VAP) is a care-related event that could be promoted by immune suppression caused by critical diseases, malignancies and cancer treatments. Low dose of hydrocortisone was proposed for modulation of immune response in the critically ill population.

Methods: In this monocentric observational study, all cancer patients mechanically ventilated for more than 48 h were included. Effect of low-dose hydrocortisone administered during the first 48 h of mechanical ventilation was evaluated applying inverse probability weighting analysis after propensity score assessment. VAP impact on 1-year mortality, ICU length of stay and mechanical ventilation duration was secondarily determined.

Results: Within this cohort, 190 cancer patients were followed. VAP was confirmed in 22.1% of cases in the early hydrocortisone group and confirmed in 42.6% of cases in the no or late hydrocortisone group. Early hydrocortisone exhibited a protective effect on the risk of VAP (OR 0.23; 95% CI 0.12–0.44; $P < 0.0001$). VAP was associated with 1-year mortality (HR 1.60; 95% CI 1.10–2.34; $P = 0.017$) and increased ICU length of stay (mean extra length of stay: 4.2 days; 95% CI 0.6–7.8).

Conclusions: Immune modulation with low-dose hydrocortisone administered in the first days of mechanical ventilation could protect from VAP occurrence in cancer patients.

Keywords: Ventilator-associated pneumonia, Neoplasms, Immunomodulation, Hydrocortisone, Propensity score

Background

Recently introduced aggressive treatments have significantly decreased the overall mortality rate in cancer patients [1]. These new approaches come at the price of a steep rise in infections and treatment-related toxicities [2]. Immune suppression with or without neutropenia is a major concern in this setting. On the other side, critical conditions found during sepsis or acute respiratory failure induce a complex immune response making severely ill patients prone to secondary ICU-acquired infections, such as ventilator-associated pneumonia (VAP) [3]. During sepsis, hydrocortisone improves the phagocytic abilities of neutrophils, decreases the blood concentration of anti-inflammatory cytokines (interleukin-10) and increases the blood concentrations of the host defence against infection (interferon γ and interleukin-12) [4, 5]. By balancing the inflammatory response, hydrocortisone might also decrease the growth and virulence of bacteria [6, 7]. In septic shock, low-dose hydrocortisone improves shock reversal irrespective to adrenal response to corticotropin [8]. Moreover, it has been shown that low-dose hydrocortisone can reduce the incidence of hospital-acquired pneumonia in intubated patients with multiple

*Correspondence: david.lagier@ap-hm.fr
[1] Intensive Care Unit, Paoli-Calmettes Institute, 232 Boulevard de Sainte-Marguerite, 13009 Marseille, France
Full list of author information is available at the end of the article

trauma [9]. Survival of cancer patients with acute respiratory failure has improved over time to about 60% [10]. Nevertheless, invasive mechanical ventilation remains associated with a 28-day mortality rate of about 50% [11]. In non-selected populations, VAP is a common hospital-acquired pneumonia and occurs in up to 30% of patients receiving mechanical ventilation for more than 48 h. The main objective of our study was to evaluate the preventive role of early treatment with low-dose hydrocortisone regarding incidence of VAP in cancer patients. The prognostic impact of VAP on 1-year mortality, mechanical ventilation duration and ICU length of stay was secondarily assessed.

Methods

Study population

In this monocentric observational study, all consecutive cancer patients requiring invasive mechanical ventilation for more than 48 h that have been admitted to our ICU between January 1, 2009, and December 31, 2013, were prospectively followed. We excluded from the study patients that needed two or more invasive mechanical ventilation periods during their ICU stay. The Paoli-Calmettes Institute Institutional Review Board approved this observational study (No. IPC-2017-077). No consent was needed in this observational study.

Diagnosis of VAP

All ventilated patients were daily screened for new respiratory or septic events. VAP was suspected if a recent and persistent infiltrate on chest radiograph was associated with at least two of the following criteria: hyperthermia ($> 38\ °C$) or hypothermia ($< 36\ °C$), purulent tracheal secretions and worsening of gas exchange. Because of its high variability and poor specificity in the onco-haematological context, leucocyte count was not taken into account. Quantitative microbiological culture of 10^6 colony-forming unit (CFU)/mL of a typical pathogen from endotracheal aspirate or 10^4 CFU/mL from bronchoalveolar lavage fluid confirmed VAP [12, 13]. Early VAP was defined as a VAP diagnosed before the 5th day of invasive mechanical ventilation. An adjudication committee (two senior ICU physicians) systematically reviewed VAP diagnosis to determine whether it meets protocol-specified criteria. It was blinded to hydrocortisone status.

VAP bundles

In our ICU, VAP prevention strategy included 30° semi-sitting position, endotracheal cuff pressure control, chlorhexidine 0.2% daily oral care and a sedation protocol based on the Richmond Agitation Sedation Scale with daily sedation discontinuation. No selective digestive or oropharyngeal decontamination was used. Enteral

nutrition was gradually implemented as early as possible. Parenteral nutrition was used if contraindication or poor tolerance to enteral route was present. Anti-acid treatment was pursued during mechanical ventilation periods irrespective of the hydrocortisone status.

Low-dose hydrocortisone treatment

In this study, low-dose hydrocortisone was usually prescribed in case of refractory septic shock with persistent arterial hypotension despite high-dose vasopressor therapy ($\geq 0.8\ \mu g\ kg^{-1}\ min^{-1}$ of norepinephrine) or as an alternative therapy in case of sepsis with previous curative corticosteroid therapy. In case of sepsis and ongoing curative corticosteroid therapy, the treatment was switched for hydrocortisone. Fifty milligrams was administered intravenously every 6 h according to our local protocol.

Data collection

All data were extracted and analysed by senior physicians using our ICU management software (MetaVision ICU, iMDsoft Inc.®, Dedham, MA, USA). As previously described [10], baseline data were recorded upon ICU admission: gender, age, cancer type, cancer stage classified in four categories (newly diagnosed, complete remission, partial remission and evolutive disease), main ICU admission purpose (septic shock, acute respiratory failure, coma and others), presence of neutropenia, history of haematopoietic stem cell transplantation (HSCT) and recent exposure to antibiotics or curative corticosteroids (during the 10 days before admission). SOFA score [14] was also reported at the time of endotracheal intubation. Several approaches implemented during the first 48 h after endotracheal intubation, including vasopressors, renal replacement therapy, substitutive steroids therapy for refractory shock, granulocyte colony-stimulating factors (G-CSF), enteral nutrition and antibiotherapy (adapted or empirical), were recorded. VAP microbiological evidences were also documented. ICU mortality was evaluated. ICU survivors were prospectively followed after ICU discharge until the end of the study and 1-year survival was determined.

Statistical analysis

Data are presented as median (interquartile range) for quantitative variables and count (percentages) for qualitative variables. Binary outcome (i.e. the occurrence of VAP) was analysed using a Chi-square test or the non-parametric Wilcoxon rank-sum test as appropriate. The multivariate analyses were performed using a logistic model. The primary outcome of the study was to evaluate the prevention of VAP using early low dose of hydrocortisone. VAP incidence was reported to the incidence per

1000 ventilator days. Effect of early low-dose hydrocortisone on incidence of VAP was studied using propensity score analysis to take into account the non-randomized design of this study. Early hydrocortisone group was defined by hydrocortisone treatment initiated during the first 48 h of invasive mechanical ventilation. Patients treated by hydrocortisone for more than 48 h before tracheal intubation were excluded from this analysis. Propensity score, which is the probability that a patient will receive low-dose hydrocortisone, was assessed using a logistic regression model with baseline covariates as explanatory variables and treatment with low-dose hydrocortisone as the outcome. An inverse probability weighting (IPW) analysis was then performed to assess the average treatment effect of low-dose hydrocortisone assessed by comparison of two pseudo-population, one where nobody would have received low-dose hydrocortisone and one where everybody would have received it. Cumulative incidence of VAP in ICU was estimated taking into accounts competing risk of discharge of ICU (either death or discharge alive).

Association between baseline variables, describing patient's condition at ICU admission or at intubation, and overall mortality was assessed by univariable analysis using Cox proportional hazard models. Multivariable analysis including variables significantly associated with death was performed using a Cox proportional hazard model with VAP as a time-dependent variable. Variable selection was based on Akaike information criteria (AIC). Since VAP is a time-dependent event, it cannot be treated as a baseline covariate. Hence, a Mantel–Byar analysis was performed to assess and graphically display the effect of VAP on 1-year mortality. To estimate extra length of stay (in ICU-discharged patients) and extra duration of intubation (in extubated patients) due to VAP, we used a multistate model that takes into account time to VAP.

Results

Between January 1, 2009, and December 31, 2013, 208 patients were included in the study. Among them, 18 have been excluded for multiple periods of invasive mechanical ventilation. Among the 190 patients included in the final analysis, 55 (28.9%) develop a confirmed VAP. Early VAP onset was found in 12 patients (21.8% of the total VAP). Microbiological data are outlined in Table 1. Substitutive corticotherapy with low-dose hydrocortisone was prescribed in 122 (64.2%) cases and was predominantly used in patients without VAP ($P = 0.003$; Table 2). The median mechanical ventilation duration was 11 (6–18) days. ICU and 1-year mortality rate were 56 and 77%, respectively (Table 3).

Table 1 Microbiological documentation depending on the timing of VAP

	Early VAP ($n = 12$)	Late VAP ($n = 43$)
P. aeruginosa	4	10
E. coli	2	6
K. pneumoniae	1	6
E. cloacae	1	3
Enterococcus sp	2	8
Staphylococcus sp	1	2
Stenotrophomonas sp	0	5
Other Gram-negative bacteria	1	3

Effect of early low-dose hydrocortisone

Nine patients received hydrocortisone for more than 48 h before tracheal intubation and were excluded from this analysis. Global VAP incidence in the 181 patients included in the analysis; incidence was 25.5/1000 ventilator days. Stratified according to cortisone, incidence was 20.3/1000 ventilator days in the group receiving early low-dose hydrocortisone and 32.7/1000 ventilator days in the group receiving no or late low-dose hydrocortisone. A prior multivariable analysis has identified early hydrocortisone treatment as the only independent variable significantly associated with the VAP occurrence (OR 0.41; 95% CI 0.2–0.8; $P < 0.01$). The propensity score was constructed using the following relevant variables: age, neutropenia and admission purpose at admission, as well as SOFA score, vasopressors, antibiotherapy (adapted, empirical, none) and enteral nutrition at the time of intubation. Standardized differences in the unweighted population and in the weighted population are shown in Fig. 1. VAP was confirmed in 22.1% of cases in the early hydrocortisone group (25 out of 113 patients) and confirmed in 42.6% of cases in the no or late hydrocortisone group (29 out of 68 patients). Using IPW analysis, early hydrocortisone exhibited a protective effect on the risk of VAP (OR 0.23; 95% CI 0.12–0.44; $P < 0.0001$, Fig. 2).

VAP prognostic impact

Considering VAP as a time-dependent covariate, univariate analysis (Table 2) revealed that VAP is not associated with 1-year mortality (HR 1.41; 95% CI 0.98–2.03; $P = 0.06$). After multivariate adjustment (Table 2), an independent and significant association is revealed between VAP and 1-year mortality (HR 1.60; 95% CI 1.10–2.34; $P = 0.017$, Fig. 3). Regarding initial vs late onset VAP, there indeed was a difference in prognosis, with late onset VAP being associated with a higher mortality [HR 1.74 (95% CI 1.17–2.58)], but early VAP being not significantly different from no VAP [HR 0.98

Table 2 Patient's characteristics

Variables	Patients without VAP (n = 135)	Patients with VAP (n = 55)	P
Male gender, n (%)	87 (64.4)	41 (74.5)	0.23
Age (year), median (IQR)	59.2 (52.2–65.8)	60.4 (50.2–67.1)	0.99
Cancer type			0.39
Haematological malignancy, n (%)	95 (70.4)	35 (63.6)	
Solid tumour, n (%)	40 (29.6)	20 (36.4)	
Cancer stage			0.91
Diagnosis, n (%)	36 (26.7)	15 (27.3)	
Complete remission, n (%)	29 (21.5)	13 (23.6)	
Partial remission, n (%)	31 (23)	14 (25.5)	
Evolutive, n (%)	39 (28.9)	13 (23.6)	
HSCT, n (%)	47 (24.7)	14 (25.4)	0.43
Admission purpose			0.32
Septic shock, n (%)	59 (43.7)	21 (38.2)	
Acute respiratory failure, n (%)	51 (37.8)	27 (49.1)	
Coma, n (%)	14 (10.4)	2 (3.6)	
Others, n (%)	11 (8.1)	5 (9.1)	
Clinical sepsis upon admission			0.042
Respiratory, n (%)	79 (58.5)	31 (56.4)	
Non-respiratory, n (%)	31 (23)	6 (10.9)	
None, n (%)	25 (18.5)	18 (32.7)	
Characteristics upon admission			
Neutropenia, n (%)	54 (40)	18 (32.7)	0.41
Antibiotherapy, n (%)	104 (77)	43 (78.2)	1
Corticosteroids (curative), n (%)	32 (23.7)	19 (34.5)	0.15
SOFA score (day of intubation), median (IQR)	11 (8–14)	11 (8–13)	0.28
Characteristics at the first 48 h of MV			
Vasopressors, n (%)	99 (73.3)	44 (80)	0.36
Renal replacement therapy, n (%)	28 (20.7)	9 (16.4)	0.55
Substitutive hydrocortisone, n (%)	96 (71.1)	26 (47.3)	0.003
G-CSF, n (%)	20 (14.8)	9 (16.4)	0.82
Enteral nutrition, n (%)	40 (29.6)	21 (38.2)	0.3
Antibiotherapy			0.09
Adapted, n (%)	41 (30.4)	11 (20)	
Empirical, n (%)	89 (65.9)	38 (69)	
None, n (%)	5 (3.7)	6 (10.7)	

HSCT haematopoietic stem cell transplantation, G-CSF granulocyte colony-stimulating factors, MV mechanical ventilation, IQR interquartile range

(0.39–2.46)]. VAP resulted in a significantly longer ICU stay for patients discharged [mean extra length of stay: 4.2 days (95% CI 0.6–7.8)] and a longer, although not significant, mechanical ventilation duration for patients extubated [mean extra duration: 1.7 days (95% CI − 1.5 to 5.0)].

Discussion

We report herein on 190 onco-haematology patients admitted to ICU and treated with mechanical ventilation over 4 years. We showed the protective effect of low-dose hydrocortisone administered in the first days of mechanical ventilation regarding VAP occurrence. An association was found between VAP occurrence and 1-year mortality. The deleterious impact of VAP on ICU length of stay was also demonstrated. To our knowledge, this is the first study reporting prognosis data with regard to VAP in the specific cancer population.

VAP is a controversial topic [15–17]. In the global ICU population, VAP incidence and attributable mortality are uncertain [18, 19]. In a systematic review of published randomized trials [20], VAP-cumulated incidence

Table 3 Predictors of 1-year mortality: univariate and multivariate analysis

Variables	Univariate			Multivariate		
	HR	95% CI	P	HR	95% CI	P
Male gender	0.89	0.64–1.24	0.49			
Age	0.99	0.98–1	0.13			
Cancer type						
Haematological malignancy	1	(Reference)	0.91			
Solid tumour	0.91	0.65–1.28				
Cancer stage						
Complete remission	1	(Reference)	0.02	1	(Reference)	0.03
Diagnosis	1.37	0.87–2.16		1.44	0.88–2.35	
Partial remission	0.82	0.50–1.33		0.98	0.57–1.68	
Evolutive	1.54	0.99–2.41		1.77	1.10–2.87	
HSCT	1.28	0.86–1.92	0.23			
Admission purpose						
Others	1	(Reference)	0.055			
Septic shock	0.96	0.54–1.71				
Acute respiratory failure	0.62	0.34–1.11				
Coma	0.66	0.31–1.43				
Clinical sepsis upon admission						
None	1	(Reference)	0.02	1	(Reference)	0.04
Respiratory	1.67	1.09–2.56		1.65	1.03–2.65	
Non-respiratory	1.91	1.16–3.15		1.78	1.01–3.15	
Characteristics upon admission						
Neutropenia	1.41	1.02–1.94	0.04			
Antibiotherapy	1.18	0.80–1.72	0.4			
Corticosteroids (curative)	1.03	0.73–1.45	0.89			
SOFA score (day of intubation)	1.10	1.06–1.15	0.0001	1.11	1.05–1.17	0.0002
Characteristics at the first 48 h of MV						
Vasopressors	1.34	0.93–1.94	0.11			
Renal replacement therapy	1.45	1.00–2.12	0.06			
Substitutive hydrocortisone	1.28	0.92–1.77	0.28			
G-CSF	1.85	1.23–2.78	0.005	1.65	1.03–2.65	0.042
Enteral nutrition	1.17	0.68–2.00	0.58			
Antibiotherapy						
Adapted, n (%)	1	(Reference)	0.83			
Empirical, n (%)	0.85	0.6–1.22				
None, n (%)	0.96	0.5–1.86				
VAP	1.41	0.98–2.03	0.06	1.60	1.10–2.34	0.017

HSCT haematopoietic stem cell transplantation, *G-CSF* granulocyte colony-stimulating factors, *MV* mechanical ventilation, *VAP* ventilator-associated pneumonia

varies from 9% to more than 40% depending on the study and the given population. This heterogeneity is mainly explained by the lack of consensual definition [17, 21] and by the variability in VAP bundles implementation rates [22, 23] in the different ICUs. In this study, we used an association of clinical and bacteriological criteria to diagnose VAP in reference to the 2005 ATS/IDSA guidelines [12]. This definition is slightly different from the definition of probable VAP according to the last CDC definition of ventilator-associated events [24], which emphasize on FiO2 and positive end-expiratory pressure adjustment in response to worsening oxygenation. However, the prognostic significance of that current CDC definition remains to be established [25]. The cumulative incidence of VAP in our cohort was 28.9%. Despite regular use of validated VAP bundles in our ICU, this remains relatively high. Cancer treatments and malignancy-related immunosuppression could explain the

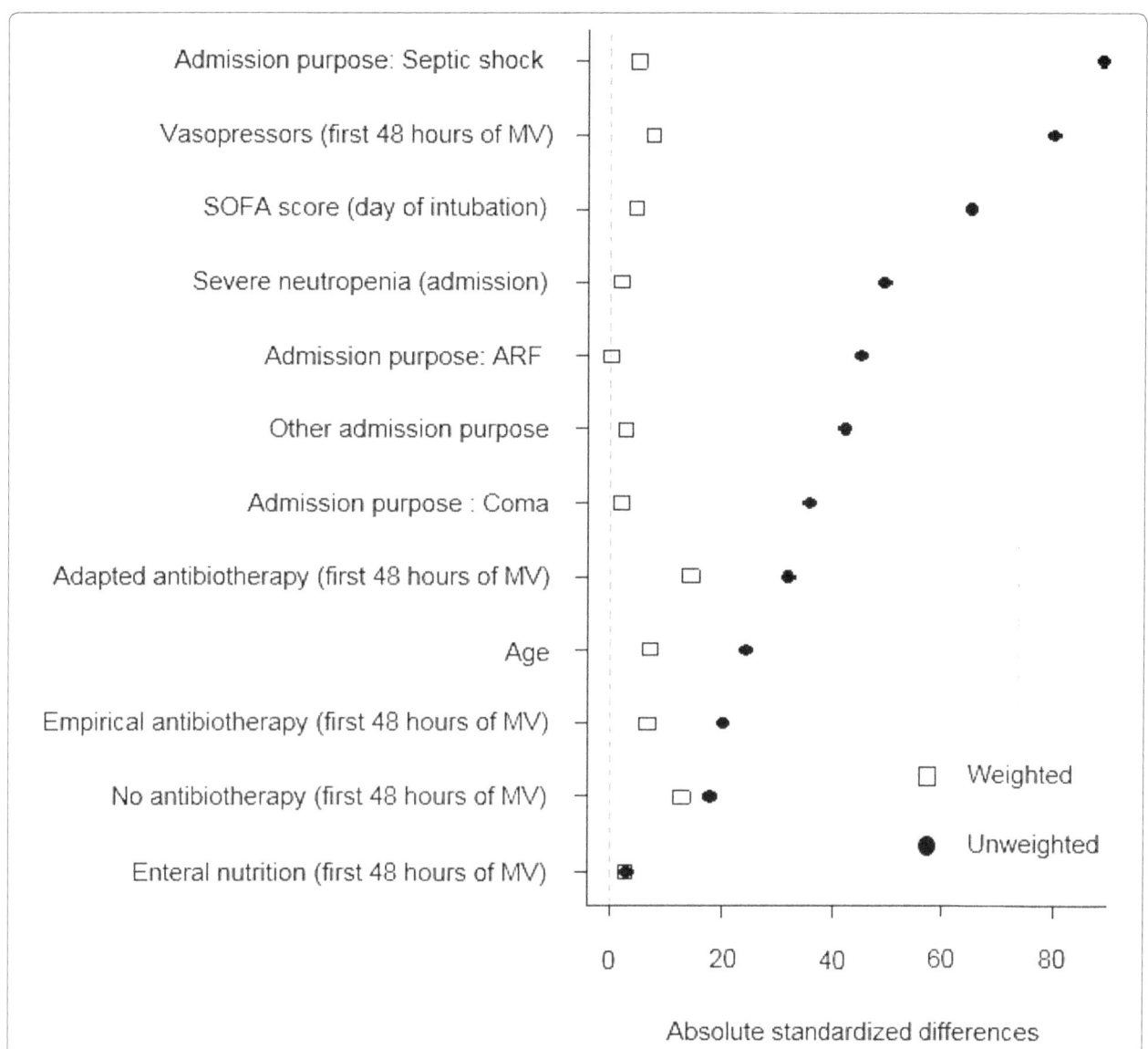

Fig. 1 Covariate imbalance (assessed by standardized mean differences) between the two groups of patients receiving and not receiving early HC in the unweighted (original) and weighted populations

higher susceptibility to develop nosocomial infections in the onco-haematological population.

Theoretically, VAP is a delayed event that happens after 48 h of mechanical ventilation. The pathophysiology of nosocomial infections combines the bacterial colonization induced by the invasiveness of general ICU cares (endotracheal intubation, catheter, etc.) and a state of susceptibility to infection [26]. It is well recognized that initial aggression induces a delayed state of profound immunodeficiency few days after the initial insult [3, 27]. More specifically, a biphasic evolution of immunological competence has been well described in sepsis [28] and trauma [29]. After an initial pro-inflammatory phase, a post-aggressive phase is characterized by a compensatory systemic anti-inflammatory state and an apoptotic depletion of immune cells [30, 31]. This delayed immunological status confers wider susceptibility to ICU-acquired infection [28] and viral reactivation. In the haematology population, ICU-induced immunodeficiency has also been described in neutropenic patients [32]. Monocyte and alveolar macrophage deactivation have been described after septic ARDS [33, 34] and could thus facilitate the occurrence of ICU-acquired infections. In order to counteract this phenomenon, low dose of hydrocortisone has been suggested to prevent post-aggressive immunosuppression. Indeed, hydrocortisone

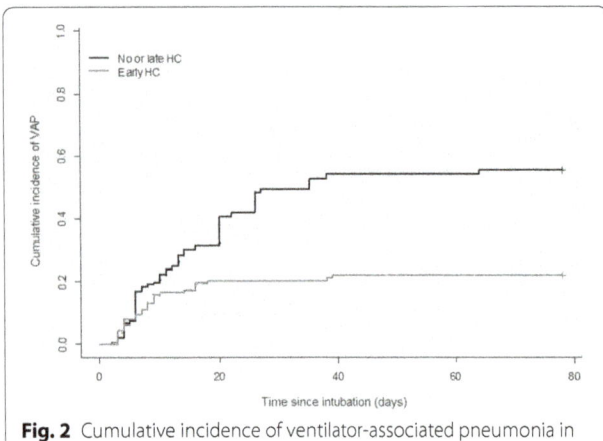

Fig. 2 Cumulative incidence of ventilator-associated pneumonia in the inverse probability of treatment weighting analysis

improves immune capacities, decreases blood concentrations of anti-inflammatory cytokines (interleukin-10) and increases host defence cytokines (interferon γ and interleukin-12) [4, 5]. However, despite positive hemodynamic effect, beneficial effect of substitutive corticotherapy on

septic shock survival remains controversial [8, 35, 36]. Last study showed that it failed to prevent the development of septic shock in the severe sepsis population [37]. The HIPOLYTE study [9] has compared low-dose hydrocortisone to placebo in the first 28 days after a severe trauma. It showed a reduction in the incidence of hospital-acquired pneumonia with 4 more ventilation-free days. Despite hydrocortisone treatment, no significant reduction in norepinephrine treatment duration was found in this study. To be effective, hydrocortisone should be started earlier as possible in order to decrease the initial pro-inflammatory response and counteract the anti-inflammatory compensation. In immunosuppressed cancer patients, we focused on potential beneficial effects of the early initiation of substitutive hydrocortisone for VAP prevention. A reverse propensity score analysis was used to control bias and population heterogeneity inherent to non-randomized observational studies. After weighing on the most pertinent covariates, we found that early hydrocortisone prescribed around the intubation time was protective against the subsequent occurrence of VAP.

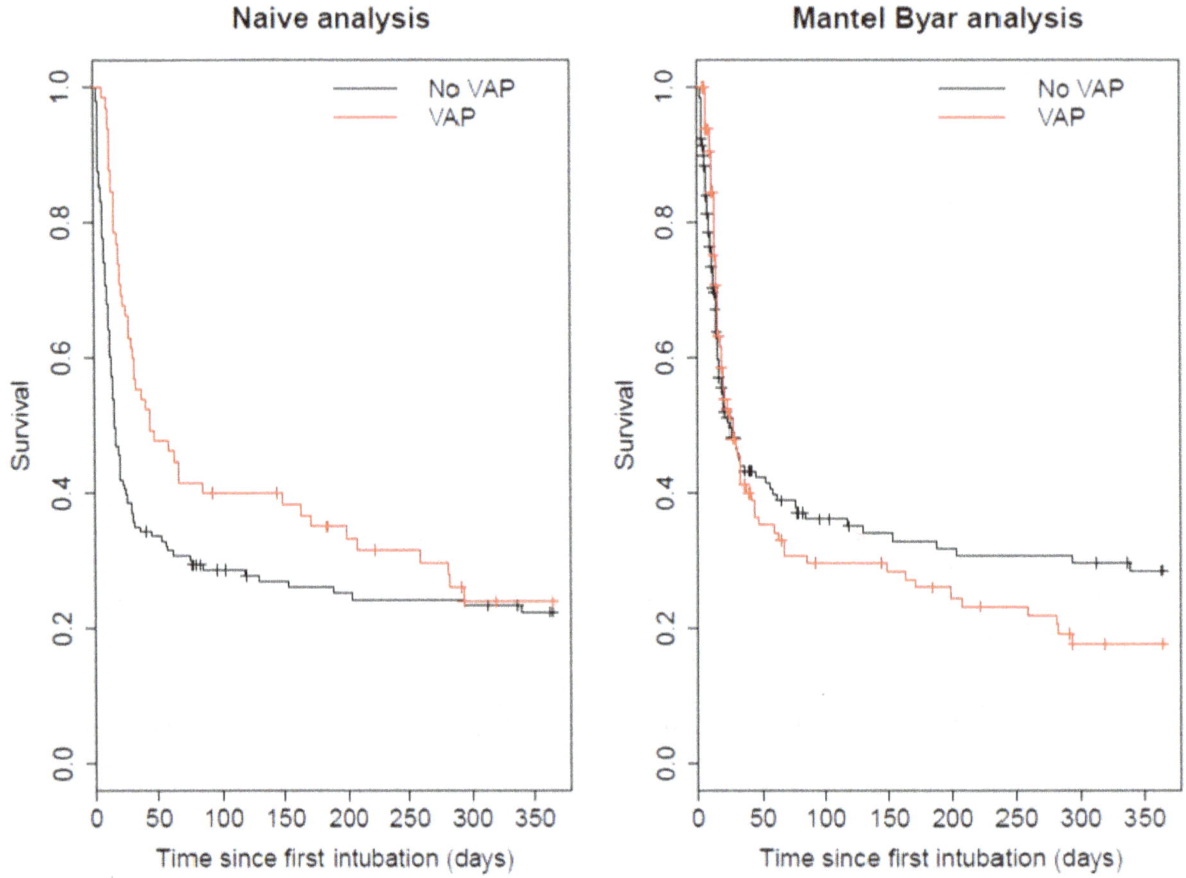

Fig. 3 One-year survival according to ventilator-associated pneumonia status: naive analysis and time-dependent Mantel–Byar analysis

VAP impact on mortality remains debated [38, 39]. The overuse of traditional crude statistical test in past studies had led to conflicting results and overestimation of attributable mortality of VAP [21]. In our work, VAP was not associated with mortality in the naive-exposed–unexposed analysis. That result is surely related to the high mortality rates in the first days of ICU admission in the critically ill cancer patients. Indeed, a majority of patients did not have time to develop VAP before dying (competing risk). On the contrary, by considering VAP as a time-dependent variable and estimating survival from the time of VAP diagnosis, we showed that VAP was significantly associated with 1-year mortality.

Our study has limitations. First, despite the use of propensity score analysis, this study is observational and residual confounding factors and biases may exist. For example, exposure to chemotherapy with or without curative corticotherapy before ICU stay has not been taking into account. However, neutropenic status was included in the baseline covariates for the propensity score construction. Second, this is a monocentric study, so it is possible that our local protocol including VAP prevention bundle, diagnosis strategies and therapeutic management could influence the occurrence and the prognostic impact of the disease. Third, adherence to VAP prevention bundle is not reported in each treatment group and could induce a bias. Finally, systemic antibiotic treatment could play a preventive role on VAP occurrence depending on its spectrum and its duration. These data are missing, but it is likely that the liberal use of broad spectrum antibiotics in the immunocompromised patients, irrespective of the hydrocortisone status, would diminish the confounding effect of these parameters.

Conclusions

We found a positive effect of early low-dose hydrocortisone treatment in preventing VAP. Immunological aspects are crucial in the development of nosocomial infections, specifically in patients prone to immunological disorders. Critically ill cancer patients could benefit from the administration of low-dose hydrocortisone in the days surrounding mechanical ventilation initiation. This interesting result should be evaluated in a future large-scale randomized controlled trial.

Abbreviations
CFU: colony-forming unit; G-CSF: granulocyte colony-stimulating factors; HSCT: haematopoietic stem cell transplantation; ICU: intensive care unit; IPW: inverse probability weighting; VAP: ventilator-associated pneumonia.

Authors' contributions
DL, LP and DM were involved in design of the work, data collection, interpretation of the results and writing of the draft. JL was involved in design of the work, full statistical analyses, writing of the draft. LCC, AS, MB, JPB and MF were involved in design of the work, data collection and manuscript revision. ML and KA were involved in design of the work, interpretation of the results and manuscript revision. All authors read and approved the final manuscript.

Author details
[1] Intensive Care Unit, Paoli-Calmettes Institute, 232 Boulevard de Sainte-Marguerite, 13009 Marseille, France. [2] Biostatistics Department, Saint Louis Teaching Hospital, AP-HP, 1, Avenue Claude Vellefaux, 75010 Paris, France. [3] Department of Anesthesiology and Critical Care Medicine, Hotel Dieu, University Hospital of Nantes, 1 Place Alexis Ricordeau, 44903 Nantes, France. [4] Department of Anesthesiology and Critical Care Medicine, Hopital Nord, University Hospital of Marseille, Chemin des Bourrely, 13015 Marseille, France.

Acknowledgements
None.

Competing interests
The authors declare that they have no competing interests.

Funding
No financial support.

References
1. Mokart D, Pastores SM, Darmon M. Has survival increased in cancer patients admitted to the ICU? Yes. Intensive Care Med. 2014;40(10):1570–2.
2. Azoulay E, Pene F, Darmon M, Lengline E, Benoit D, Soares M, et al. Managing critically ill hematology patients: time to think differently. Blood Rev. 2015;29(6):359–67.
3. van Vught LA, Klein Klouwenberg PM, Spitoni C, Scicluna BP, Wiewel MA, Horn J, et al. Incidence, risk factors, and attributable mortality of secondary infections in the intensive care unit after admission for sepsis. JAMA. 2016;315(14):1469–79.
4. Kaufmann I, Briegel J, Schliephake F, Hoelzl A, Chouker A, Hummel T, et al. Stress doses of hydrocortisone in septic shock: beneficial effects on opsonization-dependent neutrophil functions. Intensive Care Med. 2008;34(2):344–9.
5. Keh D, Boehnke T, Weber-Cartens S, Schulz C, Ahlers O, Bercker S, et al. Immunologic and hemodynamic effects of "low-dose" hydrocortisone in septic shock: a double-blind, randomized, placebo-controlled, crossover study. Am J Respir Crit Care Med. 2003;167(4):512–20.
6. Kanangat S, Meduri GU, Tolley EA, Patterson DR, Meduri CU, Pak C, et al. Effects of cytokines and endotoxin on the intracellular growth of bacteria. Infect Immun. 1999;67(6):2834–40.
7. Meduri GU, Kanangat S, Stefan J, Tolley E, Schaberg D. Cytokines IL-1beta, IL-6, and TNF-alpha enhance in vitro growth of bacteria. Am J Respir Crit Care Med. 1999;160(3):961–7.
8. Sprung CL, Annane D, Keh D, Moreno R, Singer M, Freivogel K, et al. Hydrocortisone therapy for patients with septic shock. N Engl J Med. 2008;358(2):111–24.
9. Roquilly A, Mahe PJ, Seguin P, Guitton C, Floch H, Tellier AC, et al. Hydrocortisone therapy for patients with multiple trauma: the randomized controlled HYPOLYTE study. JAMA. 2011;305(12):1201–9.
10. Azoulay E, Mokart D, Pene F, Lambert J, Kouatchet A, Mayaux J, et al. Outcomes of critically ill patients with hematological malignancies: prospective multicenter data from France and Belgium—a groupe de recherche respiratoire en reanimation onco-hematologique study. J Clin Oncol. 2013;31(22):2810–8.
11. Lemiale V, Mokart D, Resche-Rigon M, Pene F, Mayaux J, Faucher E, et al. Effect of noninvasive ventilation vs oxygen therapy on mortality among immunocompromised patients with acute respiratory failure: a randomized clinical trial. JAMA. 2015;314(16):1711–9.
12. American Thoracic S. Infectious diseases society of A. Guidelines for the management of adults with hospital-acquired, ventilator-associated, and healthcare-associated pneumonia. Am J Respir Crit Care Med. 2005;171(4):388–416.
13. Kalanuria AA, Ziai W, Mirski M. Ventilator-associated pneumonia in the ICU. Crit Care. 2014;18(2):208.
14. Vincent JL, Moreno R, Takala J, Willatts S, De Mendonca A, Bruining H, et al. The SOFA (Sepsis-related Organ Failure Assessment) score to describe organ dysfunction/failure. On behalf of the Working Group

on Sepsis-Related Problems of the European Society of Intensive Care Medicine. Intensive Care Med. 1996;22(7):707–10.

15. Borgatta B, Rello J. How to approach and treat VAP in ICU patients. BMC Infect Dis. 2014;14:211.

16. Klompas M, Platt R. Ventilator-associated pneumonia-the wrong quality measure for benchmarking. Ann Intern Med. 2007;147(11):803–5.

17. Nair GB, Niederman MS. Ventilator-associated pneumonia: present under-standing and ongoing debates. Intensive Care Med. 2015;41(1):34–48.

18. Bekaert M, Timsit JF, Vansteelandt S, Depuydt P, Vesin A, Garrouste-Orgeas M, et al. Attributable mortality of ventilator-associated pneu-monia: a reappraisal using causal analysis. Am J Respir Crit Care Med. 2011;184(10):1133–9.

19. Melsen WG, Rovers MM, Groenwold RH, Bergmans DC, Camus C, Bauer TT, et al. Attributable mortality of ventilator-associated pneumonia: a meta-analysis of individual patient data from randomised prevention studies. Lancet Infect Dis. 2013;13(8):665–71.

20. Safdar N, Dezfulian C, Collard HR, Saint S. Clinical and economic conse-quences of ventilator-associated pneumonia: a systematic review. Crit Care Med. 2005;33(10):2184–93.

21. Timsit JF, Zahar JR, Chevret S. Attributable mortality of ventilator-associ-ated pneumonia. Curr Opin Crit Care. 2011;17(5):464–71.

22. Batra P, Mathur P, John NV, Nair SA, Aggarwal R, Soni KD, et al. Impact of multifaceted preventive measures on ventilator-associated pneumonia at a single surgical centre. Intensive Care Med. 2015;41(12):2231–2.

23. Pileggi C, Bianco A, Flotta D, Nobile CG, Pavia M. Prevention of ventilator-associated pneumonia, mortality and all intensive care unit acquired infections by topically applied antimicrobial or antiseptic agents: a meta-analysis of randomized controlled trials in intensive care units. Crit Care. 2011;15(3):R155.

24. Magill SS, Klompas M, Balk R, Burns SM, Deutschman CS, Diekema D, et al. Developing a new, national approach to surveillance for ventilator-associated events. Crit Care Med. 2013;41(11):2467–75.

25. Bouadma L, Sonneville R, Garrouste-Orgeas M, Darmon M, Souweine B, Voiriot G, et al. Ventilator-associated events: prevalence, outcome, and relationship with ventilator-associated pneumonia. Crit Care Med. 2015;43(9):1798–806.

26. Peleg AY, Hooper DC. Hospital-acquired infections due to gram-negative bacteria. N Engl J Med. 2010;362(19):1804–13.

27. Angus DC, Opal S. Immunosuppression and secondary infection in sepsis: part, not all, of the story. JAMA. 2016;315(14):1457–9.

28. Landelle C, Lepape A, Voirin N, Tognet E, Venet F, Bohe J, et al. Low monocyte human leukocyte antigen-DR is independently associated with nosocomial infections after septic shock. Intensive Care Med. 2010;36(11):1859–66.

29. Asehnoune K, Roquilly A, Abraham E. Innate immune dysfunction in trauma patients: from pathophysiology to treatment. Anesthesiology. 2012;117(2):411–6.

30. Grimaldi D, Louis S, Pene F, Sirgo G, Rousseau C, Claessens YE, et al. Pro-found and persistent decrease of circulating dendritic cells is associated with ICU-acquired infection in patients with septic shock. Intensive Care Med. 2011;37(9):1438–46.

31. Monneret G, Lepape A, Voirin N, Bohe J, Venet F, Debard AL, et al. Persist-ing low monocyte human leukocyte antigen-DR expression predicts mortality in septic shock. Intensive Care Med. 2006;32(8):1175–83.

32. Mokart D, Darmon M, Azoulay E. The alveolar macrophage and acute respiratory distress syndrome: A silent actor? Am J Respir Crit Care Med. 2014;189(4):499–500.

33. Mokart D, Kipnis E, Guerre-Berthelot P, Vey N, Capo C, Sannini A, et al. Monocyte deactivation in neutropenic acute respiratory distress syn-drome patients treated with granulocyte colony-stimulating factor. Crit Care. 2008;12(1):R17.

34. Mokart D, Guery BP, Bouabdallah R, Martin C, Blache JL, Arnoulet C, et al. Deactivation of alveolar macrophages in septic neutropenic ARDS. Chest. 2003;124(2):644–52.

35. Annane D, Sebille V, Charpentier C, Bollaert PE, Francois B, Korach JM, et al. Effect of treatment with low doses of hydrocortisone and fludrocortisone on mortality in patients with septic shock. JAMA. 2002;288(7):862–71.

36. Kalil AC, Sun J. Low-dose steroids for septic shock and severe sepsis: the use of Bayesian statistics to resolve clinical trial controversies. Intensive Care Med. 2011;37(3):420–9.

37. Keh D, Trips E, Marx G, Wirtz SP, Abduljawwad E, Bercker S, et al. Effect of hydrocortisone on development of shock among patients with severe sepsis: the HYPRESS randomized clinical trial. JAMA. 2016;316(17):1775–85.

38. Nguile-Makao M, Zahar JR, Francais A, Tabah A, Garrouste-Orgeas M, Allaouchiche B, et al. Attributable mortality of ventilator-associated pneu-monia: respective impact of main characteristics at ICU admission and VAP onset using conditional logistic regression and multi-state models. Intensive Care Med. 2010;36(5):781–9.

39. Melsen WG, Rovers MM, Koeman M, Bonten MJ. Estimating the attribut-able mortality of ventilator-associated pneumonia from randomized prevention studies. Crit Care Med. 2011;39(12):2736–42.

Permissions

All chapters in this book were first published in AIC, by Springer; hereby published with permission under the Creative Commons Attribution License or equivalent. Every chapter published in this book has been scrutinized by our experts. Their significance has been extensively debated. The topics covered herein carry significant findings which will fuel the growth of the discipline. They may even be implemented as practical applications or may be referred to as a beginning point for another development.

The contributors of this book come from diverse backgrounds, making this book a truly international effort. This book will bring forth new frontiers with its revolutionizing research information and detailed analysis of the nascent developments around the world.

We would like to thank all the contributing authors for lending their expertise to make the book truly unique. They have played a crucial role in the development of this book. Without their invaluable contributions this book wouldn't have been possible. They have made vital efforts to compile up to date information on the varied aspects of this subject to make this book a valuable addition to the collection of many professionals and students.

This book was conceptualized with the vision of imparting up-to-date information and advanced data in this field. To ensure the same, a matchless editorial board was set up. Every individual on the board went through rigorous rounds of assessment to prove their worth. After which they invested a large part of their time researching and compiling the most relevant data for our readers.

The editorial board has been involved in producing this book since its inception. They have spent rigorous hours researching and exploring the diverse topics which have resulted in the successful publishing of this book. They have passed on their knowledge of decades through this book. To expedite this challenging task, the publisher supported the team at every step. A small team of assistant editors was also appointed to further simplify the editing procedure and attain best results for the readers.

Apart from the editorial board, the designing team has also invested a significant amount of their time in understanding the subject and creating the most relevant covers. They scrutinized every image to scout for the most suitable representation of the subject and create an appropriate cover for the book.

The publishing team has been an ardent support to the editorial, designing and production team. Their endless efforts to recruit the best for this project, has resulted in the accomplishment of this book. They are a veteran in the field of academics and their pool of knowledge is as vast as their experience in printing. Their expertise and guidance has proved useful at every step. Their uncompromising quality standards have made this book an exceptional effort. Their encouragement from time to time has been an inspiration for everyone.

The publisher and the editorial board hope that this book will prove to be a valuable piece of knowledge for researchers, students, practitioners and scholars across the globe.

List of Contributors

Jérôme Martin-Babau
Réanimation Médicale, CHRU de Brest – La Cavale Blanche, Bvd Tanguy-Prigent, 29609 Brest Cedex, France

Erwan L'her
Réanimation Médicale, CHRU de Brest – La Cavale Blanche, Bvd Tanguy-Prigent, 29609 Brest Cedex, France
LATIM INSERM UMR 1101, Université de Bretagne Occidentale, Brest Cedex, France

François Lellouche
Institut Universitaire de Cardiologie et de Pneumologie de Québec, Quebec, Canada

Matthieu Dorison, Jérémy Rosman and Aude Gibelin
Groupe Henri Mondor-Albert Chenevier, Centre Hospitalier Universitaire Henri Mondor, DHU A-TVB, Service de Réanimation Médicale, Assistance Publique-Hôpitaux de Paris, 51, Avenue du Maréchal de Lattre de Tassigny, 94010 Créteil Cedex, France

Damien Contou, Guillaume Carteaux, Keyvan Razazi, Christian Brun-Buisson, Armand Mekontso Dessap and Nicolas de Prost
Groupe Henri Mondor-Albert Chenevier, Centre Hospitalier Universitaire Henri Mondor, DHU A-TVB, Service de Réanimation Médicale, Assistance Publique-Hôpitaux de Paris, 51, Avenue du Maréchal de Lattre de Tassigny, 94010 Créteil Cedex, France
Groupe de Recherche CARMAS, Faculté de Médecine de Créteil, Université Paris Est Créteil, 94010 Créteil, France

Frédéric Schlemmer
Centre Hospitalier Universitaire Henri Mondor, DHU A-TVB, Antenne de Pneumologie, Assistance Publique-Hôpitaux de Paris, 94010 Créteil, France

Françoise Foulet and Françoise Botterel
Unité de Mycologie, Département de Biologie-Pathologie, Centre Hospitalier Universitaire Henri Mondor, DHU VIC, Assistance Publique-Hôpitaux de Paris, 94010 Créteil, France

Kevin J. Solverson
Department of Critical Care Medicine, Cumming School of Medicine, University of Calgary, 3134 Hospital Drive NW, Calgary, AB T2N 2T9, Canada

Christopher Grant
Department of Critical Care Medicine, Cumming School of Medicine, University of Calgary, 3134 Hospital Drive NW, Calgary, AB T2N 2T9, Canada
Division of Physical Medicine and Rehabilitation, Cumming School of Medicine, University of Calgary, 3134 Hospital Drive NW, Calgary, AB T2N 2T9, Canada

Christopher J. Doig
Department of Critical Care Medicine, Cumming School of Medicine, University of Calgary, 3134 Hospital Drive NW, Calgary, AB T2N 2T9, Canada
Department of Community Health Sciences, Cumming School of Medicine, University of Calgary, 3134 Hospital Drive NW, Calgary, AB T2N 2T9, Canada

Anahita Rouzé, Erika Parmentier-Decrucq, Benoit Voisin and Emmanuelle Jaillette
Centre de Réanimation, CHU Lille, 59000 Lille, France

Saad Nseir
Centre de Réanimation, CHU Lille, 59000 Lille, France
Faculté de Médecine, Université Lille, 59000 Lille, France

Julien De Jonckheere
Centre d'Investigation Clinique, CHU Lille, 59000 Lille, France

Farid Zerimech and Patrice Maboudou
Centre de Biologie et de Pathologie, CHU Lille, 59000 Lille, France

Julien Labreuche
EA 2694 - Santé publique : épidémiologie et qualité des soins, CHU Lille, 59000 Lille, France

Malika Balduyck
Centre de Biologie et de Pathologie, CHU Lille, 59000 Lille, France
Faculté de Pharmacie, Université Lille, 59000 Lille, France

Chun-Yu Lin and Ying-Jen Chen
Department of General Medicine and Geriatrics, Chang Gung Memorial Hospital at Linkou, Taoyuan, Taiwan
College of Medicine, Chang Gung University, Taoyuan, Taiwan

Han-Chung Hu, Kuo-chin Kao, Ning-Hung Chen, Cheng-Ta Yang and Chung-Chi Huang
Department of Pulmonary and Critical Care Medicine, Chang Gung Memorial Hospital at Linkou, Taoyuan, Taiwan
College of Medicine, Chang Gung University, Taoyuan, Taiwan

Wei-Lun Liu
Department of Intensive Care Medicine, Chi Mei Medical Center, Liouying, Tainan, Taiwan
College of Health Sciences, Graduate Institute of Medical Sciences, Chang Jung Christian University, Tainan, Taiwan
College of Medicine, Fu Jen Catholic University, New Taipei, Taiwan

Che-Chia Chang
Department of Pulmonary and Critical Care Medicine, Chang Gung Memorial Hospital at Chiayi, Chiayi, Taiwan

Hou-Tai Chang
Department of Critical Care Medicine, Far Eastern Memorial Hospital, New Taipei City, Taiwan

George Dimopoulos
Department of Critical Care, ATTIKON University Hospital, University of Athens, Medical School, Athens, Greece

Rob B. P. de Wilde, Jos R. C. Jansen, David J. van Westerloo and Evert de Jonge
Department of Intensive Care Medicine, Leiden University Medical Center, Leiden 2300 RC, The Netherlands

Hendrik J. F. Helmerhorst
Department of Intensive Care Medicine, Leiden University Medical Center, Leiden 2300 RC, The Netherlands
Department of Anesthesiology, Leiden University Medical Center, Leiden, The Netherlands
Laboratory of Experimental Intensive Care and Anesthesiology, Academic Medical Center, Amsterdam, The Netherlands

Dae Hyun Lee
Department of Nephrology, Einthoven Laboratory for Vascular Medicine, Leiden University Medical Center, Leiden, The Netherlands

Meindert Palmen
Department of Cardiothoracic Surgery, Leiden University Medical Center, Leiden, The Netherlands

Benjamin Bueno
Pediatric Intensive Care and Neonatal Medicine, Paris South University Hospitals, Assistance Publique Hôpitaux de Paris, 78, Rue du Général Leclerc, 94270 Le Kremlin-Bicêtre, France

Michaël Levy and Nolwenn Le Sache
Pediatric Intensive Care and Neonatal Medicine, Paris South University Hospitals, Assistance Publique Hôpitaux de Paris, 78, Rue du Général Leclerc, 94270 Le Kremlin-Bicêtre, France
Centre de référence Maladie Rare: Hernie de Coupole Diaphragmatique, 94270 Le Kremlin-Bicêtre, France

Mostafa Mokhtari
Centre de référence Maladie Rare: Hernie de Coupole Diaphragmatique, 94270 Le Kremlin-Bicêtre, France

Guy Fagherazzi
INSERM U1018, Center for Research in Epidemiology and Population Health (CESP), Paris South University, 94805 Villejuif, France

Gaelle Cuzon
Bacteriology-Hygiene Unit, Paris South University Hospitals, Assistance Publique Hôpitaux de Paris, Le Kremlin-Bicêtre, France

Virginie Fouquet
Centre de référence Maladie Rare: Hernie de Coupole Diaphragmatique, 94270 Le Kremlin Bicêtre, France
Pediatric Surgery, Paris South University Hospitals, Assistance Publique Hôpitaux de Paris, Le Kremlin-Bicêtre, France
School of Medicine, Paris South University, UPS11, Le Kremlin-Bicêtre, France

Alexandra Benachi
Centre de référence Maladie Rare: Hernie de Coupole Diaphragmatique, 94270 Le Kremlin-Bicêtre, France
School of Medicine, Paris South University, UPS11, Le Kremlin-Bicêtre, France

Obstetrics, Gynecology and Reproductive Medicine, Antoine Béclère Hospital, Assistance Publique Hôpitaux de Paris, Clamart, France

Sergio Eleni Dit Trolli
Pediatric Intensive Care and Neonatal Medicine, Paris South University Hospitals, Assistance Publique Hôpitaux de Paris, 78, Rue du Général Leclerc, 94270 Le Kremlin-Bicêtre, France
Centre de référence Maladie Rare: Hernie de Coupole Diaphragmatique, 94270 Le Kremlin-Bicêtre, France
Institute of Integrative Biology of the Cell, CNRS, CEA, Univ. Paris Sud, Paris Saclay University, Gif-sur-Yvette, France

Pierre Tissieres
Pediatric Intensive Care and Neonatal Medicine, Paris South University Hospitals, Assistance Publique Hôpitaux de Paris, 78, Rue du Général Leclerc, 94270 Le Kremlin-Bicêtre, France
Centre de référence Maladie Rare: Hernie de Coupole Diaphragmatique, 94270 Le Kremlin-Bicêtre, France
School of Medicine, Paris South University, UPS11, Le Kremlin-Bicêtre, France
Institute of Integrative Biology of the Cell, CNRS, CEA, Univ. Paris Sud, Paris Saclay University, Gif-sur-Yvette, France

Fekri Abroug, Lamia Ouanes-Besbes, Zeineb Hammouda, Saoussen Benabidallah, Fahmi Dachraoui and Islem Ouanes
Intensive Care Unit, CHU Fatouma Bourguiba, Research Laboratory LR12SP15, University of Monastir, 5000 Monastir, Tunisia

Philippe Jolliet
Département des Centres Interdisciplinaires et de Logistique Médicale, Lausanne, Switzerland

Stephan Ehrmann
Médecine Intensive Réanimation, Réseau CRICS-TRIGGERSEP, Centre Hospitalier Régional et Universitaire de Tours, Tours, France
Centre d'études des Pathologies Respiratoire, INSERM U1100, Faculté de Médecine de Tours, Université François Rabelais de Tours, Tours, France

Jean Chastre
Service de Réanimation Médicale, Institut de Cardiologie, Assistance Publique-Hôpitaux de Paris, Pitié- Salpêtrière Hospital, UPMC (University Pierre and Marie Curie) Paris-6, Paris, France

Patrice Diot
Centre d'études des Pathologies Respiratoire, INSERM U1100, Faculté de Médecine de Tours, Université François Rabelais de Tours, Tours, France
Pneumologie, Centre Hospitalier Régional et Universitaire de Tours, Tours, France

Qin Lu
Multidisciplinary Critical Care Unit, Department of Anesthesiology and Critical Care Medicine, Assistance Publique-Hôpitaux de Paris, Pitié-Salpêtrière Hospital, UPMC (University Pierre and Marie Curie) Paris-6, Paris, France

Pan Pan Wang
Pharmacy Department, Lakeshore General Hospital, Montreal, Canada

Elaine Huang and Charles-André Bray
Pharmacy Department, Hôpital de Verdun, Montreal, Canada

Xue Feng
Pharmacy Department, Hôpital du Sacré-Coeur de Montréal, 5400 Gouin West, Montreal, QC H4J 1C5, Canada

Anne Julie Frenette and David Williamson
Pharmacy Department, Hôpital du Sacré-Coeur de Montréal, 5400 Gouin West, Montreal, QC H4J 1C5, Canada
Faculté de Pharmacie, Université de Montréal, Montreal, Canada

Marc M. Perreault
Faculté de Pharmacie, Université de Montréal, Montreal, Canada
Pharmacy Department, McGill University Health Center, Montreal, Canada

Paul Murgoi
Pharmacy Department, McGill University Health Center, Montreal, Canada

Philippe Rico and Patrick Bellemare
Critical Care Department, Hôpital du Sacré-Coeur de Montréal, Montreal, Canada
Faculté de Médecine, Université de Montréal, Montreal, Canada

Céline Gélinas
Ingram School of Nursing, McGill University, Montreal, QC, Canada

Centre for Nursing Research and Lady Davis Institute, Jewish General Hospital, Montreal, Canada

Annie Lecavalier
Department of Adult Critical Care, Jewish General Hospital, McGill University, Montreal, QC, Canada

Dev Jayaraman
Department of Critical Care, Montreal General Hospital, McGill University Health Center, Montreal, Canada

Jeffrey B. Geske
Department of Cardiovascular Medicine, Mayo Clinic, 200 First Street SW, Rochester, MN 55905, USA

Jacob C. Jentzer
Department of Cardiovascular Medicine, Mayo Clinic, 200 First Street SW, Rochester, MN 55905, USA
Division of Pulmonary and Critical Care Medicine, Department of Medicine, Mayo Clinic, 200 First Street SW, Rochester, MN 55905, USA

Ognjen Gajic
Division of Pulmonary and Critical Care Medicine, Department of Medicine, Mayo Clinic, 200 First Street SW, Rochester, MN 55905, USA
Multidisciplinary Epidemiology and Translational Research in Intensive Care (METRIC) Laboratory, Mayo Clinic, 200 First Street SW, Rochester 55905, MN, USA

Saraschandra Vallabhajosyula
Department of Cardiovascular Medicine, Mayo Clinic, 200 First Street SW, Rochester, MN 55905, USA
Division of Pulmonary and Critical Care Medicine, Department of Medicine, Mayo Clinic, 200 First Street SW, Rochester, MN 55905, USA
Multidisciplinary Epidemiology and Translational Research in Intensive Care (METRIC) Laboratory, Mayo Clinic, 200 First Street SW, Rochester 55905, MN, USA
Center for Clinical and Translational Science, Mayo Clinic Graduate School of Biomedical Sciences, Mayo Clinic, 200 First Street SW, Rochester 55905, MN, USA

Govind Pandompatam and Ankit Sakhuja
Division of Pulmonary and Critical Care Medicine, Department of Medicine, Mayo Clinic, 200 First Street SW, Rochester, MN 55905, USA

Mukesh Kumar and Rahul Kashyap
Multidisciplinary Epidemiology and Translational Research in Intensive Care (METRIC) Laboratory, Mayo Clinic, 200 First Street SW, Rochester 55905, MN, USA
Department of Anesthesiology and Perioperative Medicine, Mayo Clinic, 200 First Street SW, Rochester 55905, MN, USA

Kianoush Kashani
Division of Pulmonary and Critical Care Medicine, Department of Medicine, Mayo Clinic, 200 First Street SW, Rochester, MN 55905, USA
Multidisciplinary Epidemiology and Translational Research in Intensive Care (METRIC) Laboratory, Mayo Clinic, 200 First Street SW, Rochester 55905, MN, USA
Division of Nephrology and Hypertension, Department of Medicine, Mayo Clinic, 200 First Street SW, Rochester 55905, MN, USA

Lu Chen and Laurent Brochard
Interdepartmental Division of Critical Care Medicine, University of Toronto, Toronto, ON, Canada
Keenan Research Centre and Li Ka Shing Knowledge Institute, St. Michael's Hospital, 30 Bond St, Toronto, ON M5B 1W8, Canada

Nuttapol Rittayamai
Interdepartmental Division of Critical Care Medicine, University of Toronto, Toronto, ON, Canada
Keenan Research Centre and Li Ka Shing Knowledge Institute, St. Michael's Hospital, 30 Bond St, Toronto, ON M5B 1W8, Canada
Division of Respiratory Diseases and Tuberculosis, Department of Medicine, Faculty of Medicine Siriraj Hospital, Bangkok, Thailand

François Beloncle
Interdepartmental Division of Critical Care Medicine, University of Toronto, Toronto, ON, Canada
Keenan Research Centre and Li Ka Shing Knowledge Institute, St. Michael's Hospital, 30 Bond St, Toronto, ON M5B 1W8, Canada
Medical Intensive Care Unit, Hospital of Angers, University of Angers, Angers, France

Ewan C. Goligher
Interdepartmental Division of Critical Care Medicine, University of Toronto, Toronto, ON, Canada

Department of Medicine, University of Toronto, Toronto, Canada
Department of Physiology, University of Toronto, Toronto, Canada
Division of Respirology, Department of Medicine, University Health Network and Mount Sinai Hospital, Toronto, Canada

Jordi Mancebo
Centre de recherche du Centre Hospitalier de l, Université de Montréal (CRCHUM), University of Montreal', Montreal, Canada
Servei de Medicina Intensiva, Hospital Sant Pau, Barcelona, Spain

Jean-Christophe M. Richard
Emergency Department, General Hospital of Annecy, Annecy, France
INSERM UMR 955 eq 13, Créteil, France

Gerie J. Glas, Janneke Horn and Marcus J. Schultz
Laboratory of Experimental Intensive Care and Anesthesiology (L·E·I·C·A), Department of Intensive Care, Academic Medical Center, Meibergdreef 9, 1105 AZ Amsterdam, The Netherlands

Ary Serpa Neto
Department of Critical Care Medicine, Hospital Israelita Albert Einstein, São Paulo, Brazil
Department of Critical Care Medicine, Faculdade de Medicina do ABC, Santo André, Brazil
Program of Post-Graduation, Research and Innovation, Faculdade de Medicina do ABC, Santo André, Brazil

Amalia Cochran and Iris Faraklas
Department of Surgery, University of Utah Health Sciences Center, Salt Lake City, UT, USA

Barry Dixon
Department of Intensive Care, St. Vincent's Hospital, Melbourne, Australia

Elamin M. Elamin
Division of Pulmonary, Critical Care, and Sleep Medicine, Department of Internal Medicine, James A. Haley Veteran's Hospital, University of South Florida, Tampa, FL, USA

Sharmila Dissanaike
Department of Surgery, Texas Tech University Health Sciences Center, Lubbock, TX, USA

Andrew C. Miller
Department of Critical Care Medicine, Clinical Center, National Institutes of Health, Bethesda, MD, USA
Department of Emergency Medicine, West Virginia University, Morgantown, WV, USA

Clément Medrinal
Normandie Univ, UNIROUEN, EA3830 - GRHV, 76000 Rouen, France
Institute for Research and Innovation in Biomedicine (IRIB), 76000 Rouen, France
Intensive Care Unit Department, Groupe Hospitalier du Havre, Avenue Pierre Mendes France, 76290 Montivilliers, France

Aurora Robledo Quesada
Intensive Care Unit Department, Groupe Hospitalier du Havre, Avenue Pierre Mendes France, 76290 Montivilliers, France

Guillaume Prieur
Pulmonology Department, Groupe Hospitalier du Havre, Avenue Pierre Mendes France, 76290 Montivilliers, France

Yann Combret
Institut de Recherche Expérimentale et Clinique (IREC), Pôle de Pneumologie, ORL and Dermatologie, Université Catholique de Louvain, Brussels 1200, Belgium
Physiotherapy Department, Groupe Hospitalier du Havre, Avenue Pierre Mendes France, 76290 Montivilliers, France

Tristan Bonnevie
Normandie Univ, UNIROUEN, EA3830 - GRHV, 76000 Rouen, France
Institute for Research and Innovation in Biomedicine (IRIB), 76000 Rouen, France
ADIR Association, Bois Guillaume, France

Francis Edouard Gravier
ADIR Association, Bois Guillaume, France

Eric Frenoy
Intensive Care Unit Department, Hôpital Jacques Monod, 76290 Montivilliers, France

Olivier Contal
University of Applied Sciences and Arts Western Switzerland (HES-SO), Avenue de Beaumont, 1011 Lausanne, Switzerland

Bouchra Lamia
Normandie Univ, UNIROUEN, EA3830 - GRHV, 76000 Rouen, France
Institute for Research and Innovation in Biomedicine (IRIB), 76000 Rouen, France
Pulmonology Department, Groupe Hospitalier du Havre, Avenue Pierre Mendes France, 76290 Montivilliers, France
Intensive Care Unit, Respiratory Department, Rouen University Hospital, Rouen, France

Hernan Aguirre-Bermeo, Marta Turella, Maddalena Bitondo, Juan Grandjean, Stefano Italiano, Olimpia Festa, Indalecio Morán and Jordi Mancebo
Servei de Medicina Intensiva, Hospital de la Santa Creu i Sant Pau, Universitat Autònoma de Barcelona (UAB), Sant Quintí, 89, 08041 Barcelona, Spain

Sophie Emilia Huttmann, Friederike Sophie Magnet, Christian Karagiannidis and Wolfram Windisch
Department of Pneumology, Cologne-Merheim Hospital, Kliniken der Stadt Köln gGmbH, Witten/Herdecke University Hospital, Ostmerheimer Strasse 200, 51109 Cologne, Germany

Jan Hendrik Storre
Department of Pneumology, University Medical Hospital, Freiburg, Germany
Department of Intensive Care, Sleep Medicine and Mechanical Ventilation, Asklepios Fachkliniken Munich-Gauting, Gauting, Germany

Faten May, Nicolas de Prost, Christian Brun-Buisson and Guillaume Carteaux
AP-HP, DHU A-TVB, Service de Réanimation Médicale, Hôpitaux Universitaires Henri Mondor, 94010 Créteil, France
Faculté de Médecine de Créteil, IMRB, GRC CARMAS, Université Paris Est Créteil, 94010 Créteil, France

Armand Mekontso Dessap and Keyvan Razazi
AP-HP, DHU A-TVB, Service de Réanimation Médicale, Hôpitaux Universitaires Henri Mondor, 94010 Créteil, France
Faculté de Médecine de Créteil, IMRB, GRC CARMAS, Université Paris Est Créteil, 94010 Créteil, France
Unité U955 (Institut Mondor de Recherche Biomédicale), INSERM, Créteil, France

Florence Boissier
Service de Réanimation Médicale, Centre Hospitalier Universitaire de Poitiers, Poitiers 86021, France
AP-HP, Service de Réanimation Médicale, Hôpital Européen Georges Pompidou, 75015 Paris, France

Mathilde Neuville
AP-HP, Réanimation Médicale et des Maladies Infectieuses, Hôpital Bichat Claude Bernard, Paris, France

Sébastien Jochmans
Faculté de Médecine de Créteil, IMRB, GRC CARMAS, Université Paris Est Créteil, 94010 Créteil, France
Département de Médecine Intensive, Groupe Hospitalier Sud Ile-de-France, Hôpital de Melun, 77011 Melun, France

Martial Tchir
Service de Réanimation, Centre Hospitalier de Villeneuve-Saint-Georges, 94190 Villeneuve-Saint-Georges, France

Carlos Toufen Junior, Roberta R. De Santis Santiago, Adriana S. Hirota, Susimeire Gomes and Carlos Roberto Ribeiro Carvalho
Divisão de Pneumologia, Cardiopulmonary Department, Heart Institute (InCor) University of São Paulo, INCOR Av. Dr. Enéas de Carvalho Aguiar, 44 Pinheiros, São Paulo, SP CEP 05403-900, Brazil

Alysson Roncally S. Carvalho
Laboratory of Pulmonary Engineering, Biomedical Engineering Program, Alberto Luiz Coimbra Institute of Post-Graduation and Research in Engineering, Federal University of Rio de Janeiro, Rio de Janeiro, Brazil
Laboratory of Respiration Physiology, Carlos Chagas Filho Institute of Biophysics, Federal University of Rio de Janeiro, Rio de Janeiro, Brazil

Marcelo Brito Passos Amato
Respiratory Intensive Care Unit, University of São Paulo School of Medicine Hospital das Clínicas, São Paulo, Brazil

Nicolas Terzi
INSERM, Université Grenoble-Alpes, U1042, HP2, 38000 Grenoble, France
CHU Grenoble Alpes, Service de réanimation médicale, 38000 Grenoble, France

Service de réanimation médicale, Centre Hospitalier Universitaire Grenoble - Alpes, CS10217, Grenoble Cedex 09, France

Romain Masson, Cédric Daubin and Jennifer Brunet
Service de réanimation médicale, Centre Hospitalier Universitaire Grenoble - Alpes, CS10217, Grenoble Cedex 09, France

Frédéric Lofaso
Université de Versailles Saint Quentin en Yvelines, INSERM U1179, Garches, France
CIC 1429, INSERM, AP-HP, Hôpital Raymond Poincaré, 92380 Garches, France
Service d'Explorations Fonctionnelles Respiratoires, AP-HP, Hôpital Raymond Poincaré, 92380 Garches, France

Pascal Beuret
Service de Réanimation, Centre Hospitalier de Roanne, 42300 Roanne, France

Hervé Normand
INSERM, U1075, 14000 Caen, France
Université de Caen, 14000 Caen, France
CHRU Caen, Service d'Explorations Fonctionnelles Respiratoire, 14000 Caen, France

Edith Dumanowski
CHRU Caen, Service d'Explorations Fonctionnelles Respiratoire, 14000 Caen, France

Line Falaize
INSERM U 1179, Université de Versailles-Saint Quentin en Yvelines, 104 Bd Raymond Poincaré, 92380 Garches, France
CIC 1429, Inserm-APHP, Hôpital Raymond Poincaré, 104 Bd Raymond Poincaré, 92380 Garches, France

Bertrand Sauneuf
Service de réanimation médicale, Centre Hospitalier Universitaire Grenoble - Alpes, CS10217, Grenoble Cedex 09, France
Service de Réanimation Médicale Polyvalente, Centre Hospitalier Public du Cotentin, BP 208, 50102 Cherbourg-en-Cotentin, France

Djillali Annane
General Intensive Care Unit, Raymond Poincaré Hospital (AP-HP), Laboratory of Inflammation and Infection, U1173, INSERM and University of Versailles SQY, 92380 Garches, France

Jean-Jacques Parienti
Unité de Biostatistique et de Recherche Clinique, Centre Hospitalier Universitaire de Caen, Avenue de la Côte de Nacre, 14033 Caen, France

David Orlikowski
Université de Versailles Saint Quentin en Yvelines, INSERM U1179, Garches, France
CIC 1429, INSERM, AP-HP, Hôpital Raymond Poincaré, 92380 Garches, France
Pôle de ventilation à domicile, AP-HP, Hôpital Raymond Poincaré, 92380 Garches, France
Service de Santé Publique, AP-HP, Hôpital Raymond Poincaré, 92380 Garches, France

Pedro Póvoa and Joana Silvestre
Polyvalent Intensive Care Unit, Centro Hospitalar de Lisboa Ocidental, São Francisco Xavier Hospital, Estrada do Forte do Alto do Duque, 1449-005 Lisbon, Portugal
NOVA Medical School, CEDOC, New University of Lisbon, Lisbon, Portugal

Ignacio Martin-Loeches, Gisela Gili, Gema Goma and Antonio Artigas
Critical Care Center, Sabadell Hospital, Corporación Sanitaria Universitaria Parc Taulí, Universitat Autonoma de Barcelona, Sabadell, Spain
CIBER de Enfermedades Respiratorias (CIBERES), Madrid, Spain

Paula Ramirez
CIBER de Enfermedades Respiratorias (CIBERES), Madrid, Spain
Intensive Care Unit, University Hospital La Fe, Valencia, Spain

Lieuwe D. Bos
Department of Intensive Care, Academic Medical Center, University of Amsterdam, Amsterdam, The Netherlands

Mariano Esperatti and Antoni Torres
CIBER de Enfermedades Respiratorias (CIBERES), Madrid, Spain
Respiratory Disease Department, Hospital Clínic i Provincial de Barcelona, IDIBAPS, Barcelona, Spain

Eugenio Berlanga and Mateu Espasa
Laboratory Department, UDIAT, Corporación Sanitaria Universitaria Parc Taulí, Sabadell, Spain

María Teresa Peláez
Anaesthesiology and Surgical Critical Care Department, Hospital Clínico Universitario de Valladolid, Avenida Ramón y Cajal, 3, 47005 Valladolid, Spain

María Heredia-Rodríguez, Esther Gómez-Sánchez, Estefanía Gómez-Pesquera, Mario Lorenzo, José I. Gómez-Herreras and Eduardo Tamayo
Anaesthesiology and Surgical Critical Care Department, Hospital Clínico Universitario de Valladolid, Avenida Ramón y Cajal, 3, 47005 Valladolid, Spain
Group of Biomedical Research in Critical Care Medicine (BioCritic), Hospital Clínico Universitario de Valladolid, Valladolid, Spain

Inmaculada Fierro and F. Javier Álvarez-González
Department of Pharmacology and Therapeutics, Faculty of Medicine, University of Valladolid, Valladolid, Spain

Juan Bustamante-Munguira
Department of Cardiovascular Surgery, Hospital Universitario de La Princesa, Madrid, Spain

José María Eiros
Group of Biomedical Research in Critical Care Medicine (BioCritic), Hospital Clínico Universitario de Valladolid, Valladolid, Spain
Department of Microbiology, Faculty of Medicine, University of Valladolid, Valladolid, Spain

Jesús F. Bermejo-Martin
Group of Biomedical Research in Critical Care Medicine (BioCritic), Hospital Clínico Universitario de Valladolid, Valladolid, Spain
Investigación Médica en Infección e Inmunidad (IMI), Hospital Clínico Universitario de Valladolid-IECSCYL, Valladolid, Spain

Sylvain Roche and Céline Bridey
CHU Nancy, Service de Réanimation Médicale Brabois, Pole Cardiovasculaire et Réanimation Médicale, Hôpital Brabois, 54511 Vandoeuvre les Nancy, France

Antoine Kimmoun and Bruno Levy
CHU Nancy, Service de Réanimation Médicale Brabois, Pole Cardiovasculaire et Réanimation Médicale, Hôpital Brabois, 54511 Vandoeuvre les Nancy, France

INSERM U 1116, Groupe Choc, Equipe 2, Faculté de Médecine, 54511 Vandoeuvre les Nancy, France
Université de Lorraine, 54000 Nancy, France

Abrice Vanhuyse
INSERM U 1116, Groupe Choc, Equipe 2, Faculté de Médecine, 54511 Vandoeuvre les Nancy, France
Université de Lorraine, 54000 Nancy, France
CHU Nancy, Département de Chirugie Cardiaque Brabois, Pole Cardiovasculaire et Réanimation Médicale, Hôpital Brabois, 54511 Vandoeuvre les Nancy, France

Damien Mandry
Université de Lorraine, 54000 Nancy, France
CHU Nancy, Département de Radiologie, Hôpital Brabois, 54511 Vandoeuvre les Nancy, France

Renaud Fay and Nicolas Girerd
INSERM, Centre d'Investigations Cliniques- 9501 and CHU de Nancy, 54511 Vandoeuvre les Nancy, France

David Lagier, Laura Platon, Laurent Chow-Chine, Antoine Sannini, Magali Bisbal and Jean-Paul Brun
Intensive Care Unit, Paoli-Calmettes Institute, 232 Boulevard de Sainte-Marguerite, 13009 Marseille, France

Marion Faucher and Djamel Mokart
Intensive Care Unit, Paoli-Calmettes Institute, 232 Boulevard de Sainte-Marguerite, 13009 Marseille, France

Jérome Lambert
Biostatistics Department, Saint Louis Teaching Hospital, AP-HP, 1, Avenue Claude Vellefaux, 75010 Paris, France

Karim Asehnoune
Department of Anesthesiology and Critical Care Medicine, Hotel Dieu, University Hospital of Nantes, 1 Place Alexis Ricordeau, 44903 Nantes, France

Marc Leone
Department of Anesthesiology and Critical Care Medicine, Hopital Nord, University Hospital of Marseille, Chemin des Bourrely, 13015 Marseille, France

Index